SPARE PARTS

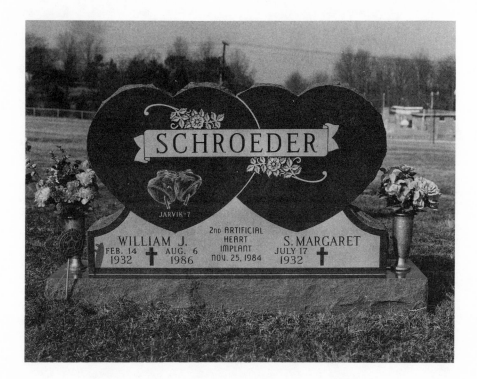

SCHROEDER

JARVIK-7

WILLIAM J.
FEB. 14 ✝ AUG. 6
1932 1986

2ND ARTIFICIAL
HEART
IMPLANT
NOV. 25, 1984

S. MARGARET
JULY 17 ✝
1932

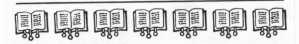

Donated by

C. Mason

1994

SPARE PARTS

Organ Replacement in American Society

RENÉE C. FOX and
JUDITH P. SWAZEY

with the assistance of Judith C. Watkins

New York   Oxford
OXFORD UNIVERSITY PRESS
1992

Oxford University Press

Oxford   New York   Toronto
Delhi   Bombay   Calcutta   Madras   Karachi
Kuala Lumpur   Singapore   Hong Kong   Tokyo
Nairobi   Dar es Salaam   Cape Town
Melbourne   Auckland

and associated companies in
Berlin   Ibadan

Copyright © 1992 by The Acadia Institute

Published by Oxford University Press, Inc.,
200 Madison Avenue, New York, New York 10016

Oxford is a registered trademark of Oxford University Press

Library of Congress Cataloging-in-Publication Data
Fox, Renée C. (Renée Claire), 1928–
Spare parts : organ replacement in American Society / Renée C. Fox
and Judith P. Swazey ; with the assistance of Judith C. Watkins.
p. cm.   Includes bibliographical references and index.
ISBN 0-19-507650-8
1. Transplantation of organs, tissues, etc.—United States—Moral
and ethical aspects.   2. Transplantation of organs, tissues, etc.—
Social aspects—United States.   3. Heart, Artificial—History.
4. Heart, Artificial—United States—Moral and ethical aspects.
I. Swazey, Judith P.   II. Title.
[DNLM: 1. Artificial Organs—trends—United States.   2. Heart,
Artificial—history—United States.   3. Organ Transplantation—
psychology.   4. Organ Transplantation—trends—United States. WO
660 F793s]
RD120.7.F68   1992
362.1'9795'00973—dc20
DNLM/DLC
for Library of Congress   91-39727

9 8 7 6 5 4 3 2 1

Printed in the United States of America
on acid-free paper

As we leave the field, we dedicate this book to Peter Swazey and Willy De Craemer for their encouragement, understanding, and endurance; to our mothers, Henrietta Fox and Louise Pound Krayer, for all that they have given us over the years; and to our very special friend, Doris Kahnhauser, whose life and death taught us so much and helped to inspire this book.

Acknowledgments

Throughout the course of researching and writing this book we have received invaluable help from many sources. We extend our deepest thanks to many people involved in organ replacement who, over the years, have so generously and freely shared their knowledge and experience with us. The first phase of our work—and our initial journey into the field to study the artificial heart experiment—was supported by grants from the James Picker Foundation and Medicine in the Public Interest; we thank them, as well as the National Science Foundation and the National Heart, Lung, and Blood Institute, for their subsequent support of our study of the rise and fall of the Jarvik-7 artificial heart.

Among the many people whose counsel and encouragement helped us complete our work, we are particularly indebted to Professor George J. Annas, Dr. Rachelle Hollander, and Dr. Elizabeth Knoll. We are also grateful to Marjorie Dahl, Janet Meryweather, and Martha Rosso for their tireless and expert work in preparing the various stages of the manuscript—and for believing that someday a book would emerge.

Finally, we are indebted both literally and figuratively to The Acadia Institute in Bar Harbor, Maine, for housing and supporting the writing and rewriting of this book.

We gratefully acknowledge permission to quote materials from the following sources:

J. Childress, Ethical criteria for procuring and distributing organs for transplantation; H. Hansmann, The economics and ethics of markets for organs; C. Havighurst and N. King, Liver transplantation in Massachusetts: public policymaking as morality play; J. Prottas, The organization of organ procurement;

R. Rettig, The Politics of organ transplantation: a parable of our time; P. Schuck, Government funding for organ transplants. In *Organ Transplantation Policy: Issues and Prospects,* edited by J. F. Blumstein and F. A. Sloan, Copyright © 1989, Duke University Press. Reprinted by permission.

C. Siebert, The rehumanization of the heart. Copyright © 1990 by *Harper's Magazine.* All rights reserved. Reprinted from the February issue with special permission.

L. Altman, Surgeon's move highlights controversial trends; Utah surgeon moving heart implant program to Kentucky; Cause of recipient's death is undetected until too late; 4,000 in U.S. now live with another's heart; Artificial heart in turmoil; Great success with drug in transplant of organs; The limits of transplantation: how far should surgeons go?; Tracking a new drug from the soil in Japan to organ transplants; With new boldness, surgeons create patchwork patients; Researchers prepare for first human tests of an artificial lung; FDA approves use in tests of pump to aid failing heart. P. Boffey, Panel appeals for funds in artificial heart work. Gina Kolata, Complication occurs in liver transplants; First liver transplant from a living donor; Lungs from parents fail to save girl, 9, and doctors assess ethics. A. Quindlen, The heart's reasons. T. Trucco, Sales of kidneys prompt new laws and debate. The Dracula of medical technology (editorial). Heart patient steps forward grateful for extended life. Medicare coverage is approved for liver transplant operations. New liver transplant recipient in "outstanding" recovery. Patient a father, a neighbor, and a "fighter." Symbion board ousts Jarvik. Copyright © 1984–91 by The New York Times Company. Reprinted by permission.

J. D. Reed. Organ transplant. Reprinted by permission; copyright © 1970 The New Yorker Magazine, Inc.

L. Herskowitz. With latest death, criticism of artificial-heart program. Reprinted with permission from The Philadelphia Inquirer.

M. Mayfield, DeVries believes in more "Bionic Bills." Copyright © 1986, *USA TODAY.* Reprinted with permission.

M. Gladwell, FDA recalls artificial heart used in historic transplants. Copyright © 1990, The Washington Post. Reprinted with permission.

Photo by Robert McCarty. Courtesy of The Park Ridge Center for the Study of Health, Faith, and Ethics, Chicago.

We also wish to thank the following for permission to quote materials: *The Atlanta Journal/The Atlanta Constitution* and Mike King, *Bangor Daily News, Deseret News, Louisville Courier-Journal, Louisville Times, The New England Journal of Medicine, Pittsburgh Post Gazette, Pittsburgh Press, Salt Lake City Tribune,* and *Second Opinion.*

Contents

Introduction:
Rebuilding People

This book is concerned with some of the major developments in the field of organ replacement that occurred in the United States over the course of the 1980s and the beginning of the 1990s. It centers on significant medical and social changes in the transplantation of solid organs and on the development and clinical testing of the Jarvik-7 artificial heart, which took place during this period, with special emphasis on how these biomedical events were related to the political, economic, and value climate of American society.

In many respects, *Spare Parts* is an outgrowth and a continuation of the collaborative research begun in 1968, about which we have written in many papers and in two editions (1974 and 1978) of a previous book, *The Courage to Fail: A Social View of Organ Transplants and Dialysis.* When we began our collaborative work in the fall of 1968, we never imagined that the world of organ replacement and its medical, societal, and cultural ramifications would occupy so much of our professional lives for more than two decades. Our years of research and writing have involved us in firsthand studies at centers throughout the United States as well as in Europe, the People's Republic of China, and even on a tiny coral atoll in the Pacific Ocean.[1] These journeys into the field began when the late Dr. Emmanuel G. Mesthene, director of the Harvard University Technology and Society Program, asked us to examine the long-range implications for American society of new and emerging biomedical technologies. As we considered possible topics in light of our professional backgrounds, interests, and research styles, we agreed that we would focus on an area of biomedical innovation that was sufficiently advanced to permit in-depth empirical study through fieldwork and the analysis of primary and secondary sources.

Within this framework, we selected organ transplantation and chronic dialysis as case studies of therapeutic innovation. Our choice of these interconnected topics was influenced by our prior knowledge of and interest in them. From 1951 to 1954 Renée Fox, a sociologist of medicine, had been a participant observer on the metabolic research ward (F-Second) of Boston's Peter Bent Brigham Hospital. During those years the "experiment perilous" work of the clinical investigators on this ward included pioneering clinical research on the artificial kidney and human kidney transplantation (Fox 1959).[2] Judith Swazey, trained in biology and the history of science and medicine, had spent 1966–68 as a member of the Technology and Society Program research group, which was involved in exploration of the social, ethical, legal, and policy implications of various current and prospective biomedical developments; she had found transplantation and dialysis particularly absorbing and illuminating (Mendelsohn et al. 1971). We also selected these therapeutic innovations as the subject for what we originally thought would be a onetime, intensive study because they met our criterion of being sufficiently developed for us to conduct empirical research rather than a speculative, futuristic, "what if" inquiry. During the mid-1960s, when we launched our research, the replacement of various body parts by human and man-made substitutes was attracting increasing medical and public attention. To many—as heralded in a 1965 photo-essay in *Life* magazine—the growing ability to "rebuild people" dramatically exemplified the "control of life" being ushered in by the new knowledge and techniques of science and medicine (Control of life 1965).

Chronologically, *Spare Parts* begins where *The Courage to Fail* leaves off. The transplantation of human organs and the deployment of dialysis and artificial hearts have undergone numerous biomedical and sociocultural developments since the 1960s. Despite the changes that have occurred, however, the principal phenomena and themes we identified in *The Courage to Fail* are still of central importance. Indeed, we believe that with the passage of time these themes have become more, rather than less, contemporaneous. The largest, most enduring significance of transplanting organs and of devising artificial ones to take their place still resides in the triple themes of uncertainty, gift-exchange, and the allocation of scarce material and nonmaterial resources, in their interrelations, and in the ways they open onto metaquestions of life and death, identity and solidarity, and purpose and meaning. Biomedical progress has been made in transplantation surgery, immunosuppressive therapy, and the technology of artificial organs. Even with this progress, though, the fact stubbornly persists that the basic problems associated with such interventions are concerned with forestalling the rejection reaction and the adverse biocompatibility responses they trigger in the human body. Although there are many respects in which the transplantation of organs has become more therapeutic and less experimental, the experiment-therapy dilemmas they entail are as pronounced and complex as ever. The gift-exchange and allocation of scarce resources dimensions of organ transplantation have been catapulted into greater prominence through a convergence of factors that range from an escalating shortage of organs due to the increased scale and scope of the transplantation endeavor to new questions about the social and moral import of the gift evoked by changes in the value climate of American society.

However, *Spare Parts* is not simply or primarily a sequel to *The Courage to Fail*. Its title, chosen in part to contrast with the connotations of *The Courage to Fail*, reflects our increasingly troubled and critical reactions to the expansion organ replacement has undergone during the past decade—its magnitude, its scope, and the medical and cultural fervor by which it has been driven. The number, variety, and combination of solid organs and other body parts transplanted during the 1980s, along with the array of extracorporeal and implanted devices in regular use, being tested, or being designed has brought our society closer to the world of "rebuilt people" (Control of life 1965) classically portrayed in science fiction, in which humans are more and more composed of transplanted parts of one another, and of "man–machine unions" that "prosthetize" humans and humanize man-made organs (Asimov 1976). It is the "spare parts" pragmatism, the vision of the "replaceable body" and limitless medical progress, and the escalating ardor about the life-saving goodness of repairing and remaking people in this fashion that we have found especially disturbing.

Our disquietude about these developments is integral to the contents and outlook of *Spare Parts*. Not only has it been a prime mover in the writing of this book; it has played a crucial role in our resolve to make it our final major work on organ replacement. For as we explain in our closing chapter, after 23 years of joint, frontline research in this area (for RCF, 40 years in toto of such involvement), we have decided that the time has come for us to leave this sphere of inquiry.

This book is not an exhaustive or even-handed work about every form of organ replacement or all advances that occurred in the field during the 1980s and early 1990s. For example, it deals more extensively with solid organ than with tissue transplants, and it examines developments in liver transplantation in greater detail than those involving other organs. Furthermore, although several chapters are devoted to the artificial heart, the artificial kidney is only passingly considered. The choices we made when selecting materials and about the relative emphases we assigned them were shaped by empirical and analytical considerations. For instance, we did not feel impelled to write an updated, revised version of the extensive account of dialysis that we published in *The Courage to Fail* for inclusion in this book because, in our judgment, the issues surrounding this mode of treatment for end-stage renal failure have not changed substantially during the past decade (Levinsky and Rettig 1991a). In contrast, the rich data we generated through our firsthand study of the experimental implantations of the Jarvik-7 artificial heart during the 1980s, their powerful human condition symbolism, and their dramaturgic relation to cardinal American values, beliefs, and institutions led us to accord a central place in the book to what we came to think of as this "desperate appliance."

Spare Parts is written largely in a narrative, ethnographic style, with thickly descriptive, verbatim, and atmospheric detail essential to a societal and cultural interpretation of organ replacement. The primary data on which the book is based are qualitative materials, collected via participant observation and in situ interviewing in a variety of medical milieux and through the content analysis of our vast collection of relevant medical journal, newspaper and magazine articles, and a number of television scripts. The book also contains some quantitative data on such matters as the performance of organ transplants of various types, their outcome and their costs; on organ donation and the "supply" of transplantable organs and tissues it provides; and on the persons who are waiting to receive organs.

In Part I (Chapters 1–4) we examine some of the important biomedical advances and events in organ transplantation during the 1980s and their social and cultural concomitants. Much of what happened in the field of transplantation was triggered by the discovery of cyclosporine, a major new immunosuppressive drug. The "advent" of cyclosporine precipitated a "transplant boom." The greater ability of cyclosporine (compared to that of its predecessors) to forestall the body's immune system from defensively rejecting tissue and organ transplants as "foreign" emboldened physicians and medical centers to enter the field, to transplant a wider spectrum of organs—singly and in various combinations and clusters—and to perform a greater number of retransplants. What was euphorically hailed as a "golden era of transplants" was tempered only by the few clinical moratoria that were eventually called on certain experimental forays and by the gradual and reluctant recognition of the side effects and limitations of cyclosporine.

The expansion of organ transplantation and the medical and social exuberance that fostered it greatly increased the problems associated with procuring enough organs for the growing lists of transplant candidates. What was now perceived as a serious "organ shortage" and a crisis about how to most fairly allocate scarce organs generated a variety of medical, philosophical and ethical, economic and political, and social strategies to obtain more "gifts of life" and to decide who should receive them. This state of affairs contributed to significant alterations in the gift-exchange matrix of organ transplantation. It played an important part in ending some of the informal taboos that had previously restricted live organ donor transplants and reduced the wariness with which most transplant teams approached them. The "supply-and-demand" problems associated with transplants also catalyzed serious consideration of "rewarded gifting"—of compensating donors and donor families in order to provide them with greater "incentives" to contribute organs. In the free-enterprise, market-oriented economic and political context of the 1980s and early 1990s, the concept of transplantable body parts as commodities gained considerable momentum. Serious arguments were advanced for what some lawyers, economists, and policy analysts called the "marketification" or "commodification" of "the gift of life," inspiring proposals to solve the organ "shortfall" by means such as a futures market in HBPs (human body parts).

While one part of "the medical commons" (Hiatt 1975) was concerned about transplantation supply, demand, and allocation issues, another part of the common focused on the mounting expenses incurred by transplantation and the merits of restraining them. In the "cost containment" atmosphere of the 1980s and 1990s, and in the face of entrenched federal government resistance to assuming additional financial responsibility for the delivery of medical care, the question of how to pay for the burgeoning number and range of transplants grew more urgent and more political. Economics and political pressures, as well as medical indicators and outcomes, became major ingredients in the process by which "medical consensus" was reached on the experimental or therapeutic status of procedures such as pediatric and adult liver transplants.

As the 1980s ended and the 1990s began, all portents suggested that the events and issues characterizing transplantation since the introduction of cyclosporine would not only continue but that history might be repeating itself. In October 1989 the press announced the "stunning success" and the "miraculous" properties and promise of another new immunosuppressive drug, FK 506, which was described a month later by Dr. Thomas Starzl and his colleagues in *The Lancet* (Altman 1989a,c; Starzl et al. 1989; Transplants and miracles 1989). Based on their first trials with FK 506 in 14 liver, kidney, and pancreas recipients, an ecstatic Starzl, who had been one of cyclosporine's chief clinical investigators and champions, described the new agent as "a wonder drug, a miraculous drug, one of those drugs that comes along once in a lifetime" (Altman 1989a).

In Part II (Chapters 5–7) the focus of the book shifts from organ transplantation to the story of the rise and fall of the Jarvik-7 artificial heart in the United States, its relation to a complex of American social institutions and cultural patterns, and its bearing on an ensemble of social control issues associated with therapeutic innovation and the patient-oriented clinical research it entails. This sociomedical case study, which turns around the four permanent Jarvik-7 artificial heart implants performed by Dr. William DeVries from 1982 to 1985, is based on the field study we conducted at the University of Utah in Salt Lake City, where the Jarvik-7 heart was developed and the first human implant was done, and at the Humana Hospital Audubon in Louisville, Kentucky, where DeVries carried out his final three implants of the device. In recounting and analyzing this story we also drew heavily on its presentation by the media, paying due attention to the implications of the extraordinary coverage it was accorded, to the version of the tale related by the print and electronic media, and to the language, imagery, and symbolism they used to do so. We were especially interested in identifying and exploring the distinctively American features of the artificial heart experiment that shaped the experiment's trajectory—including the roles that the cultural meanings of the heart, the influence of Mormonism, and the experiment's academic and corporate connections played in relation to its medical and ethical deficiencies as well as its achievements.

Chapter 8, which constitutes Part III of this book, is not only a final chapter in the editorial and chronological sense of the term; it is also a more personal conclusion. It contains our reflections on the turning point we have reached after so many years of intimate contact with the field of organ replacement. Our decision to leave this field, as we explain, is due not only to the cumulative participant-observer "burnout" we have experienced. It is also motivated by our deepening social and moral concerns about the increasing zeal with which the procurement and transplantation of human organs and the quest to develop and implant artificial ones is being pursued. Allowing American medicine and the society of which it is a part to become too caught up in repairing and rebuilding people through organ replacement—while health care continues to be defined as a private consumption rather than a social good in American society, and while millions of people do not have adequate or even minimally decent care— speaks to a values framework and a vision of medical progress we find medically and morally untenable.

We hope that our final message will be heard and, although not expressed in the conventional form of policy recommendations, will contribute to a more contemplative, culturally thoughtful approach to organ replacement in American society.

Organ Transplantation: Patterns and Issues in the 1980s

Of Wonder Drugs, the Transplant "Boom," and Moratoria

The "Advent" of Cyclosporine

At the end of the 1970s and early 1980s transplanters exuberantly hailed the "advent" of a new immunosuppressive drug, cyclosporine. Hundreds of medical journal articles described it as the most "important," "unique," "interesting," "remarkable," "exciting," "powerful," "effective," "superior" agent yet discovered in the effort to combat rejection. Indeed, it played a determining role in the dramatic rise in the number of organ transplantations carried out during the decade, which was continually reported by the mass media and professional literature.[1]

Cyclosporine is a fungal metabolite discovered in 1972 by J. F. Borel at the Sandoz Pharmaceuticals Corporation. Its development moved from laboratory studies on animals to pilot clinical trials on a small number of patients in 1978. The drug exhibited what appeared to be such felicitous and relatively nontoxic immunosuppressive action that in 1981 *The New England Journal of Medicine* published an editorial-essay celebrating the "Cosmas and Damian"-like promise cyclosporine offered.

> To achieve this miraculous skill remains the exclusive goal of workers in transplantation. . . . Today, consistently successful cadaveric transplantation appears to be more within our grasp than at any time since chemotherapeutic immunosuppression . . . was introduced . . . nearly 20 years ago. The advent of cyclosporin A offers hope that the legendary success of the two third-century patron saints of the healing profession will become a *fait accompli* of modern medical practice. (Kahan 1981, p. 280)

By 1989, only six years after it had received marketing approval from the Food and Drug Administration (FDA), cyclosporine had become a drug that was "almost universally given to transplant recipients" alone or in combination with other immunosuppressive agents (Ballantyne et al. 1989, p. 53), and its clinical applications had been experimentally extended to a widening range of autoimmune disorders. With respect to its initial and primary use, the transplant community judged that the new drug had "contributed substantially" to the "ever-expanding number" of transplants "because of improved survival and decreased postoperative morbidity" and thus had played a preeminent role moving organ transplantation "from an experimental operation to an accepted mode of treatment for many end-stage heart, lung, liver, and renal diseases" (Ballantyne et al. 1989, p. 53).

Given its impact on organ transplantation, it is not surprising that one of the striking features of most of the published medical reports on cyclosporine has been the upbeat, sometimes almost millennial "wonder drug" kind of language with which its therapeutic properties have been described. Numerous toxic side effects of cyclosporine have been progressively cited, including the appearance of lymphomas, especially in the gastrointestinal tract; acute and chronic nephrotoxicity; hypertension; hepatotoxicity; hirsutism; anemia; neurotoxicity; endocrine and neurological complications; and gastrointestinal distress (Kahan 1989). These effects were at first characterized as "unforeseen" and "surprising." They were largely attributed either to the continuing search for the optimal dose of the drug or to the complications caused by the "lethal diseases" from which the patients receiving it suffered, rather than to cyclosporine itself. Slowly and seemingly reluctantly, this generalized tendency to extol cyclosporine and to explain away or minimize its limitations and drawbacks gave way to more balanced statements about its negative as well as its positive attributes. Thus, for example, a 1989 article, "Cyclosporine-Induced Hyperuricemia and Gout," ended with a philosophical statement that stands in sharp contrast to the relatively unqualified enthusiasm expressed in the earlier outpourings.

> [T]he ancient disease of gout has appeared as an important cause of morbidity in modern organ-transplant recipients. Our studies of cyclosporine-induced hyperuricemia and gout emphasize that advances in modern technology are a double-edged sword. The beneficial properties of cyclosporine that prolong the survival of allografts are accompanied by adverse consequences—nephrotoxicity and decreased renal clearance of uric acid. (Lin et al. 1989, p. 291)

There have been, as well, more reflective and cautionary statements about the efforts to experimentally extend the scope of cyclosporine's use for the treatment of autoimmune diseases. Commenting on a trial of the drug for chronic inflam-

matory bowel disease, for example, Sachar called for more "pharmokinetic ingenuity" and other "constructive approaches" that can make cyclosporine more
than "just another overused immunoregulatory fad (a drug in search of a disease)" or "an unacceptable toxic agent (a drug worse than the disease)" (Sachar
1989, p. 895). The several stages in the therapeutic innovation cycle through
which cyclosporine has passed since the 1970s have been shaped by the social
attitudes and values of the physicians involved in its testing and use, as well as
by more strictly biomedical factors. It is especially apparent in the "accentuate-
the-positive" attitudes that research physicians displayed during the clinical trials of cyclosporine and its expanding use as soon as it was approved by the FDA.
The range and severity of a drug's side effects often are not thoroughly elucidated
during animal testing and investigational studies with human subjects, and they
may not be recognized and defined until an agent has been used for several years
in many patients. The fact that cyclosporine is often given in combination with
other immunosuppressive drugs rather than alone, immunologists pointed out,
also has "obscured . . . the delineation of [its] toxicity" (Kahan 1989, p. 1730).
Thus, as Starzl and Fung wrote in 1990 after more than a decade of extensive
clinical use and study, "the full profile of cyclosporine action is incomplete," and
"[a]side from its immunosuppressive qualities, the spectrum of seemingly unrelated cyclosporine activities is bewildering" (Starzl and Fung 1990, p. 2686).

These factors notwithstanding, there is no inherent biological or pharmaco-
logical reason why recognition of the beneficial properties of cyclosporine should
have preceded identification of some of its negative characteristics, or at least the
expectation that such characteristics existed. Nor should transplanters have been
"surprised" or "disappointed" when they encountered these untoward side
effects. Underlying this pattern was the belief in the existence of a utopian,
magic-bullet kind of therapy and the hope that they had found it in cyclosporine
because it selectively inhibited immune responses as compared to the generalized immunosuppression induced by azathioprine and adrenal corticosteroids.
Moreover, there was a "desperately optimistic" wish to be able to "save" the
organs and lives of the gravely ill patients who were also their research subjects.
As one transplant surgeon put it, "it was necessary to hope for better immunosuppressive drugs" (personal communication).

At the end of the decade, *The New England Journal of Medicine* published a
comprehensive review of cyclosporine by a leading authority in transplantation
immunology, Barry D. Kahan, who had authored the journal's "Cosmas and
Damian" editorial in 1981. In the review, Kahan briefly summarized the therapeutic effects of cyclosporine, which had "revolutionized the field of organ
transplantation" (Kahan 1989, p. 1730). After detailing what was known and
unknown about the drug's mechanism of action and its immunological and
nonimmunological side effects, Kahan's assessment of the drug's prospects

soberly acknowledged that it had not, after all, enabled transplanters to match "the legendary success of the two third-century patron saints of the healing profession" (Kahan 1981, p. 280).

By July 1991, the medical profession's acknowledgment of the frequency and seriousness of cyclosporine's side effects had reached the point that *The New England Journal of Medicine* devoted a clinicopathological conference (CPC) to them. The CPC dealt with a patient who had died from the effects of a malignant lymphoma that was described as "typical" of those "arising in a transplant recipient treated with cyclosporine." The case discussion ended with a cautionary statement.

> The principal point made by this case is that the immunosuppressive agents available for the treatment of rejection are very potent and very nonspecific, and this type of unfortunate outcome is the occasional result of the overuse of these drugs. In cases of kidney transplantation we must be very careful about the amount of these agents that we use, because renal transplantation is not a lifesaving procedure. We shall continue to see such complications, particularly in recipients of extrarenal grafts, until we develop more specific immunosuppression. (Kirkman and Ferry 1991, p. 194)

Thus as the 1990s began, transplanters recognized that although cyclosporine had "made possible the transplantation of cadaveric . . . organs with an effectiveness scarcely dreamed of a decade ago" (Starzl and Fung 1990, p. 2686), they must still pursue the quest for more selectively effective and less toxic immunosuppressive agents. Furthermore, after what would soon be a decade of treating organ recipients with cyclosporine, the transplantation community was engaged in intensive discussion about the use of this powerful immunosuppressive agent as "indefinite therapy." Central to the debate was the question: Could the renal toxicity precipitated by cyclosporine be sufficiently well managed with lower doses and careful monitoring to justify its long-term use, or did the cumulative renal injury cyclosporine caused mean that a way must be found to progressively withdraw patients from it, rather than continuing them on it indefinitely as maintenance therapy?[2] (Randall 1990, pp. 1794, 1797). This controversy occurred within the context of the early clinical trials taking place with FK 506, the code name for a new immunosuppressive drug that appeared to be so promising it was already being hailed, like cyclosporine before it, as transplantation's "miracle drug."

Their enthusiasm about FK 506 and about other new immunosuppressive agents (such as rapamycin and monoclonal antibodies) notwithstanding, physician-investigators still thought that "one of the major questions remaining in clinical transplantation is whether it will be possible to induce states of antigen-specific unresponsiveness, so that true [graft] tolerance is achieved with little or no long-term drug therapy." For "[a]lthough improved short-term success rates do translate into better long-term survival, the exponential rate of graft loss over time in patients with HLA mismatches has not changed over the past two decades" (Carpenter 1990, p. 1226).

The Expansion of Organ Transplantation

The discovery and pervasive use of cyclosporine, coupled with the evolution of surgical and organ procurement techniques, were the key biomedical factors that led to what the transplant community termed a "boom" or "explosion" in the range, number, and combinations of tissues and solid organs that were transplanted from the early 1980s through 1990. More than 2,000 multiple-organ transplants were performed during the 1980s, often in desperate efforts to ameliorate or cure a growing variety of diseases including genetic disorders, birth defects, diabetes, and cancer (Altman 1989d). The most common multiple-organ transplants were pancreas–kidney–duodenum combinations for patients with end-stage renal failure from type 1 or juvenile diabetes, and heart–lung transplants in infants and adults. Other combinations of organs that were "harvested" from donors and grafted into recipients were double-lungs, liver–heart, liver–kidney, heart–liver–kidney, and the radical "cluster transplants" of organs including, in various combinations, the stomach, small intestine, colon, pancreas, and liver for children with short-gut syndrome and secondary liver failure and for adults dying of hepatic, pancreatic, or duodenal carcinoma.

The number of solid organ grafts (singly, in combinations, and as first and retransplant procedures) also escalated. The quasimoratorium on heart transplants that existed in 1970, for example, ended at the close of 1983, when cyclosporine was approved for general use. Since then, the number of heart transplant programs and procedures in the United States and worldwide has increased dramatically. On a global scale, it was estimated that of the more than 6,000 heart transplants carried out by 1988, 80 percent took place within the 4-year period from 1984 to 1988. In 1989 there were 1,673 cardiac transplants performed in the 131 American hospitals with heart transplantation programs approved by the federal government for Medicare coverage, compared to just 172 heart transplants undertaken by only 12 programs in 1983 (*ACT Newsline* 1989; Miscellanea Medica 1990). As many as 8,886 kidneys, 2,160 livers, 412 pancreases, 89 lungs, and 70 heart–lungs also were transplanted in the United States during 1989 (Miscellanea Medica 1990). The boom triggered by cyclosporine is seen, too, in the fact that 90 percent of the liver transplants done in the United States by the end of 1988 had been performed since 1984 for more than 60 distinct diseases (Starzl et al. 1989a).

According to the most recent figures from the transplant registry maintained by the United Network for Organ Sharing (UNOS), the period 1985–90 saw a substantial growth in the number of the six most frequent solid organ transplants: kidney, heart, heart–lung, liver, and pancreas. As success rates improved with the availability of cyclosporine and more medical teams and centers entered the transplant field, the total number of these six grafts mounted from 9,176 in 1985 to 15,164 in 1990 (Cate and Laudicina 1991, p. 2). The number of these and other transplants has been limited by the supply of donor organs. As organ grafts and their success rates have increased, so too has "competition" for patients at the growing number of transplant centers, "with older and older and sicker and sicker patients . . . now considered 'suitable' candidates" (Annas 1988, p. 621). Concomitantly, as the volume of patients on waiting lists steadily expands, the number of cadaveric organ donors in the United States has plateaued at about 4,000 persons a year for the past 3 years (Peters 1991, p. 1302).

Efforts to meet the growing demand for organs (see Chapter 3) took various forms that involved significant alterations in the ways transplants have been defined as "gifts of life." The organ shortage also spawned innovations in the procedures and techniques for utilizing organs, including the development of segmental, or "reduced size," liver transplants (implanting a liver lobe from a cadaveric or live donor into a child recipient smaller than the donor), and "split-liver" transplantation (dividing the liver and implanting its lobes into two recipients). The supply–demand problem also motivated surgeons to try "domino-donor" operations, in which hearts removed from patients with terminal pulmonary disease who undergo a heart–lung transplant are implanted into other individuals with end-stage cardiac disease (Baumgartner et al. 1989). Toward the end of 1989, it was reported that at least one transplant team (at the University of Western Ontario in London, Canada) was testing the use of damaged cadaveric hearts they had surgically repaired as temporary "bridge" transplants to keep patients alive until more intact, stronger, or better-matched donated hearts became available (Altman, 1989b).

The Experiment-Therapy Status of Organ Transplantation

Many physicians involved in transplantation have judged that heart and liver transplants, like kidney transplants before them, are no longer experimental procedures but have become successful therapies. This assessment, disseminated by the mass media as well as within the profession, has helped to augment both the growing clinical demand for transplants and the problems of organ scarcity. Although claims to this effect have had self-fulfilling prophecy repercussions, the objective experimental-therapeutic status of the three most established forms of organ transplantation and the status of more recent procedures such as lung transplantation are not simple or clear-cut.

Human kidney, liver, heart, and lung transplants were initiated, respectively, in 1951, 1963, 1967, and 1981. Their clinical histories show that multiple factors are involved in determining the extent to which such innovations are investigational or treatment modalities (both per se and relative to each other) and in influencing the speed at which they traverse the experiment-to-therapy spectrum. As we pointed out in *The Courage to Fail*, therapeutic innovation, rather than being conceptualized and discussed in dichotomous and static terms as either "experiment" or "therapy," should be viewed as a dynamic process or continuum that usually moves from animal experiments to clinical trials with gravely or terminally ill patients beyond the help of conventional treatments to, if warranted, use with less and less critically ill patients (Fox and Swazey, 1978a, ch. 3). Single indicators, such as patient morbidity or mortality, the number of times a new drug, device, or procedure has been tried, or the length of time it has been used, do not determine an intervention's location on the spectrum. This is one reason physicians do not have standardized, clear-cut terms to designate the developmental stages of a new therapy and why they often use elaborate, equivocal, emotionally charged language to characterize its clinical status. As the history of organ transplantation shows clearly, this classificatory aspect of the experiment-therapy dilemma is an issue whose import goes far beyond semantic preciousness or academic hairsplitting. Evaluation of the status of a particular procedure is a primary criterion for deciding on whom and under what circumstances it may be justifiably used and—of increasing salience to patients and physicians—whether its costs will be reimbursed by health insurance.

When they are viewed comparatively along the experiment-to-therapy spectrum, kidney transplants are the most therapeutically advanced, followed by heart, liver, and lung transplants. Significant progress has been made in the short-term outcome of all three of these transplants. They are currently associated with an overall 85 percent 1-year "success rate" in the United States, defined as the survival and the relatively healthy functioning of the transplanted organ and the patient who received it. In some of the nation's most respected transplantation programs, this rate has reached 95 percent. These figures, along with the growing number of heart and liver transplantation programs,[3] are indicators of the fact that during the 1980s heart, liver, and kidney transplants moved further away from the experimental end of the continuum and closer to the established therapy pole.

This momentum notwithstanding, solid organ transplants are still done only on patients who have reached the point of critical illness in the end-stage diseases from which they suffer. Organ recipients continue to be drawn mainly from the group of terminally ill cases the first patients to undergo transplants personified (like the earliest human subjects of other "experiment perilous" therapeutic innovations). Furthermore, the progress made in dealing with acute rejection that has prolonged the survival of transplant recipients and their donor organs has led to an increased incidence of long-term or chronic rejection, which physicians regard as the most troublesome biomedical limitation of transplantation at this time. Although there are numerous patients whose transplanted organs have remained viable for many years, more than 50 percent of all kidney transplants are rejected within 10 years. In the case of other organs, such as the heart, as many as one-third to one-half of the transplants are rejected after 5 years even in the most respected programs (King 1988, p. 2). The only current solution for this ill-understood immune response is to provide patients with other organs to take the place of the ones their bodies are gradually and inexorably rejecting. In this form, then, the same basic problem of uncertainty persists that has been central to organ transplantation since its inception: "the innate and unrelenting intolerance of individuals to grafts of other people's tissues and organs" (Billingham 1969, p. 1020). It also remains the chief biological deterrent to transplants achieving fully nonexperimental, conventional therapy status. Nonetheless, we have observed continuing tendencies for many laypersons to assume that the rejection reaction occurs only in instances where donor and recipient are poorly matched and for the transplant community to avoid discussing the inevitability of eventual organ rejection in all cases where donor and recipient are not genetically identical twins.

In addition to chronic rejection, another problem for long-term transplant survivors is that they are prone to develop or redevelop the very life-threatening medical conditions that made them candidates for an organ graft in the first place. For example, coronary artery disease in transplanted hearts has become a major clinical problem and "the principal cause of death among transplant recipients after the first post-transplantation year" (Schroeder and Hunt 1991, p. 1806). At present, the only way to deal with advanced coronary artery disease grafts is to do a retransplantation. "Unfortunately, the survival rates are not as good as those achieved after the first transplantation, and . . . the incidence of another development of coronary artery disease in the graft appears to be high" (Schroeder and Hunt 1991, p. 1806).

The fact that many more teams and hospitals were transplanting organs during the 1980s than during the 1970s was not only indicative of a more therapeutic, less experimental stage of development; there also was a "jumping on the bandwagon" aspect to it that threatened to undermine the progress that had been made in the transplantation success rate. For example, a report by the U.S. Congress Government Accounting Office issued at the end of 1988 revealed that 91 of the country's then 131 heart transplant programs performed fewer than 12 transplants that year—the minimum number the 1986 Task Force on Transplantation recommended based on its conclusion that there is a "positive rela-

tionship between the number of heart transplants performed and patient outcomes" (*ACT Newsline* 1989). This lack of what the doyen of academic surgery
and organ transplantation Francis D. Moore termed "field strength" (Moore
1989, p. 1484), may have accounted for the rise in the 30-day mortality rate
among heart transplant recipients, from 7.5 percent in 1986 to 10.5 percent in
1987, "the first increase in 5 years" (King 1988, p. 2).

To a striking and, in our opinion, troubling degree, the process through which
the experiment-therapy status of organ transplantation is determined and cod-
ified also became more politicized during the 1980s. It was dramatically apparent in the context of the Consensus Development Conference on Liver Transplantation held in Bethesda, Maryland, in June 1983, under the co-sponsorship
of the National Institutes of Health (NIH) and their Office of Medical Applications of Research.[4] Social scientists Gerald Markle and Daryl Chubin have aptly
described this particular conference as "a public performance of democracy,
which [had] all the trappings of theater but the unmistakable mark of backstage
politics" (Markle and Chubin 1987, p. 2).

Not only was the meeting carefully choreographed; its outcome was a fore-
gone conclusion. Throughout the conference, with the exception of one participating expert, the panel refused to deal directly with the question of how experimental or therapeutic liver transplantation was. Working a semantic alchemy
over the question, they claimed that it was a political and economic "policy issue
. . . integral to government and funding" rather than a "scientific" matter and
therefore should be dealt with by agencies such as the Health Care Financing
Administration and Congress' Office of Technology Assessment, not by medical
professionals. The panel also eschewed any direct discussion of the costs of transplantation and of who pays for it on the justifiable grounds that this question
was "nonscientific." Yet the most important implicit issues of the conference—
in fact one might say its hidden agenda—were precisely these two sets of issues
and their interconnections.

> If liver transplantation was deemed an experimental procedure by the consensus
> panel, then third-party payment was unlikely. However, if it was classified as a ther-
> apy with all the trappings of success, i.e., impressive survival rates and enhanced
> quality of life, then a government subsidy for the procedure would be warranted.
> (Markle and Chubin 1987, pp. 20–21)

In the end, the final consensus statement of the conference read as follows.

> After extensive review and consideration of all available data, this panel concludes
> that liver transplantation is a therapeutic modality for endstage liver disease that
> deserves broader application. However, in order for liver transplantation to gain its
> full therapeutic potential, the indications for and results of the procedure must be

the object of comprehensive, coordinated, and ongoing evaluation in the years ahead. This can best be achieved by expansion of this technology to a limited number of centers where performance of liver transplantation can be carried out under optimal conditions. (National Institutes of Health 1983a)

Using carefully chosen, evasive language such as "therapeutic modality," "full therapeutic potential," and "limited . . . expansion of this technology" to avoid taking an outright position on how experimental or therapeutic liver transplantation currently was, the panel nonetheless came down strongly on the therapeutic side of the issue. In so doing, it not only provided an explicit rationale for extending the clinical use of the procedure but an unspoken yet understood legitimation for covering the costs of liver transplantation as a therapy.[5]

Indeed, as is discussed more fully in Chapter 4, paying for the high individual costs of a transplant and postoperative care has been one of the chief motivators for efforts to define various procedures as therapeutic rather than experimental or investigative. For example, in a March 1990 editorial in *The New England Journal of Medicine* entitled "Lung Transplantation Comes of Age," Stanford transplanters James Theodore and Norman Lewiston noted that "the median cost of a heart–lung transplantation is $240,000 for initial care and approximately $47,000 a year for follow-up medication and care," adding that "many insurance companies still consider lung transplantation an investigational treatment and are unwilling to provide it as a benefit" (Theodore and Lewiston 1990, p. 773).

In tacitly arguing that lung transplantation, which includes heart–lung, single-lung, and double lung grafts, should be covered by insurers, Theodore and Lewiston refrained from declaring unequivocally that it had reached the status of a conventional therapy during the few years since it became a "clinical reality" in 1981. Rather, they carefully characterized lung transplantation as a "useful procedure" that will never "be a panacea for pulmonary ills" but, "like the transplantation of other major organs," may benefit "selected patients when other treatments have failed" (Theodore and Lewiston 1990, pp. 772, 773–774). This characterization of the clinical status of lung transplantation and why it merits insurance coverage was based on a 55 percent survival rate for 51 single-lung recipients and a 57 percent survival rate for 57 double-lung transplant patients as of 1988, and "actuarial survivals" of "70 percent for 1 year, 66 percent for 2 years, and 60 percent for 3 years" for the 450 heart-lung transplants done from 1986 to 1988 (Theodore and Lewiston 1990, p. 773).

The transplanter-editorialists judged that "[t]hese results represent good news and a source of optimism for the hundreds of patients with cardiopulmonary or pulmonary disease who might benefit from such surgery," but they also recognized—invoking the caution voiced in 1989 by Dr. Francis Moore about cluster transplants—that "not all patients are suitable candidates, and desperate clinical situations do not in themselves constitute appropriate indications" (Theodore and Lewiston 1990, p. 773). Furthermore, the editorializers conceded, patients who are medically eligible for a lung transplant face an array of potentially devastating problems. Added to the scarcity of donor organs and costs are mechanical problems such as pleural bleeding and stenosis in the newly transplanted lung, the "worrisome" twin threats of acute rejection and infection, and, particularly after a heart–lung transplant, "the insidious development of severe obstructive lung disease in a matter of weeks." Given what they judged to be the postexperimental "useful procedure" status of lung transplantation at the end of the 1980s, Theodore and Lewiston define eligible candidates as "anyone with lung disease who is sick enough to need the operation, well enough to survive the waiting period of several months for a donor organ, fit enough to survive the surgery, and courageous enough to deal with the complex postoperative care" (Theodore and Lewiston 1990, p. 773).

A Multiplicity of Clinical Moratoria

While some types of transplants evolved toward the therapeutic pole of the experiment-therapy spectrum, other more experimental and controversial efforts to obtain and implant organs and tissues were attempted that engendered various types of clinical moratoria. As we have used the term, a clinical moratorium is the suspension or sharp curtailment, rather than permanent cessation, of the use of an experimental procedure on patients. Although it is a recurrent phenomenon in the process of therapeutic innovation, it is especially associated with "desperate remedies" research with patients and the problems of uncertainty and the experiment-therapy dilemmas that such research entails. For this reason, moratoria are more likely to take place during the early human experimentation phase of the clinical research process, when the only persons on whom it is considered ethically acceptable to try an uncertain, risky new drug, device, or procedure are consenting, gravely ill patients for whom there is no other therapeutic alternative. Under the circumstances, the death of these human subjects is a likely result of the trials, rather than any palpable improvement in their medical condition or their sustained survival. In turn, such outcomes acutely raise the question of whether it is scientifically and morally justifiable for the research physicians conducting such "failed experiment[s] perilous" to continue them, or the rational and right thing to do is to cease and desist, at least until there is a greater biomedical likelihood of "success" (Fox 1959; Swazey and Fox 1970; Swazey et al. 1986).

The multiplicity of clinical moratoria and of moratorium-relevant phenomena that developed around transplantation during the 1980s included experimental efforts in cardiac xenotransplantation, multiple abdominal organ transplants in children, the transplantation of adrenal gland tissue into the brain of patients with Parkinson's disease, and attempts to use anencephalic newborns as organ donors to help alleviate the scarcity of transplantable organs for infants. Additionally, as we discuss in Chapters 5 and 6, the 1980s saw the dramatic beginning and muffled ending, for now, of the clinical phase of experimental attempts to permanently replace the heart with a man-made device.

Baby Fae

On October 26, 1984, pediatric heart surgeon Leonard L. Bailey and his associates at Loma Linda University Medical Center in California implanted a heart from a 7-month-old baboon in a newborn human infant with hypoplastic left heart syndrome (HLHS), a spectrum of fatal congenital cardiovascular malformations with which about 10,000 babies are born each year in the United States. "Baby Fae," as the recipient of the cardiac xenotransplantation came to be known to the public through the extensive media coverage of her case, died 20 days later, having undergone rapidly progressive rejection of her baboon heart. In the medical journal article that he published on this case, Bailey affirmed that the "data derived from this first clinical trial suggest that cardiac xenotransplantation for the management of neonatal HLHS is a reasonable investigative option [that] deserve[s] further exploration,"[6] and that future "protocol changes . . . should result in extended graft and patient survival" (Bailey et al. 1985, pp. 3321, 3329). Nevertheless, partly as a result of the great medical and public furor the implant created, Bailey has not yet attempted another xenotransplantation. Instead, he seems to have concentrated on developing a surgical procedure for doing human heart transplants on infants with HLHS. Over the period 1985 to 1988, he performed this operation on 19 babies less than 6 months of age. At the end of September 1988, 15 of these children were still alive, and one was nearly 3 years old (Goldsmith 1988, pp. 1671–1672).

Anencephalic Donors

Leonard Bailey and his colleagues in the Department of Pediatrics called a second moratorium in July 1988. This time it involved suspending the highly controversial protocols under which Loma Linda had become, for a time, the only medical center in the United States with an active program for using anencephalic infants, born with most of the brain absent other than its stem, as organ sources for infants and young children awaiting transplantation.

The Loma Linda program took place against a 25-year history of sporadic kidney and heart transplants with anencephalic donor organs, occasioned by "the difficulties in obtaining adequate numbers of infant cadavers with artificially supported vital functions" (Shewmon et al. 1989, p. 1773). Providing organs from anencephalic infants attracted interest because it might, even marginally, help meet the supply–demand imbalance and because, it has been argued, it responds to the "repeatedly expressed desire of parents to donate their [anencephalic] infants' organs and bring something positive out of otherwise tragic pregnancies" (Peabody et al. 1989, p. 334). According to a May 1990 report by a special medical task force constituted to develop a consensus on medical issues concerning the infant with anencephaly, Loma Linda was one of 25 institutions that had attempted to use organs from anencephalic infants for transplantation. In toto, the task force identified 80 anencephalic infants who had been involved in transplantation protocols, but "for various reasons, 39 of these infants were not used as sources of transplanted organs. Of the remaining 41 infants, 37 provided kidneys, 2 provided livers, and 3 provided hearts for transplantation. . . . Eleven renal, no hepatic, and one cardiac transplantation were reported as successful" (Medical Task Force on Anencephaly 1990, p. 673).

Although 95 percent of live-born anencephalic infants usually die within 7 days, verifying neurological criteria for brain death in such infants is difficult, especially if they are being maintained on ventilatory support to keep their organs viable for transplantation. This difficulty, coupled with the growing demand for small transplantable organs that has accompanied progress in neonatal and pediatric transplantation, has led to proposals to define anencephalic infants as living "nonpersons" or to revise the Uniform Anatomical Gift Act or the Uniform Determination of Death Act to make it ethically and legally permissible to harvest their organs while they are still spontaneously breathing (Annas 1987; Shewmon et al. 1989; Truog and Fletcher 1989). There have been strong moral and legal objections, however, to the idea and implications of using still-living infants, anencephalic or not, as organ sources. Thus the Loma Linda protocol called for removing organs from anencephalic infants only after brain death had been diagnosed and pronounced.

The Loma Linda team ended their project after they had made 12 consecutive failed attempts to obtain solid organs from anencephalic infants over a 7-month trial period. In a report on their experience, the chief neonatologists described how, under the first protocol they used from December 1987 to April 1988 six anencephalic infants underwent resuscitation and intensive care from birth (Peabody, et al. 1989). Only one of these babies met the criteria of brain death within the seven-day limit set by Loma Linda's protocol "in order to prevent indefinite prolongation of the dying process in the infant." The other five infants had persistent brain-stem activity, even after they were extubated and put on customary comfort care (hydration, nutrition, and temperature supports); eventually all died from cardiac rather than brain death. Because it appeared that intensive care had "interrupt[ed] the natural dying process," the next six infants were treated under a different protocol from May to July 1988, which entailed customary care until signs of imminent death developed, when ventilatory support and other aggressive treatments were initiated. Three infants were put on life supports, but once again only one of these babies met brain death criteria within 7 days.

In the end, not even the organs of the two infants who met the brain death criteria were used for transplants. The reasons for not using the organs were the blood types and state of health of waiting infants, the size of the organs needed, and "the fear of transplantation centers that they would become involved in the controversy over donation of organs from anencephalic infants, potentially jeopardizing their transplantation programs" (Peabody et al. 1989, p. 350). This frustratingly disappointing outcome, the combined anguish of watching the babies live longer than expected and watching them die, the discomfort and pain of relating to their parents, and coping with the medical, media, and bioethical notoriety that the program attracted were stressful for the staff (Abraham 1988). All these elements were involved in the starkly understated conclusion reached by the Loma Linda group and in the moratorium they based on this conclusion.

> [S]ome other mechanism for increasing the donor pool of solid organs for infants must be sought. . . . Our data suggest that it is not feasible, within the restrictions imposed by current requirements of total brain death, to procure from anencephalic infants a substantial number of hearts and livers for transplantation. (Peabody et al. 1989, p. 350)

Cluster Transplants

On January 14, 1989, through the medium of an announcement/interview issued by the Associated Press, transplant surgeon Thomas E. Starzl called for a temporary halt of the multiple-organ abdominal transplants on children he had performed. He stated that he and his University of Pittsburgh colleagues now wanted to wait a year—"looking ahead to getting better methods of controlling organ rejection"—before doing any more of these procedures.

> I think we have failed here in what we really wanted to do . . . . We don't quite yet have the capability of bringing it off in a predictable and reliable way. . . . It's merely an acceptance of reality. But it certainly isn't a turncoat approach. . . . What we don't want to do is draw a curtain on this, but to realize that we probably need better tools. (Pittsburgh surgeon seeks hiatus 1989)

This statement was made 1 week after the death of Rolandrea Dodge, a 3-year-old Navajo child born with intractable secretory diarrhea. On November 29

Starzl had supervised the team headed by surgeon Satoru Todo who implanted a new liver, pancreas, part of a stomach, and small and large intestines into "Rolly." The Pittsburgh group had previously carried out similar en bloc transplantations of the stomach, small intestine, colon, pancreas, and liver in two children with the short-gut syndrome and secondary liver failure. The first one was done in August 1983, on a 6-year-old white girl who survived the operation but died in cardiac arrest and intractable hypertension 30 minutes after she arrived in the intensive care unit. The second operation was conducted in November 1987 on a 3-year-old black girl, Tabatha Foster, who became well known to the American public through the press coverage of her 193 days of postoperative survival. Although there was no evidence of graft rejection or of graft-versus-host disease in her case, she died of an Epstein-Barr virus-associated lymphoproliferative disorder that caused biliary obstruction and lethal sepsis, which Starzl and his associates thought may have been due to "overimmuno-suppression" to prevent rejection that was "too intensive" (Starzl et al. 1989c, p. 1456). Because of what they believed they had learned from Tabatha Foster's case and because Rolandrea Dodge, unlike Tabatha, did not have scars from previous abdominal surgery, "hopes for the success of [Rolly's] operation were high," according to Satoru Todo (Goldsmith 1989, p. 1397). Yet her death from lymphoproliferative disease 6 weeks after her "organ cluster" transplant was similar to that of Tabatha, and her survival time was much shorter. Rolly's death under these circumstances triggered Starzl's public statement that he and his colleagues had decided to wait a year before undertaking another such transplant.

Two months after announcing this moratorium, a full clinical and research report on their first two multiple abdominal viscera procedures was published by Starzl, Todo, and associates in *The Journal of the American Medical Association (JAMA)*. The article (which did not include the case of Rolandrea Dodge) ended with an affirmation about what the operation in these two children, especially Tabatha Foster, had achieved and with the intimation that the Pittsburgh group, albeit "cautiously," would be inclined to try again.

> The most important conclusion from our longest surviving patient was that she came tantalizingly close to truly long-term survival with a functioning gastrointestinal tract. There were no mortality factors that were beyond rational explanation nor any management adjustments that require therapeutic tools that are not now available. It seems inevitable that further cautious trials of multi-visceral and/or intestinal transplantation will be made. (Starzl et al. 1989c, p. 1457)

The medical news section of the same *JAMA* issue contained a report on the "new direction" in transplantation of multiple organs into the abdomen that Starzl had already taken. Since June 1988, he revealed, his surgical team had performed numerous transplants of multiple abdominal viscera on 13 adults near death from hepatic, pancreatic, or duodenal carcinoma. Satoru Todo, the surgeon who headed the Pittsburgh team that did many of these procedures, was quoted as saying that the 11 patients who had survived the operation were apparently free of cancer, "one for as long as 6 months," and these results "are the reason Dr. Starzl is so encouraged." Linking these visceral transplants to the experimental operations previously performed on Tabatha Foster and Rolandrea Dodge, Starzl himself made a more tentatively positive claim: "Those failures spawned these seeming, at least early, successes" (Goldsmith 1989, p. 1397).

In addition to Starzl's communications, this issue of *JAMA* also had an article by a transplantation group in Chicago on the en bloc liver, stomach, duodenum, pancreas, jejunum, and ileum transplants they had performed on two infants (Williams et al. 1989). Accompanying these reports was an editorial by the venerable surgeon, Francis D. Moore. A pioneering surgeon-researcher in his own right, Moore was no stranger to what he has called the early, "black years" phase of therapeutic innovation (Moore 1968) and to the great uncertainty, risk, "desperate attempts," and high mortality rate that are inherent to it. Recognizing these factors, Moore commended the Pittsburgh and Chicago teams and the patients and their families for the "suffering and trials [they] weathered," and he praised the physicians for their "surgical enthusiasm," and the "elements of inspiration and leadership" they displayed in their work (Moore 1989, p. 1483). Having said this, however, Moore went on to make a passionately critical statement about the "desperate remedies phenomenon" to which he believed the physicians who operated on and cared for these dying children might be succumbing.

> We often read in the medical literature that some patient was so desperately ill that almost anything was welcomed by the patient, the family, and the physicians. This sort of hyperbolic "desperate remedies" pressure . . . should be looked on with skepticism. There must be some likelihood of success before the desperate remedy becomes more than a desperate search for an opportunity to try a new procedure awaiting trial. . . . One must expect appropriate restraint until a research group has shown that there is a real likelihood of success in application of this procedure. (Moore 1989, p. 1484)

Because he believed that "there must be a rationale on which the desperately ill patient may be offered not merely pain, suffering, and cost, but also a true hope of prolonged survival (without lymphoma)," Moore wrote that "there can be no question that this procedure should be withheld from other patients for the immediate future, until such time as these two research groups (or others working in this field) have perfected an animal model. . . . An animal model needs to

be developed if for no other reason than to study the nature of the lymphoma."
He concluded the editorial by exhorting the operating teams to return to the laboratory and not perform this procedure on patients again until through "extensive laboratory work" on an animal model they could show that "there [was] a
palpable likelihood of success" (Moore 1989, p. 1484).

Six months later Starzl published a reply to several letters to the editor of
JAMA about his team's transplantations of abdominal viscera (Starzl 1989). He
admitted that the first child on whom they had performed the procedure, who
died immediately afterward, had been "too ill to have survived, even with a perfect operation. This was evident in retrospect [he continued], since the autopsy
findings reported in our article included diagnoses not established prospec-
tively." Starzl neither conceded that it was wrong to have tried the procedure on
this child nor justified having done so. Without directly referring to Moore's
comments, Starzl made a laconically poignant statement about what had
impelled him and his colleagues to operate on the little girl: "No one who saw
this beautiful child could resist the instinct to save her." In the same letter,
though, Starzl expressed respectful gratitude for the counsel and encouragement
he had repeatedly received from Moore.

> The use of related transplant procedures to treat extensive abdominal tumors . . .
> was reported before the American Surgical Association in April 1989 and discussed
> by Moore, whose advice and comments throughout the years have been unfailingly
> wise and supportive. Eight of the . . . adult recipients are alive after 3 to 9 months,
> all out of the hospital without known recurrence of tumor.

Woven into this carefully composed paragraph was Starzl's implicit acknowledgment of Moore's prior recommendation that a moratorium be called on further multiple-organ abdominal transplants for the treatment of abdominal
malignancies in adult patients. However, as we shall discuss, spurred on by the
promise of FK 506 and other new antirejection agents, Starzl's efforts to "salvage" adults with lethal malignancies continued.

Brain Tissue Implants

The 1980s ushered in a series of ground-breaking clinical trials of tissue transplants into the brain for a variety of disorders involving damage to the central
nervous system (Gill and Lund 1989). The graft that caused the most initial
excitement was adrenal medullary tissue transplanted into the right caudate
nucleus in patients with advanced intractable Parkinson's disease. (Parkinsonism is one of the most common neurological diseases, affecting more than 1 million persons in the United States, many of whom are over 60 years of age.) The

procedure and its therapeutic promise burst onto the medical scene in 1987 with a published report by a team of neurologists in Mexico City about the dramatic and continued improvement in the tremor, speech impairment, and difficulties in balance in two patients incapacitated with Parkinson's disease on whom this operation had been performed (Madrazo et al. 1987a). Their first report was immediately followed by several others that contained similar findings on a larger series of patients and provided corroboration by another researcher who independently examined their patients and found such impressive postoperative improvement that in some cases antiparkinsonian medications could be significantly reduced or even discontinued (Madrazo et al. 1987b).

These publications created so much excitement that several months later, at the 1987 Schmitt Neurological Sciences Symposium, the presentation by a member of this Mexican team eclipsed all the other papers delivered.

> The centerpiece was a presentation by Rene Drucker-Colin, of the Hospital de Especialidades Centro Medico "La Raza," Mexico City, who showed a videotape of some of his implant patients before and after surgery. Although none of the patients were restored to normal after the procedure, one man who had been rendered virtually immobile by the disease eventually became well enough to return to his home, where he ran a small farm. Others showed degrees of recovery almost as dramatic.
>
> The intensity of applause at the close of the presentation demonstrated the admiration that much of the audience felt for Drucker-Colin and his pioneering Mexican colleagues. In addition to research neuroscientists, the audience included large numbers of neurosurgeons who had come to Rochester specifically to assess the prospects of doing the implant operation themselves. (Lewin 1987, p. 245)

In fact, by the time this meeting took place, four neurology centers in the United States were conducting clinical trials of the procedure; 15 other U.S. hospitals were contemplating doing so; and a total of 29 patients with Parkinson's disease in North America (Canada and the United States) had already received adrenal medullary transplants (Lewin 1987). At the same symposium, another less publicly noticed oral and videotape presentation was made by Shou-shu Jiao of the Beijing (China) Institute for Neuroscience, about the positive results he and his colleagues had obtained in doing a comparable procedure on three patients who had been virtually immobilized by Parkinson's disease (Jiao et al. 1987). The Mexican team's report at this meeting was enthusiastically picked up by the American media and given wide and prominent coverage, catapulting the adrenal medullary grafts into a relatively brief "wonder procedure" phase.

In a number of respects, the dynamics of the early clinical trials of this procedure and the moratorium-relevant patterns that accompanied them differed significantly from those surrounding the cases of xenotransplantation, anencephalic infant organ donation, and multiple-organ abdominal transplants. To begin with, despite all the excitement that the Mexican group's pioneering venture and their first results engendered, from the outset the overall professional response was bivalent. As *Science* writer Roger Lewin noted at the Schmitt Neurological Sciences Symposium, many of the neurosurgeons there reacted to the Mexican group's presentation with an "it works, so let's get on with it" response. In contrast, "many of the research neuroscientists were more cautious, saying, 'it's not clear what's going on here, so let's get some more information'" (Lewin 1987, p. 245).

Once American and Canadian medical teams launched their own trials, it soon became apparent that another bifurcation existed between those involved in the field. A consistent difference quickly emerged concerning the magnitude of the symptomatic improvements that were observed by the Mexican and Chinese teams on the one hand and by their American and Canadian counterparts on the other. The results obtained by the North Americans were "encouraging but quantitatively different." Unlike the Mexicans and the Chinese, they "did not see the 'excellent amelioration of most of the clinical signs of Parkinson's disease.' Furthermore, the improvements occurred in [their] patients while they were receiving stable doses of both levodopa and dopamine agonists [antiparkinsonian medications], and during this period these doses could not be decreased in [their] patients," as both the Mexican and Chinese groups had been able to do. In addition, "medical complications were frequent and severe" (Goetz et al. 1989, pp. 339–340).

Compared to the other sets of early clinical trials we have examined, it is striking how much cooperation immediately developed between the various teams pioneering the transplantation of adrenal medullary tissue for Parkinson's disease and how systematically and collaboratively they have worked together to study and evaluate this therapeutic innovation and to explain the important and tenacious differences in their results. For example, the neurological sciences and neurology departments of Rush–Presbyterian–St. Luke's Medical Center in Chicago, the University of South Florida in Tampa, and the University of Kansas in Kansas City organized a three-center protocol to test the efficacy and safety of the procedure, reproducing the technique described by the Mexico City team and assessing baseline disability in patients and postoperative changes according to standardized scales and methods for evaluating Parkinson's disease. It involved collaboration not only between the three study centers but also with the head of the Mexican group, who allowed them to review selected videotapes of his patients (Goetz et al. 1989b). Still another cohort of researchers from Chicago, Atlanta, and Edmonton, Canada collaborated to evaluate the new procedure and its postoperative effects. They had occasion to go to China to directly examine patients with Parkinson's disease on whom the operation had been performed in Beijing (Tanner et al. 1989).

This kind of national and international scientific and clinical collaboration between teams has helped to mitigate and control the "desperate remedies" impulses of investigators participating in the early experimentation with adrenal medulla transplants in patients with Parkinson's disease. Their ardor was rapidly superseded by a "proceed-with-care" approach. Rather than a complete moratorium, a hard braking action was applied to transplants for Parkinson's disease. The physician-investigators involved in this therapeutic innovation showed a mutual desire to conduct their studies within the framework of a good and shared research design. They also accepted the neuroscientists' conviction that the implantation of tissue into the human brain should go forward "very cautiously until the appropriate fund of basic knowledge is acquired and evaluated" (Gill and Lund 1989, p. 2676). They agreed that the complications the transplant patients were developing postoperatively were so serious that, at this stage, the procedure should take place only in hospitals with the multidisciplinary expertise to effectively manage these complications. The fact that the first recipients of adrenal medulla transplants were severely disabled adults, rather than "the tiny, lovely, desperately ill dying children" (Moore 1989, p. 1484) on whom Starzl performed his en bloc abdominal transplants or Bailey his cardiac xenotransplantation, also insulated the adrenal implant trials from some of the emotional forces that drove transplanters in these other fields.

From 1987 to 1989, the multicenter research groups in the United States and Canada progressively arrived at a working consensus about the experiment-therapy status of adrenal medullary transplantation for Parkinson's disease and the implications of this evaluation for their course of action. At this juncture, they concluded, the results of the trial of the procedure warranted "cautious optimism."

> We do not think that the procedure we have examined will be the ultimate surgical technique used to test the efficacy of adrenal medullary transplantation in Parkinson's disease. We still view all transplantation procedures in Parkinson's disease as investigational. Despite the morbidity, we have seen significant benefits (though not nearly of the magnitude described by Madrazo) in patients who otherwise could not be improved through the manipulation of standard and experimental antiparkinsonian drugs. Laboratory studies have suggested a number of technical modifications that may enhance the clinical benefits and reduce the risk. Because of the prolonged improvements that we have demonstrated in this initial trial and the prospects for newer adaptations, we continue to express cautious optimism for neurotransplantation in Parkinson's disease. (Goetz et al. 1989a)

To our knowledge, there has been only one published call for stopping the performance of the procedure altogether—issued by three members of the University of Miami School of Medicine faculty in the form of a letter to the editor of *The New England Journal of Medicine* (Weiner et al. 1989). They pointed out that the so-called positive findings reported by Goetz et al. in their multicenter study that had engendered "cautious optimism" were accompanied by "significant morbidity, [and a] mean hospital stay of 34 days." Nor did "the procedure alter the objective assessment of the patients' parkinsonian disability." It was highly likely that "a placebo effect" was operating here, they argued, and for these reasons "the results of this study should not lead to 'cautious optimism' but to 'prudent pessimism.'" They ended their statement with an outright call for a clinical moratorium: "The minor and perhaps placebo-influenced positive results reported in this study do not justify further use of this procedure in patients with Parkinson's disease."

Thus, although seen as a whole the ever-expanding field of organ transplantation continues to become less experimental and more therapeutic, its evolution has not been a homogeneous or straight line progression. The transplantation of various organs, combinations of organs, and tissues is in different stages of development. Moreover, as has been the case since the first clinical trials of kidney transplants during the mid-1950s, the transplantation endeavor is still characterized by periodic moratoria and postmoratorium re-beginnings, along with de novo advances.

The dynamics of the transplantation-associated moratoria that took place during the 1980s seem to be sociologically more complex than those we have observed and studied in the past. To begin with, they have occurred in a "multiple" rather than a "singleton" fashion[7] due in part to the increases in the numbers and types of transplants being performed. In addition, the process by which these moratoria developed stands in sharp contrast to the simple, one-man fashion in which, for example, Eliot Cutler personally decided to call a halt to further clinical trials of mitral valve heart surgery in 1929 after experiencing a mortality rate of 80 percent in ten operations (Swazey and Fox 1970). The various transplantation moratoria of the 1980s are more intricate, too, than the collective and cumulative moratorium on human heart transplants that began in 1969 and ended during the early 1980s with the advent of cyclosporine. To a greater extent than these previous moratoria, those associated with transplantation during the 1980s have been galvanized not only by sentiments and social pressures coming from within the medical profession but also by the influence of the mass media, opinions of members of the lay public in their roles as participants in organizations concerned with the conduct of research on human subjects, and the growing authority of a professional community of bioethicists that emerged at the end of the 1960s (Fox 1989; Fox and Swazey 1984).

The Coming of FK 506

The type of collective optimism with which the transplant community greeted cyclosporine and the structured ways in which they gradually recognized and acknowledged its side effects and, more soberly, assessed its benefits and limitations are not unique to that drug's history. In our own research, for example, we have found that comparable "wonder drug" patterns characterized the discovery and clinical introduction of earlier immunosuppressive agents, the steroids ACTH and cortisone, and the first major psychotropic drug, chlorpromazine (Fox 1959; Swazey 1974). Similarly, as we discuss in Chapter 5, one factor in the decision to initiate human testing of the Jarvik-7 artificial heart was the hope that the human body would be as, or more, tolerant of this foreign object than the bodies of laboratory animals had been, much as transplanters had once hoped that the human heart would be more "privileged" with respect to rejection than other organs.

It was thus with a strong sense of familiarity that, during the last months of 1989, we read the first press and medical journal accounts of the discovery and early clinical results of a "miraculous" new immunosuppressive agent, FK 506: The reportage by both journalists and physicians contained the same elements of virtually unrestrained exuberance that had been woven into the first assessments of other ardently sought therapies, albeit with a few more cautionary notes than for the initial appraisals of cyclosporine when it burst upon the transplant scene a decade earlier.

The relatively rapid movement of FK 506 from its identification as a possible immunosuppressive agent in 1984 to its first experimental uses with patients in February 1989 was due primarily to Dr. Thomas Starzl, who has long been both acclaimed and criticized in medical circles for his relentless efforts to develop transplant techniques and to test means to overcome the rejection reaction. In 1988, scanning the list of presentations for a meeting in Helsinki, Finland, Starzl's attention was caught by the title of a paper by a Japanese scientist, Takenori Ochiai, of Chiba University. Dr. Ochiai was scheduled to give a preliminary report on the immunological properties of a fungal microbe discovered in soil samples by researchers at Fujisawa Pharmaceutical Company as part of their search for compounds that would either suppress or increase the activity of the immune system. Starzl decided to attend the conference to hear this first report about this agent, called FK 506. Based on what he heard, Starzl "said he developed an instinctive feeling that FK 506 could be a breakthrough drug, and several days after the presentation he flew to Fujisawa's headquarters in Osaka with an associate, Dr. Satoru Todo, to get samples" (Altman 1989c).

Starzl was one of two prominent transplant surgeons who obtained samples of FK 506 and rapidly began in vitro and animal testing to assess its safety and efficacy. The other surgeon was Roy A. Calne in Cambridge, England, who, like Starzl, had been one of the principal clinical developers of cyclosporine. In a 1987 issue of *Transplantation Proceedings*, Calne's team at Cambridge and Starzl's group at the University of Pittsburgh reported on the results of their animal studies with FK 506. As *New York Times* reporter Dr. Lawrence K. Altman observed, "In one of those twists that makes scientific competition so fascinating, the British and American teams drew opposite conclusions from similar lines of research" (Altman 1989c).

From their studies of the drug in dog and baboon kidney transplant recipients, the British investigators judged that FK 506 was too toxic to scientifically and ethically warrant tests on humans (Thiru et al. 1987). Starzl's group, in turn, tested FK 506, alone and in combination with cyclosporine, in rats, dogs, and baboons who had received, variously, heart, kidney, and liver transplants. They reached a different conclusion about its "potential clinical value" (Starzl et al. 1989b, p. 1000). The Pittsburgh investigators found that FK 506's toxicity varied from species to species, and that in terms of effectiveness it prolonged the survival of grafts in animals beyond that obtained with cyclosporine alone. "In every animal model, at every level, in every organ, FK 506 won," Starzl proclaimed (Werth 1990, p. 58).

Based on their results, the Pittsburgh transplant group decided to initiate clinical testing of FK 506.[8] Given the results of that first trial, scientists have credited Starzl "with saving FK 506 from being discarded," although at the time, as he later told reporter Lawrence K. Altman, he "faced 'a chorus of boos' from colleagues at scientific meetings who said that he had insufficient evidence to begin testing the drug in humans" (Altman 1989a,c).

Even though they differed from Calne's group in just how hazardous they thought FK 506 might be in humans, the Pittsburgh group did not expect it to be a harmless agent because, in Starzl's words, "These drugs come close to the primitive meaning of cellular physiology. If they didn't, they wouldn't be effective" (Randall 1990, p. 1797). Based on this rationale, the Pittsburgh team took the unusual step of bypassing the phase 1 tests that FDA regulations usually require for investigational new drugs. They "did not feel justified in conducting potentially dangerous pharmacokinetic studies in normal volunteers." "Instead," Starzl and his colleagues reported in their first clinical paper on FK 506, "the agent was given, in the first instance, to patients in desperate plight because their liver grafts were being rejected despite conventional immunosuppression" (Starzl et al. 1989b, p. 1000).

Whether intentionally, the nature of this justification for the way clinical test-ing of FK 506 was initiated and the language used to convey it evoked Moore's editorial discussion of "desperate remedies" for "desperate cases." Other phrases in *The Lancet* paper on FK 506 also revealed how Starzl and his associates were defining the purpose of this first human trial, including their own passionate desire to avert the deaths of the "gravely ill" patients whom they had trans-planted and retransplanted. They described their investigative protocol as "the FK 506 rescue protocol" under which the drug was first administered to 10 patients as "salvage therapy" to "rescue" the organs—and in some instances the lives—of individuals with rejection and/or nephrotoxicity, two of whom had been listed with the national organ procurement network for "emergency retran-splantation."

> The hepatic grafts that were undergoing rejection had been in place for 12 days to 6½ years. Four of the ten patients had already undergone retransplantation one to four times. . . . Patients 2 and 9, whose livers could not be salvaged with FK 506, received new grafts (their sixth and second liver, respectively) under FK 506 and low dose steroids. (Starzl et al. 1989b, pp. 1000–1001)

In addition to the two "rescue protocol" patients who received "fresh" liver grafts, two also received kidney transplants because they were in renal failure "at the time of the switch from cyclosporin to FK 506." The last four patients in the series of 14 received FK 506 not as a "salvage" attempt but as a "primary anti-rejection treatment" for their first liver transplants (as well as kidney and pan-creas grafts in one case) because they were defined as "high-risk recipients" on whom it was ethically justified to try the experimental agent.

The Pittsburgh group reported three major sets of findings from this first human test with FK 506 concerning the new agent's use in combination with cyclosporine, its immunosuppressive efficacy, and its safety. Based on in vitro and animal tests, they had anticipated that FK 506 would be used synergistically with cyclosporine in patients. In their first cases, however, they found that FK 506 "may have increased the toxicity of cyclosporin, possibly by raising its blood concentration" which "discouraged us from trying combined therapy" (Starzl et al. 1989b, pp. 1004, 1001). Used alone or with low doses of steroidal immuno-suppressives, however, FK 506 was "so potent and free of side-effects" that it seemed to realize Starzl's first "instinctive feeling" that it "could be a break-through drug."

As of September 14, 1989, Starzl's group reported, the "fate" of the liver grafts in the ten patients given "rescue treatment" with FK 506 was as follows: Seven livers were "salvaged," two were successfully replaced, and one patient had died despite a "replacement attempt." Thus far, they stated, the four primary liver transplants had "also performed flawlessly," and the patient who had received a pancreas was "insulin-free 1 month postoperatively;" two of the three transplanted kidneys were functioning "well," and the third kidney had been removed because of infection.

Given the problems of acute and chronic toxicity caused by other immunosuppressive drugs, Starzl and his colleagues were understatedly jubilant at being able to report that, at least for the time they had studied their patient-subjects, FK 506 was "remarkably free" from unwanted side effects when administered intravenously or orally. Although they recognized that longer-term studies of its effects at different dosages were needed, these early results suggested to them that FK 506's "therapeutic window may well be wide" (Starzl et al. 1989b, p. 1004).

As frequently happens in the communication of what are considered to be "breakthrough" scientific findings or medical therapies, both the press and the transplant community were aware of Starzl's results with FK 506 well before his report was published in *The Lancet* and before he delivered a paper on its clinical performance at a European Transplantation Society meeting in Barcelona, Spain on October 31, 1989. In contrast to the measured tones considered appropriate to professional publications, Starzl, other transplanters, and journalists were far more unrestrainedly optimistic in their media statements. News of the drug's "stunning success," for example, received front page coverage in the *New York Times* on October 18 (Altman 1989a). In this story, Altman stated that *The Lancet* report on the first 14 patients would soon be published, but he noted in the lead paragraph that, to date, Starzl's group had tested the drug on more than 100 patients. Word of the drug's potency and apparent lack of serious short-term side effects, Altman recounted, already had led transplant physicians at other medical centers to refer "dying patients to Dr. Starzl," who "has repeatedly called FK-506 'a miraculous drug, a wonder drug, one of those drugs that comes along once in a lifetime.'"

Not only were many patients coming to Pittsburgh because it was the only center using FK 506, but Starzl was so convinced of the superiority of this immunosuppressive agent that he was intent on giving it to as many transplant recipients as possible. Patients began to refuse to be transplanted without FK 506, Starzl reported at the Barcelona meeting. "We were faced with a practical dilemma in continuing to work in a controlled manner with the drug," he stated. "By summer," he alleged, "we were experiencing a patient revolt" (Werth 1990, p. 60). What ensued was a protracted struggle between Starzl and the Institutional Review Board (IRB) of the University of Pittsburgh Medical Center over their insistence that he proceed with caution in his use of FK 506 for kidney transplant recipients, who as a group had done relatively well on cyclosporine. The IRB recommended that Starzl conduct a series of controlled clinical trials with these patients, blindly assigning FK 506 and cyclosporine to alternate patients. Starzl refused to follow this protocol on the grounds that it was wrong to deprive patients of FK 506. Finally, in January 1990, a compromise was reached. The IRB agreed to allow Starzl to carry out unblinded randomized trials in which researchers would know who was receiving FK 506 and who cyclosporine, and they would have the built-in flexibility of switching a patient who was not faring well on cyclosporine to FK 506.

By February 1, 1990, Starzl subsequently reported, FK 506 had been used with low doses of steroids for 36 kidney, 151 liver, and 14 heart, lung, or heart–lung transplants. "All of the thoracic organ recipients and more than 90 percent of the liver recipients are alive," he wrote, and the kidney recipients, "who represented an unusually complex and difficult collection of cases, have a graft survival rate of 80 percent, with a patient mortality rate of 3 percent." "Overall," Starzl declared, "the low mortality, high graft survival, good graft function rates, and relative nondependence on steroids reflect a large and safe therapeutic window for FK 506" (Starzl and Fung 1990, p. 2686).

Knowing full well the time it took for cyclosporine's acute and chronic side effects to be recognized, Starzl told Altman in the fall of 1989 that "it would be stupid to think that the possibility of infections, cancer, nervous system damage or other hidden hazards are not there with FK 506. . . . It's the central question and we are hoping the incidence of such complications won't be a big one" (Altman 1989a).

By May 1990 Starzl was cautiously acknowledging that "the side effects of FK 506 tend to affect the same organ systems as cyclosporine, although frequently not to the same extent and sometimes not in the same direction." The new agent's diabetogenic and neurotoxic effects, unpublished data showed, were the same as those of cyclosporine, but FK 506 "may be less nephrotoxic . . . usually does not produce hypertension, reduces instead of increases serum cholesterol levels, and has little effect on serum uric acid levels. It does not [like cyclosporine] cause gingival hyperplasia or coarsening of the facial features and, instead of hirsutism, there may be hair loss" (Starzl and Fung 1990, p. 2686).

Although they realize that FK 506 will have some degree of adverse effects, Starzl and other transplant surgeons and immunologists have predicted that FK 506 will usher in a "new era" of transplant surgery and, as had been envisioned and tried with cyclosporine, the treatment of autoimmune diseases. Starzl, for one, promptly saw FK 506 as enabling increased numbers of multiple organ transplants and began to use the drug for such patients in November 1989. For transplant patients more generally, he and others anticipate shorter, less complicated, and therefore less costly postoperative hospitalization, as well as a posttransplant course with fewer of the serious or lethal complications and expensive monitoring tests that are assoicated with cyclosporine. If FK 506 proves to be as effective and safe as Starzl's early tests indicate, its proponents realize that it may increase the demand for transplants and thereby exacerbate the already acute shortage of organs. However, Starzl sees two ways that the organ supply problem might also be ameliorated by FK 506. First, he believes, the drug may lead to a resurgence of research on cross-species (animal to human) transplants, like the ill-fated Baby Fae xenograft performed by Bailey in 1984. Second, and more immediately, he believes that FK 506 may contribute to a reduction in the number of retransplants, which are done in about 20 percent of liver transplants patients treated with cyclosporine with a 50 percent mortality rate. This reduction, Altman commented, which might occur for other organs as well, "could allow people on waiting lists to receive many of those organs now used for [retransplants]" (Altman 1989a, p. B7).

At the dawn of FK 506's entrance into clinical use, Starzl, who performed the first liver transplant in 1963, is unabashedly excited about the new drug. His feeling for FK 506, he has said, "is different than for anything else ever before and represented a movement toward what I thought was unrealizable" (Altman 1989a, p. B7). Only time and experience will tell whether FK 506 is the all-powerful, relatively benign "wonder drug" that Starzl and others had expected cyclosporine to be, or if once again the initial assessments of a sought after new drug are to be skewed by the "hope springs eternal" ritualized optimism that often accompanies the early phase of discovery and favorable initial human testing. Starzl, for one, is firmly convinced that this time such optimism is warranted: "As a pathfinder, I have never had to retract any publication," he said with reference to his work on FK 506, "and at age 63 I don't want my reputation all washed away with one mistake" (Altman 1989a, p. B7).

In fact, FK 506 and its ramifications are central foci of the research in which Starzl is engaged at this juncture in his career. Since 1986 he has gradually withdrawn from what he terms his "activities as a technical surgeon," participating now "only in cases with unusual problems, or in operations which have not yet been completely worked out" (Starzl 1990). Within the context of the Transplantation Institute recently formed at the University of Pittsburgh, he plans to devote a considerable amount of research time and attention not only to the use of FK 506 in managing the rejection reaction, but also to the role that it might play in reducing the need for transplantation. For, according to Starzl's reasoning, a "significant fraction of patients who need transplantation of the kidney, liver, and heart have had these organs destroyed by so-called autoimmune diseases. With many of these conditions, the disease causing the organ destruction is produced by distortion or overactivity of the same immunologic processes that cause graft rejection." These processes "can be controlled or stopped by agents such as FK 506," Starzl asserts (Starzl 1990). What is more, he believes, aside from the autoimmune diseases, which "lead to the destruction of the commonly transplanted organs," other medical disorders such as the skin disease psoriasis, regional enteritis affecting the bowel, rheumatoid arthritis, multiple sclerosis, and recent-onset juvenile diabetes are "potential candidates for a treatment trial with FK 506" (Starzl 1990).

Thomas Starzl believes that devoting the rest of his professional life to transplantation and "its influence on the practice of medicine" through research undertakings of this kind is something he owes to unforgettable patients such as Stormie Jones, "the tow-headed, happy little girl" born with an inherited cholesterol defect. It was on Stormie whom he performed the world's first heart–liver transplantation on St. Valentine's Day 1984, when she was 6 years old, followed by a second liver transplant in 1988. She died on November 11, 1990, at the age of 13, after rejecting her heart graft. "We cannot confer immortality with our feeble efforts to help people," Starzl declared at the memorial service held on November 29, 1990, at the Children's Hospital of Pittsburgh for Stormie Jones and other deceased child patients. "We wanted more for her," he concluded, "but this was not to be.... [I]t would betray our memory of such patients to use their loss to excuse abandonment of efforts to move ahead" (Starzl 1990).

Organ Transplantation as Gift Exchange

The donor who offers a part of his body for transplantation is making an inesti-
mably precious gift. The acutely ill patient who receives the organ accepts a price-
less gift. The giving and receiving of a gift of enormous value, we believe, is the most
significant meaning of human organ transplantation. This extraordinary gift
exchange, moreover, is not a private transaction between the donor and the recipient. Rather, it takes place within a complex network of personal relationships that
extends to the families, the physicians, and all the members of the medical team
who are involved in the operation. Within the network of these relations, a complex
exchange occurs through which considerably more than the organ is transferred.
(Fox and Swazey 1978a, p. 5)

This statement about the gift-exchange dimension of organ transplantation and
its more than medical significance opened both the first and second editions of
The Courage to Fail, published during the 1970s. Despite all the biomedical and
social changes that have ensued within and around the field of organ replacement since then, these "gift of life" aspects of seeking, giving, and receiving a
human organ remain intrinsic to the dynamics and meaning of transplantation.
It is for this reason that organ transplantation continues to be one of the most
sociologically intricate and powerfully symbolic events in modern medicine.
The increased frequency of organ transplants and their greater routinization in
certain regards have not eliminated the gift elements from these surgical and
medical acts or reduced their effects on donors, recipients, and their families.
Indeed, as will be seen in Chapter 3, the persistence of a gift framework for organ
transplantation surprised and perplexed some of the market-oriented economists and policy analysts whose advice about how to increase the supply of

donor organs was sought during the 1980s. For them, it was a "peculiar" characteristic that has helped to keep transplantation outside of the "competitive, market-driven approach to health care" (Blumstein and Sloan 1989, pp. 1–2).

Transplantation has been defined by the medical profession and society at large as a "gift of life" since the first human organ grafts were performed during the mid-1950s. Initially, the notion of the gift was used metaphorically, with little awareness or analysis of its implications. Only gradually, through clinical experience and interpretive input from psychiatrists, social workers, and social scientists, did the psychological, social, and cultural meaning and repercussions of the gift-exchange aspects of transplantation become more apparent and better understood (Fox et al. 1984).

Marcel Mauss' Gift-Exchange Paradigm

"The theme of the gift, of freedom and obligation in the gift, of generosity and self-interest in giving reappear in our society like the resurrection of a dominant motif long forgotten," wrote the renowned French sociologist Marcel Mauss in his classic essay on *The Gift* (Mauss 1954, p. 66). To a remarkable degree, organ transplantation has carried with it the moral and societal import Mauss attributed to the gift. On more microdynamic levels, it has been shaped by the triple set of "symmetrical and reciprocal" obligations that, according to Mauss, govern all gift exchange, no matter how spontaneous and expressive it may appear to be. These are the entwined obligations to offer and give, to receive and accept, and to seek and find an appropriate way to repay. Failure to live up to any of these obligations, Mauss pointed out, produces major social strains that affect the giver, the receiver, and those associated with them. In Mauss' words, "To refuse to give . . . like refusing to accept . . . is a refusal of friendship and intercourse. . . . The obligation of worthy return is imperative [too]. Face is lost forever if it is not made . . ." (Mauss 1954, pp. 11, 41).

Mauss also emphasized that gifts have "emotional" and symbolic as well as "material" value and meaning. In this sense, he said, the gift and the obligations attached to it are "not inert." Rather, "the spirit of the thing given" and received is "alive and often personified." It "pertains to a person" and because it does, it creates a "sort of spiritual bond" between donor and recipient (Mauss 1954, pp. 10–11). These anthropomorphic connotations of the gift have proved to be as characteristic of the modern medical scientific and technological milieux in which the giving and receiving of organs through transplantation takes place as of the settings in "primitive" and "archaic" societies that were the contexts of Mauss' study. Even though what is given and received in organ transplantation is literally a living part of a person, transplant teams were at first startled by the animistic experiences that many donors, recipients, and their families seemed to undergo in response to this exchange. Their conceptions of the modern and the scientific did not prepare them for such "magical" reactions to this "gift of life."

Obligations to Give Organs

Applying Mauss' gift-exchange paradigm to organ transplantation illuminates many of the distinctive psychological and social phenomena that donors, recipients, their families, and the transplant team mutually encounter. To begin with, even though the American organ donation system has been organized around the cardinal societal principles of voluntarism and freedom of choice, in the type of situations where transplants are performed, prospective donors and their families are subject to strong inner and outer pressures to make such a gift. In the case of live organ transplants, which usually involve the donation of a kidney by a member of the recipient's family of origin, a parent, sibling, or child is gravely ill with end-stage renal disease. However scrupulous the transplant team may be about not urging close biological kin of a candidate-recipient to offer themselves as donors, they are nonetheless purveyors of the biomedical fact that a live kidney transplant from such a relative, who is a "good tissue match," is likely to have a better prognosis than a cadaveric transplant from a nonrelated donor. That is, there is a higher statistical probability that the rejection reaction engendered by all transplants except those between genetically identical twins will not occur as immediately or severely, and that the transplanted organ will function for a long period of time, enabling the recipient to feel relatively well and to enjoy a reasonably good quality of life. Under these immunological circumstances, no matter what efforts the medical team may make to protect the members of a prospective recipient's family from feeling coerced or self-coerced, the pressure to offer this gift of life is powerful.

Above and beyond the biomedical reasons that favor a live kidney donation, its symbolic meaning virtually obliges every family member at least to consider making such a gift. The integrity, intimacy, and generosity of the family and each of its members are involved in their individual and collective willingness to give of themselves to a terminally ill relative in this supreme, life-sustaining way. So compelling is this act, in which so much is at stake, that "the majority" of live donors make an "immediate decision" to offer their kidney "upon hearing of the need, without rumination or further investigation"—a decision so "instantaneous" that it is often taken before the transplant team has had time to launch a process of informed consent (Fellner and Marshall 1968, 1970; Simmons et al. 1977, pp. 154–158, 241–250).

The medical team, usually directed by a surgeon-transplanter, plays a gate-keeping role in determining who, if any, among the family members offering to donate their kidney is in fact selected to do so. In addition to histocompatibility testing, the eligibility screening that a prospective live donor undergoes involves psychological and social considerations. Such considerations include questions about the donor's motives for giving of himself or herself in this way and about the cross-pressures and degree of ambivalence the donor is undergoing; concomitantly there is an evaluation of how the organ exchange will be handled within the family if the recipient keeps the kidney, rejects it, or dies. Because they recognized the extraordinary forcefulness and meaning of the obligation to give an organ in this situation, most transplant teams thought it desirable to institute certain mechanisms to protect candidate donors, recipients, and their family unit against some of the harmful consequences of the pressures on them. The most common of these protective arrangements has been the generally tacit adoption of a policy of telling donors who are excluded on psychological or social grounds that they are not "compatible" with the recipient. Here, medical professionals have stretched the language of immunology, extending it to cover nonbiological factors in an effort to protect the potential live donor, the recipient, and their family from what is judged to be the damaging effects that a relative's ineligibility to give an organ for nonphysical reasons might have on them. Some moral philosophers have criticized this practice on the grounds that, however insightful and beneficently intended it may be, manipulating biomedical language in this metaphorical fashion constitutes lying to all concerned (Bok 1978).

It would be easy to assume that because cadaveric organs come from persons who are unrelated and unknown to recipients, such donations are relatively free from inner and outer gift-giving pressures. Nevertheless, under the circumstances in which the option of donating cadaver organs arises, families may feel emotionally and spiritually constrained to make such a gift of life when this prospect is presented to them by an organ procurement team. Most cadaver organs are obtained from young, healthy persons, who have been fatally injured in a vehicular accident or who have taken their own lives. These sudden and unexpected deaths are especially tragic and fraught with problems of meaning. In the face of this sort of death, the grief-stricken family may be forcefully pushed to donate their young relative's organs by their intense need to make redeeming sense out of what they would otherwise experience as morally and existentially absurd. In so doing, it is not uncommon for family members to depict the young donor as an outstandingly humane and generous person and to associate the gift of his or her organs with the admirable things that she or he would have done for others if permitted to live out a normal life span.

Obligations to Receive Organs and Patients' Reservations About Accepting Them

The candidate-recipient who is offered a live or cadaver organ is subject to strong, complementary pressures to receive it for the very reasons Marcel Mauss' analysis of the gift set forth. Whatever the potential recipient's reservations may be about a transplant, great reluctance or outright refusal to accept the life-saving gift that is offered symbolically implies a rejection of the donor and of the donor's relationship to the recipient.

There appear to be several recurrent sets of reasons for recipients' disinclination to accept the kind of gift of life a donated organ represents. First, in the case of live organ donation, the recipient may not want the donor, who is a close relative, to undergo the degree of discomfort, danger, or sacrifice a transplant entails; or the recipient may feel that because the relations between them are already so tangled or strained receiving an organ from this individual would make the situation even more emotionally complicated and difficult. Second, whether the proffered organ comes from a live relative or a deceased stranger, the recipient may be heavily burdened by the realization that it is such an extraordinary gift that he or she will never be able to repay it. Third, the recipient may have great concern or apprehension about absorbing a donated part of another known or unknown individual into his or her body, person, and life.

> Eventually, Dr. Emerson got Mrs. Amico to admit that a related donor did exist— her father. But Mrs. Amico did not want her father to give her a kidney. She could not bear to be indebted to him for such a gift. When the father came to the hospital for donor-compatability tests, he was described by Dr. Richards as a "sixty-seven-year-old fossil, in training to be a donor by dieting and so forth." The psychiatrist working with the transplant team told the group that he hoped nothing would preclude the father's serving as donor, for the act would be "the high point of his life," the first time he and his daughter had ever been close. When Mrs. Amico learned how much her father really cared for her, she was deeply moved. This reconciliation between Mrs. Amico and her father, who turned out to be a "reasonably good tissue match," provided the solution for the transplant team. Mrs. Amico was finally placed on the transplant "ready list." (Fox and Swazey 1978a, pp. 10–11)

> When Michelle Kline's brother saw a video tape of her being crowned Miss Pennsylvania this past June, he remarked, "We looked good up there on stage." Stan Kline was not simply expressing family pride in his sister's wonderful accomplishment; he was literally telling the truth. On February 2nd, 1988, Michelle Kline received a kidney transplant. The donor was her brother, Stan. . . . "Not a single day goes by when I don't think about how lucky I am," [she says].
> Ironically, Miss Kline did not always feel that lucky. . . . After the operation, she

refused to speak to her brother. She found that she resented that he had given her one of his kidneys, had tremendous guilt, felt it was "just another decision made for me by my family" during her 10-year battle with kidney disease. . . . (American Council on Transplantation 1989)

I know only a little about the donor [of the kidney I received]. They [the medical team] told me a little too much, and yet not enough. . . . She was a little girl, nine years old, who was killed in an automobile accident. . . . When certain of my friends learned that I had received a kidney from a little girl, they made jokes about it, saying that maybe I'd get back the youth and virility that I hadn't had for a long time. This so upset and disgusted me that I broke off all relations with these people. . . . But there was another patient, a woman who received a kidney at the same time that I did from the same little girl. We have become brother and sister. That is because our kidneys came from the same donor. . . . The transplants have created something between us: brotherly love, or what have you. . . . (Fox 1978, p. 1166)

The reactions of these recipients to the prospect and to the actual experience of receiving a donor's organ illustrate some of the forms in which transplantation has evoked buried, often animistic feelings that many people have about their vital organs and the integrity of their body. Among the preconscious sentiments that these recipients seem to share is the belief that some of the psychic and social, as well as physical, qualities of the donor are transferred with his or her organ into the person in whom it is implanted. "My blood has adopted a child who shuffles through my chest carrying a doll," wrote J. D. Reed in a poem about the "girls' heart" that a cardiac transplant recipient "wears" (Reed 1970). The sense that part of the donor's self or personhood has been transmitted along with the organ is likely to be most pronounced with cardiac transplants. Although on the surface recipients regard the heart they have received as just an organ, albeit one that is especially crucial to the ongoing of life, on deeper levels many respond to it as if it were a repository and emanation of the donor's quintessence.

The characteristic interest recipients of cadaver organs and their kin express in knowing what kind of a person the donor was (for example, the donor's sex, age, ethnicity, marital status, education, occupation, religion, character, and life history) and what sort of a family to which he or she belonged is related to this same phenomenon, as is the eagerness of donor families to learn something about the recipients and their families to whom a living part of their deceased relative has been given. Surgeon and author Dr. Richard Selzer, in a short story, "Whither Thou Goest," about the quest of a widow who had contributed her husband Sam's organs for transplantation, to find and visit his heart and the man who had received it, has dramatically portrayed the anthropomorphic nature of these needs.

She had been dreaming, and in her dream, she saw two men lying on narrow tables next to each other. One of them was Sam; the other she could not see clearly. . . . Both of the men were stripped to the waist, and their chests were open in the middle, the two halves raised like cellar doors. A surgeon was there, dressed in a blue scrub suit, a mask and a cap. As she watched, the surgeon reached into Sam's chest and lifted forth his heart, held it up like some luminous prize. At that moment, Hannah could see into the chests of both men, see that they were both empty. Then the surgeon turned away from Sam and lowered the incandescent, glowing heart into the chest of the other man who promptly sat up, put on his shirt and walked away.

What was instantly made clear to her . . . was that she must go to find that man who was carrying Sam's heart. If she could find him, and listen once more to the heart, she would be healed. She would be able to go on with her life. . . .

The kidneys, liver and lungs, she decided, were hidden deep away in the bodies of those who had received them. How could she possibly get to them? The corneas just didn't seem right. She didn't think she could relate to a cornea. That left the heart. A heart can be listened to. A heart can be felt. And besides, there had been her dream. She would seek to follow the heart. But then there was that man, that other, who had lain on the table next to Sam and whose face she had not been able to see. What if he refused her, mistook her intentions? No, she would explain it to him, write it all in a letter, and then he would agree. He would have to. (Selzer 1990, p. 25)

During the early years of human organ transplants, medical teams were inclined to reveal the identities of the donors of cadaver organs, their recipients, and their families to one another, and to provide them with details about each other's backgrounds and lives. Physicians believed that these intimate participants in the acts of giving and receiving that transplantation entails were entitled to such knowledge. Moreover, they thought that it would enhance the meaning of the transplant experience for the recipient and recipient's family and afford consolation and a sense of completeness to the donor family. However, with the passage of time and increased clinical experience, transplant teams became more wary about the information they conveyed. A little-discussed policy of anonymity surrounding cadaver transplants gradually developed. The transplanters were discomfited by the way in which recipients, their kin, and donor families personified cadaver organs, and about how many of them not only arranged to meet but tried to become involved in each other's lives as if they were indebted and related to one another. These interactions were major factors that led most transplant units to establish the normative practice of not telling the recipient about the donor or the donor's family about the recipient.

Most of the patients we've transplanted . . . know . . . I went [to procure a donated heart], so they try to pry information out of me. "What was my donor like? How old was he? Where did he come from?" You really try to remove yourself from that.

Mostly we tell them the age and the sex and that's all. And sometimes we tell them where the person was from. But nothing more.

We've had instances where the donor family has gotten in touch with the recipient family; sometimes that's good and sometimes that's bad. Mostly we think its bad. Donor families think that when they donate something, certainly the heart—the loved one lives on in some way. But a donation is gift. When you give somebody a gift, you don't ask them, "How's my chess set that I gave you? How's the basketball I gave you?" The same is true with organs. We don't want people saying, "How's Johnny's heart? Are you taking good care of it?" Some people feel that just because you have their brother's heart in you, they have some influence over your life. And we don't like to foster that feeling at all. We like to keep them very removed from each other. (Yaloff 1990, pp. 55–56)

Obligations to Receive Organs and Surgeons' Reservations About Live Donations

Transplant surgeons have always been ambivalent about encouraging gifts of organs by living donors, about accepting them when they are offered, and about their role in excising organs from living donors in order to implant them in waiting recipients. On the one hand, surgeons appreciate the immunological advantages for handling the rejection reaction that a well-matched live organ transplant may have over a cadaveric one. Their professional commitment to doing everything possible to prolong the lives of their gravely ill patients strongly inclines them to welcome the availability of organs from live donors. They also attach high value to the loving and selfless generosity they believe ideally impels a live donor to make such an extraordinary gift.

Nevertheless, throughout the first several decades of the clinical history of organ transplantation (from the mid-1950s until the early 1980s) transplanters restricted live vital organ donations to the kidneys because they are paired organs, and with few exceptions they required that the live kidney donor be either a parent, sibling, or child of the potential recipient. In our kinship system, during adulthood spouses, rather than parents, children, or siblings, are defined as our closest relatives. Transplanters, however, did not regard husbands and wives as eligible donors for one another ostensibly because (due to the incest taboo that regulates the choice of marriage partners) they are not biologically related.

The deep reluctance of transplant teams to consider using a kidney from a biologically unrelated donor, whether a spouse, adopted child, kin-like friend, or stranger, was powerfully brought home to us during a family and team meeting we attended during the late 1970s. The meeting was convened to discuss the possibility of a live donor transplant for a dialysis patient whose "case" we had followed for many years, both out of professional interest and because she and her family were our close friends. With the nervousness and anxiety patients and families usually feel during such encounters, Doris, her siblings, and her three children talked with each other and the transplant physicians about the pros and cons of a transplant and the feelings of family members about being a donor candidate. Suddenly, her youngest daughter broke into the conversation to ask, "Dr. B, why can't I give my mother a kidney?" Without hesitation, Dr. B responded: "Karen, you can't be a donor because you're adopted. You're not related to your mother." He and his colleagues then continued their discussion, without responding to the stricken expressions and tears on the faces of Karen and Doris. The physicians seemed oblivious to the fact that what they considered to be a scientific statement about Karen's ineligibility to be a live donor had been devastating to her and to Doris because it had negated their mother–daughter relationship along with the gift Karen had lovingly offered to make.

The refusal of transplanters to consider anyone who was not a member of the recipient's family of origin as a possible living donor was based on more than recognition of the role of genetic relatedness in histocompatibility and their desire to create optimal immunological conditions for the recipient's body to accept and retain the implanted organ. Their disquietude about the motivation of the live organ donor—about how wholesome and "pure" it really is—has also been involved. In the biologically oriented, particularistic view held by many transplant surgeons, such a donation is most likely to be an act of "healthy altruism derived from genuine moral concern" (Bevan 1971) if the person making this gift is a close "blood relative" of the individual who receives it. Yet, establishing these conditions for performing a live donor transplant has never completely allayed their anxieties and doubts about whether the donor's motives are sufficiently sound and lofty to justify the transplant team's use of their organ. In part, these concerns are a projection of transplant surgeons' own deep-seated misgivings about "inflict[ing] irreversible damage on a healthy person" (Fellner and Schwartz 1971). In a largely unspoken way, they have always been profoundly uneasy about the fact that transplanting an organ from a living donor requires them to aggressively violate the basic moral tenet of their profession to do no harm by seriously wounding an individual who is neither sick nor a conventional patient—albeit on behalf of someone who is mortally ill and has sought their help.

Obligations to Repay the "Gift of Life" and the "Tyranny of the Gift"

At the center of organ transplantation is a gift of surpassing significance—in the words of philosopher Hans Jonas, a "supererogatory gift . . . beyond duty and claim" (Jonas 1970, p. 16). Paradoxically, it is an offering that so perfectly epitomizes one of the ultimate Judeo-Christian values of our society—the injunction to give ourselves to each other in ways that include our strangers as well as our brothers and sisters—it transcends what is ordinarily asked or expected of us. The sublime meaning of what is exchanged, along with the literal and figurative sense in which a living part of the giver comes to reside and function inside the recipient, usually creates a strong bond between the donor, the recipient, and their families. The sense of oneness and ennoblement they often experience as a result of the life-giving and life-receiving acts in which they have participated can greatly enrich them, emotionally and spiritually.

As Marcel Mauss could have foretold, though, what recipients believe they owe to donors and the sense of obligation they feel about repaying "their" donor for what has been given, weigh heavily on them. This psychological and moral burden is especially onerous because the gift the recipient has received from the donor is so extraordinary that it is inherently unreciprocal. It has no physical or symbolic equivalent. As a consequence, the giver, the receiver, and their families may find themselves locked in a creditor-debtor vise that binds them one to another in a mutually fettering way. We have called these aspects of the gift-exchange dimensions of transplantation, "the tyranny of the gift" (Fox 1978, pp. 1168–1169; Fox and Swazey 1974, pp. 20–32 and 133; 1978b, pp. 812–813; Fox et al. 1984, pp. 56–57).

There are numerous ways in which the "tyranny" of this unrepaid and unrepayable gift of life can be expressed and experienced. In the case of a live kidney transplantation, for example, the donor may exhibit a great deal of "proprietary interest" in the health, work, and private life of the close relative who has received his or her organ, on the emotional grounds that, "After all, it's my kidney.... That's me in there" (Crammond 1967, p. 1226). In turn, the great indebtedness recipients may feel to the parent, sibling, or child whose life-saving kidney they carry may make it difficult for them to maintain a reasonable amount of psychic distance and independence from the donor. It is not uncommon for a recipient who needs more freedom from the donor but feels too guiltily beholden to him or her to negotiate it, to take the drastic step of completely breaking off the relationship. In the case of Michelle Kline, cited previously, she and her kidney donor-brother were reconciled and reunited once she had self-reliantly achieved her goal of becoming Miss Pennsylvania and a top finalist in the Miss America contest.

> In the audience, her brother Stanley watched, knowing it was the kidney he had donated 17 months before that allowed her to be there that night.
>   "It was the first time I have seen him since the transplant," Miss Kline confesses. "We had an extremely emotional meeting, hugging each other and crying. He told me he had tears in his eyes when I sang the aria [in the talent portion of the Miss

America competition]. He said, 'How could I not be proud when I knew it was my kidney up there that allowed you to sing?'" . . . (Top 10 finish in Miss America Pageant 1989)

However, as a letter we received from a reader of one of our publications poignantly attests, not all attempts of living donors and recipients to free themselves from the bondage that a transplant can create end this happily.

As a 1975 kidney donor, I was interested to read your piece on transplants . . . , particularly as it related to the complexities of the "gift exchange" ritual. . . . the donor is lured into a kind of smugness in the face of never-ending awe for the courage of his contribution, and the recipient is forever frustrated by trying to find an adequate response. In my case, while my sister continues to live a productive and reasonably healthy life, my "gift of life" was very much at the expense of a previously close relationship. . . . (Personal communication, September 18, 1986)

Recipients of cadaveric organ transplants also suffer from the magnitude of the gift they have received and from its unrequitable nature. For example, the man whose testimony we mentioned about the kidney he had received from a 9-year-old girl felt hauntingly unified with the bereaved mother of this child and helplessly unable to comfort or thank her for the sacrificial gift she had made.

Ever since the transplant, I have a recurrent dream. It's not about the little girl, but about her mother, or at least I assume that it's her mother. For all I know she, too, may have died in the same accident as her daughter. But in my dream, I see this woman, all dressed in black, with a black veil over her face. She is crying, and she has a reproach in her eyes. I try to communicate with her, to console her, but I can't. Because there is a pane of glass between her and me: a pane just like the one that was in the isolation room where I was hospitalized during the first days after the transplant. . . . (Fox 1978, p. 1166)

Behind an eternal barrier of soundproof glass, the face of the donor's mother remained perpetually veiled to this man. But the need of other recipients and their families to express their gratitude to the deceased donor's relatives, along with their desire to know more about the person from whom the organ has come, may impel them to make personal contact with the donor family and to become involved in their life. Correspondingly, the import of what has been given may not only drive close relatives of a cadaver donor to seek out the recipient but also, especially with heart transplants, to relate to this person as if he or she embodied the living spirit of the donor. However painful it may be for recipients and their families to be united with their organ donors' kin, they are likely to feel obligated to yield to them because of their ineffable sense of indebtedness for the gift they have received through death. These reactions are depicted in the denouement of Selzer's story, "Whither Thou Goest," when after prolonged resistance the man who received the heart of Hannah's husband, Sam, finally agrees to let her come and listen to it beat for just one hour. ("It is such a small thing, really, to ask in return for the donation of a human heart," she had written in one of a series of imploring letters that she had sent to him).

> The house was in darkness, every shade and blind having been drawn and shut. It had a furtive, tense look which was exactly what she saw on the face of the man standing before her. . . .
>
> Hannah followed him into a small room, a den furnished with a sofa, an uphol-stered easy chair and a television set. One wall was lined with bookshelves. She guessed that he had spent his convalescence in this room.
>
> "It's your show," he said. "How do you want me?" When she didn't answer, he reached up with both arms and pulled the T-shirt over his head.
>
> "I suppose you want this off," he said. Then for the first time Hannah saw on his chest the pale violet stripe that marked the passage of her husband's heart into this man. . . .
>
> "Best I think, for you to lie down flat," she said. "I'll sit on the edge and lean over." . . .
>
> "How are you going to listen to my heart without a stethoscope?" . . .
>
> "I'm going to listen with my ear." . . . "I have very good hearing," she said because he looked dubious as though he might call the whole thing off. But he didn't, and lay back down staring straight up at the ceiling and with his arms at his sides as though he were still a patient at the hospital waiting for some painful pro-cedure to be done. . . .
>
> Oh, it was Sam's heart, alright. She knew the minute she heard it. She could have picked it out of a thousand. It wasn't true that you couldn't tell one heart from another by the sound of it. This one was Sam's. . . . And Hannah settled and gave herself up to the labor of listening. . . . (Selzer 1990, pp. 26, 30)

Alterations in the Theme of the Gift

Throughout the 1960s and 1970s, as described in Chapter 2, transplant teams were highly aware of the gift-exchange dimensions of organ transplantation, its more than biomedical meaning, and the psychic and social effects of the symbolic power of giving and receiving an organ. They were particularly concerned about the emotional and familial pressures to give an organ from living donors and about how both cadaveric and live transplantations could lead donors, recipients, and their kin to become enmeshed in relationships that were painfully complicated by their creditor-debtor and anthropomorphic components.

Transplant teams responded to these phenomena by instituting certain procedures they believed would prevent or alleviate some of the psychological and social harm to which donors, recipients, and their families were subject. Most notable among these procedures were (1) the practice of telling potential live donors excluded on psychological or social grounds from giving a kidney to a relative that they were not "compatible" with the recipient; and (2) the establishment of a policy of not divulging the identities of donor families and the recipients of cadaver organs to one another. Although the policy of anonymity surrounding cadaver transplantation was primarily intended to protect donors and donees against some of the "tyranny of the gift" side effects that such transplants can engender, it may have helped transplant teams to maintain "emotional stability" by insulating them from "the stories of the donors" and the tragic ways in which they died (Annas 1988, p. 621), and from close encounters with the animistic, magic-infused thinking about transplanted organs in which the givers and receivers of cadaveric organs often engage.

The 1980s brought a number of significant changes in the ways the medical community and the American public thought about the gift of a transplantable organ and in how they acted in relation to their conception of it. To begin with, although the organ transplantation system in the United States continued to be based on what was now called "encouraged altruism" and the term "gift of life" was lavishly applied to the act of organ donation, much less attention was paid to the human dynamics of the gift-exchange aspects of transplantation than in the past. In part this was due to a latent assumption that gained ground (an erroneous assumption, in our opinion): that because transplantation had become more commonplace and routinized in some respects, it was no longer evoking the powerful positive and negative gift-associated reactions in donors, recipients, and their families that it had in the past. To the extent that "internal pressures" associated with the giving and receiving of an organ were mentioned at all, there was a tendency to regard them as inevitable, even normal, and therefore not worrisome. A "self-fulfilling prophecy" pattern was involved here. Partly because what physicians often termed these "psychosocial" aspects of transplantation were not considered as problematic as they were previously, psychiatrists and psychiatric social workers were not as likely to be active members of transplant teams. Because they were not, the gift-exchange concomitants of transplantation were less likely to be perceived.

At the same time, rather inconsistently, some of these supposedly commonplace attributes of organ transplantation were not only singled out as worthy of special note; they were perceived and presented as moving and inspiring events that affirmed the "miracles" wrought by the "gift of life." For example, the need of donor families to meet and come to know the persons who had received the cadaver organs that they had contributed and to have physical contact with the part of their deceased relative that lived on inside the recipient's body and existence was romantically portrayed in works such as medical writer Lee Gutkind's *Many Sleepless Nights,* which chronicles the world of a transplant group and its donors and recipients.

> Dick Becker, Richie's father, has never gotten used to the death of his only son, to whom he was so faithfully devoted. . . . This unfortunate and pervasive reality was especially apparent one Sunday in Charlotte, North Carolina, when I brought together, all in one room, Richie Becker's parents, Dick and Sharon, along with the recipient of Richie's heart and lungs, Winkle Fulk, and her husband Dave. . . . At the end of the evening, just as we were about to say goodbye and return to the motel . . . Dick Becker stood up in the center of the living room of his house, paused, and then walked slowly and hesitantly over toward Winkle Fulk. . . . He eased himself down on his knees, took Winkle Fulk by the shoulder and simultaneously drew her closer, as he leaned forward and placed his ear gently but firmly first between her breasts and then at her back. Everyone in that room . . . was suddenly and silently breathless, watching as Dick Becker listened for the last time to the absolutely astounding miracle of organ transplantation: the heart and lungs of his dead son

Richie, beating faithfully and unceasingly inside this stranger's warm and living chest. (Gutkind 1988, pp. 356–359)

One of the major reasons for the tendency during the 1980s to play down the macabre invasiveness and suffering such a coming together of a donor family and a recipient can entail and to play up its redemptive qualities was the growing preoccupation with the shortage of transplantable organs and the ways this shortage could be ameliorated. As we have seen, the decade was marked by a substantial expansion in the volume and types of transplants and retransplants, the number of hospitals engaged in doing these procedures, and the number of patients on waiting lists.

To the mounting distress of organ procurement agencies and transplanters, these increases occurred in the face of a plateauing of cadaveric donors at a 3-year average of 4,000 per year and a slight decline in living donors. The total number of organ donors in the United States during 1989 and 1990, according to UNOS data, was 5,797 and 6,145 respectively. The number of patients on waiting lists for the principal types of transplant (kidney, heart, heart–lung, lung, liver, and pancreas), however, grew from a total of 19,173 in 1989 to 22,008 in 1990 (Cate and Laudicina 1991, pp. 2, 4). What transplant surgeon Thomas G. Peters calls the "alarming number of patients who die waiting" for a transplant has led to the organ shortage being defined as a "public health crisis" (Peters 1991, p. 1302; Randall 1991, p. 1223). An estimated 30 percent of those waiting for a heart or liver transplant, for example, die before an organ can be procured. The situation for the oldest and most often performed transplants—kidneys—is captured by the following approximate figures (Randall 1991, p. 1223).

- Individuals added to waiting list for cadaveric kidney transplantation each month: 1000
- Individuals taken off waiting list each month: 800 (200 die or develop disqualifying medical problems, 600 receive transplants)
- Total monthly increase to waiting list: 200
- Current donors each month: 300
- Additional donors needed monthly to break even: 100 (assuming that each donor can provide kidneys for two recipients)
- Additional donors needed monthly to significantly reverse crisis: 300

In the context of the growing organ shortage "crisis," the theme of organ transplantation as a gift of life was framed and addressed primarily as a social policy problem of supply and demand. Exhortations to "make a miracle" happen through organ donation were accompanied by a structured forgetting of some of the darker emotional and existential implications of what it involved.

Efforts to augment the supply of organs included, first, a renewed and increased interest in the use of living donors. This increase resulted in an expansion of the kinds of live donor transplants surgeons were willing to perform and significant redefinitions by the transplant community of how, for purposes of giving and receiving an organ, donors and recipients can be "related" to each other. Second, there were increasingly active and large-scale campaigns to recruit future donors, urging people to "make a miracle" by giving a gift of life and to legally signify their willingness to have their bodily parts used for transplantation after their death through the provisions of the Uniform Anatomical Gift Act. In addition to public appeals, those concerned with an organ shortage, the reasons for it, and the means by which more organs could be obtained directed their attention to the medical professionals involved in the procurement process, focusing on how the doctors' and nurses' attitudes and behavior that were seen to hamper donations could be altered. Each of these strategies for remedying the shortage of organs involved alterations in the theme of the gift. As we shall see in this chapter, however, the most profound change of all was the serious consideration given to the "commodification" and "marketization" of bodily parts for transplantation.

Who Are My Kin? Who Are My Strangers? Live-Donor Kidney Transplants

One set of phenomena involving gift-exchange microdynamics did continue to concern transplant physicians in the 1980s, as they sought means to obtain more organs. It was the use of living donors for kidney transplants, which they had always found worrisome and controversial for the reasons discussed in Chapter 2. Their reservations and apprehensions caused some prominent transplant surgeons, such as Thomas Starzl, to take a strong stand against living donations.

> "The death of a single well-motivated and completely healthy living donor," [Starzl] has declared, "almost stops the clock worldwide. The most compelling argument against living donation is that it is not completely safe for the donor." (Morrow 1991, p. 57)

Nonetheless, kidney transplantation with living donors continued to be performed, especially in the United States. According to one study conducted during the 1980s, "rather than becoming extinct, living donors [were] still the preferred source of kidneys" in most of the 83 American transplant centers surveyed, "despite the improvement in cadaveric transplantation resulting from the use of cyclosporine" (Spital et al. 1986).

In a 1986 medical journal article, Andrew S. Levey and his colleagues proposed that the use of living kidney donors should be expanded by "reclaim[ing] a discarded opportunity." On both medical and ethical grounds they advocated kidney transplants from unrelated living donors "for patients in whom transplantation is recommended but for whom neither a living related donor nor a cadaveric donor is available." Levey et al. contended that the risks to the donor were "minimal" and that the benefits to donors could be "considerable," increasing their "self-esteem and sense of worth . . . regardless of the success of the transplantation." Indeed, they suggested, transplants from unrelated living donors might "also be considered as an alternative to cadaveric transplantation for selected patients in whom a planned transplant operation would provide an advantage—i.e., those who would benefit from donor-specific transfusions or other pretransplantation immunosuppression, those who require pretransplantation bilateral nephrectomies, and those who choose to avoid the long wait for a cadaveric organ" (Levey et al. 1986, p. 916).

It was the latter situation—the fact that the supply of cadaver organs was not great enough to meet the growing demand for them—that emboldened a number of medical centers to undertake transplants of kidneys from unrelated live donors during the 1980s. In effect, until then something akin to a collective taboo against performing this type of graft had existed among transplant physicians. However much "trepidation" they experienced each time a nephrectomy was done on a related donor, they nonetheless thought it could be ethically justified because of the understandable and admirable "altruism," "self-sacrifice and love" that motivated many "close blood relatives" to give of themselves in this fashion. Physicians, however, did not react the same way to unrelated donors, whose reasons for engaging in "the whole complex act of donation" they considered more enigmatic, possibly psychopathological, or driven by the prospect of receiving money for a kidney through organ brokerage arrangements that had developed (Council of The Transplantation Society 1985, pp. 715–716; Danovitch 1986, p. 714).

> Dr. Levey and his colleagues are proposing . . . that after various safeguards are observed, we permit and even encourage [living] kidney donation from a stranger to an unknown recipient. I find their proposition objectionable and unacceptable. Such donations would not be an act of love, and it is unclear to me what the prospective donor's motivation would be, if not financial. Human ingenuity knows no bounds, and in our fortunately free society it would be exceptionally difficult to be convinced of the purity of the motives of a "living stranger donor." (Danovitch 1986, p. 714)

Despite such misgivings, the use of kidneys from biologically unrelated donors began to yield to pragmatic considerations during the early 1980s. A new term appeared in the medical literature: "emotionally related donors," meaning persons whose relationship to recipients was analogous to biological relatedness. Several professional associations, such as the American Society of Transplant Surgeons and The Transplantation Society, proposed that the use of kidneys from this category of live donors be allowed: "With the assurance of relative success, it does not seem unreasonable that in selected instances, donation from unrelated persons, particularly a spouse or individual with a close relationship and intense interest in the welfare of the recipient, should be permitted" (Council of The Transplantation Society 1985, p. 715). In 1985 the Council of The Transplantation Society issued a set of "guidelines for the donation of kidneys by unrelated living donors" that legitimated their use "exceptionally when a satisfactory cadaver or living related donor cannot be found." These normative recommendations expressed continuing concern about the motives of such donors, the recognition and protection to which they were entitled for such "a gift of extraordinary magnitude," and the ever-present danger "in the current climate of commercialization" that, particularly in the case of "living stranger donors," the covert buying and selling of organs might be involved.

> It must be established by the patient and transplant team alike that the motives of the donor are altruistic and in the best interest of the recipient and not self-serving or for profit. In the best interests of all concerned, the motivation and medical suitability of the donor should be evaluated by physicians independently of the potential recipient, the recipient's physicians, and the transplant team. An independent donor advocate should be assigned to the unrelated donor to ensure that informed consent is made without pressure, to enhance personal attention given to the donor throughout the entire donation period, to ensure official expressions of gratitude, and to aid with subsequent problems and difficulties. In all instances, and especially in the exceptional case where the emotionally related donor is not a spouse or a second degree relative, the donor advocate would ensure and document that the donation was one of true altruism and not self-serving or for profit. . . . It should be clearly understood that no payment of the donor by the recipient, the recipient's relatives, or any other supporting organization, can be allowed. (Council of The Transplantation Society 1985, p. 716)

By 1988, enough "emotionally related" donor procedures had been done that centers could begin reporting on their outcomes. Between 1981 and 1988, for example, one program had performed 40 living-unrelated donor renal transplants, from "23 wives, 7 husbands, 6 friends, and 4 individuals related by marriage." On the basis of this experience, the group concluded that "living-unrelated renal transplants [were] an acceptable alternative to cadaver transplants, with excellent graft and patient survival" (Pirsch et al. 1988).

The Debut of Live-Donor Liver and Lung Transplants

At the close of the 1980s, in the atmosphere produced by the acceleration in the number and range of transplants performed, the mounting sense of crisis over the organ shortage, and the increased support given to live-donor kidney transplants, liver transplantation with living donors was tried for the first time in the United States. The initial recipients were two infants with biliary atresia (a congenital, usually fatal condition in which ducts that carry bile from the liver are blocked), each of whom was surgically implanted with a liver lobe from a parent. On November 27, 1989, Alyssa Smith, a 21-month-old girl received the left lobe from the liver of her mother, Teresa Smith. Eleven days later, 15-month old Sarina Jones underwent the same operation, with her father, Robert Jones, serving as the living donor. In both cases, the physicians involved were members of a transplantation team at the University of Chicago Medical Center, and the implants were done by surgeon Christopher E. Broelsch. The capacity of the liver to regenerate provided the anatomicophysiological rationale and justification underlying these transplants. Physicians predicted that the live donors' long-term hepatic function would not be affected because their livers would grow back to normal size and that the transplanted liver lobes would grow along with the normal development of the child-recipients.

The team's aim was not only to demonstrate the technical feasibility and clinical value of the implantation of a hepatic lobe obtained from a living parent-donor. If the transplants proved successful, they hoped to launch a living-donor program that would spread throughout the pediatric liver transplantation field and would reduce the "up to 50 percent nationwide" mortality rate among infants and young children with advanced liver disease who, "because of the shortage of [cadaver] donors . . . die awaiting transplantation" (Singer et al. 1989, p. 620).

Although the Chicago transplant team acknowledged that the operation was technically difficult, they defined it as a "therapeutic innovation" rather than as an "experiment." They did so on several grounds. To begin with, as they stated, the techniques for the transplantation of hepatic lobes they employed were not new; they had been developed and previously used for "reduced-size" liver transplantation (implanting a cadaveric liver lobe into a recipient smaller than the donor) and for "split-liver" transplantation (dividing a larger liver from a cadaveric donor and implanting the lobes into two recipients). Furthermore, the team pointed out, the survival rates of 80 percent for cadaveric reduced-size transplantation and 79 percent for split-liver transplantation were "comparable" to that obtained with more "conventional, cadaveric whole-liver transplantation" (Singer et al. 1989, p. 620). Nor was the Chicago group the first to do such transplants, they reported. Surgeons in three other countries—Australia, Brazil, Japan—had recently "attempted the operation on desperately ill children [in liver failure] as emergency procedures" (Kolata 1989b, p. B9). In those four cases, according to Dr. Peter Whitington, the university's chief of pediatric transplantation, the four donors and three of the four recipients were alive as of December 1989; one recipient had died of "unrelated complications." However, Whitington stated, "There's no way we could do [emergency operations] in the ethical environment here in the United States. But they demonstrate that this is a procedure that can be done" (Cotton 1990, p. 13).

In a sense, the most radical medical and ethical feature of these initial transplants was that rather than trying them "first in the sickest patients, as a 'desperate remedy'," which is usually the case with innovative therapies, the Chicago team deliberately chose to perform the transplantations "in infants with advanced liver disease who [were] not critically ill but who [would] certainly require a liver transplant within 3 months to survive" (Singer et al. 1989, p. 620). In an article concerning the ethics of liver transplantation with living donors, published by the Chicago group in *The New England Journal of Medicine* several months before doing the procedure, they explained that they were taking this bold medicoethical step for two reasons: First, "the pressure on the donor is reduced because the need to make a decision under emergency circumstances is obviated." Second, "since a living donor is placed at some risk," the team considered it "more appropriate ethically to select a recipient with a higher chance of survival . . . ; [i]nfants who are "not critically ill with advanced liver disease represent such recipients [and also] do not have the mortality and morbidity associated with waiting for a cadaveric liver" (Singer et al. 1989, pp. 620–621).

In its own right, the drafting and publication of this article was an innovation. It grew out of a working paper the transplant physicians, in collaboration with clinical ethicists, wrote and circulated for comment after holding a "year long series of seminars and discussions that were open to the entire university community." In turn, a revised version of the paper became the basis for the proposal the team submitted to their Institutional Review Board. Publishing a paper derived from these documents constituted another step in the "prospective research-ethics consultation" the team believed should take place before their first trials of this "innovative therapy." The publication, they thought, would allow them to extend their anticipatory dialogue about a possibly controversial clinical research protocol to a readership that was not confined to their own medical institution and university (Singer et al. 1989, pp. 620–621). Opening themselves up in this way to possible widespread professional criticism of the ethical aspects of living-donor transplants in advance of performing one was a courageous act, but in certain respects it was also protective. It enabled the Chicago group to go on record and sound out the reactions of a vast professional readership under the prestigious mantle if not the *imprimatur* of a distinguished medical journal.

In the end, however, the article elicited little formal response. No editorial accompanied it in the issue in which it appeared[1]; and to the surprise of the editors they received only one letter in response to the article and to the first two liver transplants subsequently performed by the Chicago group (personal communication). The letter to the editors was a supportive one. It "applaud[ed]" the "courage" and "ingenuity" of the "pioneering" step taken by the Chicago team and concurred with their view that although intricate ethical issues were involved in this new liver transplantation procedure its benefits outweighed its risks. The letter writers' one criticism-tinged suggestion was that the Chicago group ought to include the prospective parent-donor as a key participant in the final decision about donation: "How can we exclude from the process the person most affected by it?" (Spital and Spital 1990, pp. 549–550).

We found it especially striking that there was no published commentary on at least two facets of the Chicago group's article: (1) their statement about the "psychological benefit" parents would derive from being donors; and (2) their discussion of how informed consent for the procedure would be obtained on behalf of the infant recipients. In the words of the article:

> As a parent of the recipient, the prospective donor has a powerful motive to participate. If transplantation succeeds, the donor has the extreme satisfaction of having saved the life of the child. Even if transplantation fails, the donor may take comfort in the knowledge of having done everything possible to save the child (Singer et al. 1989, p. 620)

There is no mention of the intricacy of the gift relationship that is created between organ donors and recipients; of the strains and conflicts, as well as the satisfactions and fulfillments, involved for the participants themselves and for the family unit to which they belong; or should the child die, how emotions about the death may be complicated by the extra bond created between donor and recipient or by the donor's sense of having contributed a flawed or inadequate gift of life. The authors did allude to the fact that "the donor may feel considerable internal pressure to donate, because he or she knows that otherwise the recipient may die," but they dismissed "such pressure" as "unavoidable" and "not unique to liver transplantation." They added moralistically that the "need to balance selfishness and altruism is a universal feature of family relationships" (Singer et al. 1989, p. 621). It is as if the Chicago team believed that no psychological or social shadows could possibly hover over this parental act of "doing everything possible to save the child"; that there was nothing physically or emotionally distinctive about a mother or father giving a child a part of their liver; that it was an act identical to, and no more risky than, being the living donor of a kidney, which was also conceived to be nonproblematic; and that, in any case, the team expected that the process of obtaining the consent they had carefully designed would act as a safeguard, screening out any prospective parent-donors whose "powerful motivation to participate" was not sufficient to expunge all other feelings.

The same kind of "no problem" sentimentality characterized the authors' comments on the fact that because the recipients of liver lobe transplantations would be infants, consent would involve a "proxy decision maker" who might also be the parent-donor of the transplant. In the Chicago team's psychological and moral view, "Although this situation may influence the decision maker's readiness to give consent, . . . from the perspective of the recipient, it validates the decision maker's good faith, because a proxy who is willing to accept some personal risk to benefit the recipient will also represent the recipient's best interests" (Singer et al. 1989, p. 621). We are not only impressed by what seems to us to be the psychosocial and ethical speciousness of the assumptions underlying this analysis by the Chicago group, but also by the fact that neither the *Journal*'s editors nor its readers challenged them.

Alyssa Smith and her mother and Sarina Jones and her father all survived the transplant operations. However, in the course of removing the segment from the lobe of Mrs. Smith's liver that was implanted in Alyssa, the surgeons accidentally nicked her spleen, which they had to remove as a result. In interviews Dr. Broelsch granted the press soon after he had completed the surgery, he was reported as saying that this was a "major complication" (Bass 1989, p. 75), and that it had given him "the sickest feeling to have trouble with the first patient" (Voelker 1989, p. 34). Although he was "very pleased" with the outcome of the operation, Broelsch stated that it was nonetheless "a dangerous procedure," carrying "more risks than people would calculate or anticipate" (Kolata 1989a, p. C10).

In contrast, although Sarina Jones' transplantation was delayed by a bacterial infection she had contracted, her immediate postoperative status was described as "literally outstanding," and her father's condition as doing "remarkably well." Broelsch indicated that the surgery had been "very difficult" because of the necessity to remove signs of bacterial infection from Sarina's body, and that she would have to be monitored closely for several days because of the possibility that infection might recur (New liver transplant recipient in "outstanding" recovery 1989).

By the end of December the donor-parents and the two child-recipients had been discharged from the hospital, and the Chicago group was evaluating potential donors and recipients for another transplant operation. Their plan, it was said, was to "perform 20 living-donor liver transplants in children who are more critically ill . . . during the next year" (Voelker 1989, p. 34).

These two living-donor liver transplants and their sequelae were given prominent biomedical and human interest attention by the media. Although journalists scrupulously reported the technical problems and surgical complications the transplants entailed, the press coverage on the whole was acclamatory. The "nation's first" liver transplants from a living donor, it was declared, "usher[ed] in what [was] widely expected to be a new era in transplantation." If the procedures succeed, they "could completely change the nature of pediatric liver transplants" and constitute "a first step in transplants of other organs from living donors" (Kolata 1989a, p. B9). However, the postoperative claims made by the Chicago team that appeared in the press were more restrained; and the strongly felt medical and moral concerns voiced by a few prominent transplant surgeons about the risks to which live liver transplants would subject parent-donors were cited in several news stories. For example, in the *American Medical News'* account of a "self-portrait" conference held by the University of Chicago team about their liver transplantation program the weekend after Alyssa Smith's surgery, Broelsch was reported to be "undoubtedly . . . gratified at the success of the living-donor surgical technique he developed. But even he says [the article continued] its potential for easing the shortage of donor liver grafts for infants may have been overstated. . . . For the time being, he said, a more bountiful source of organs will be the [cadaveric] split-liver procedure" (Voelker 1989, p. 34). The article further related that "liver transplant pioneer Thomas Starzl . . . scheduled to speak [at this conference] about the new anti-rejection drug FK-506, urged transplant surgeons across the country to act with the utmost caution before attempting to duplicate the Chicago team's accomplishment" (Voelker 1989, p. 2). In a press interview with Dr. Calvin R. Stiller, head of transplant surgery at the University of Western Ontario, about his experimental work using cadaveric organs from older donors, he too expressed reluctance about undertaking or encouraging living-donor liver transplants: "There are donors currently not being used because of age," he said. "Better we find out whether they are usable and, if necessary, take the lobes out of those and put them in small children" (Altman 1989b).

It is interesting that pathmaking transplantation surgeons such as Starzl and Stiller, who are so audacious in other respects, should be admonitory about living-donor transplants and disinclined to perform them. It seems that they still experience "ambiguity of conscience" over the "unmitigated conflict" about live-kidney donors that the early transplanters experienced because "a procedure [was] adopted in which a perfectly healthy person is injured permanently in order to improve the well-being of another" (Moore 1964, p. 391; Ramsey 1970, p. 173).

By the fall of 1990, the Chicago team's continuation of parent-to-child liver lobe transplants was becoming a subject of controversy within the transplant community. There was a heated debate about the procedure at the XIIIth International Congress of the Transplantation Society. The objections to living-related liver donation that were voiced at this meeting were published in *Transplantation Proceedings*. The author, Dr. R. W. Busuttil, director of UCLA's liver transplant program, questioned the Chicago group's contention that living-related liver transplantation is "equal to or superior to cadaver transplantation" and that the completion rate for donors is "likely to be as low" as that for live kidney donors. He also expressed serious doubts about whether a parent can be "expected to make an informed, uncoerced free choice when asked to consider donating an organ to his or her dying child" (Busuttil 1991, p. 44).

These reservations about parent-to-child live liver donations do not seem to have deterred transplanters from trying to save the life of a dying child by doing comparable lung-lobe grafts. In May 1991 a University of Minnesota team went even further than the Chicago group when they performed two successive live-donor lung-lobe transplants on 9-year-old Alyssa Plum: first, from her father and then, when it did not provide the little girl with enough lung capacity, another transplant from her mother. During the second procedure, Alyssa died of heart failure (Kolata 1991a). In a press interview, Dr. R. Morton Bolman, who performed the surgery, stated that "it would be premature to condemn living-donor lung transplants," but he also said he thought less experienced medical centers should not attempt the operation. "'If this has a chilling effect [he added], I think that's appropriate'" (Kolata 1991a).

All the issues posed by parent-to-child liver transplantation were involved in Alyssa Plum's lung transplants and in the living-donor lung transplants previously performed on two other recipients. In addition, the fact that both of Alyssa's parents served as donors opened up new issues about the moral limits of altruism and sacrifice. "If I didn't give Alyssa a chance at life," her mother testified, "I didn't know if I could live with myself" (Morrow 1991, p. 57). However understandable and laudable this parental motivation may be, one has only to look at the *Time* magazine photograph of Mr. and Mrs. Plum and their only surviving child, 6-year-old Travis, to see these questions portrayed. The two parents are sitting side by side, holding a framed picture of their deceased daughter. Standing slightly behind his mother, with his right hand resting on her shoulder, is Travis—the son who might have lost one or both of his parents if their gifts of life had eventuated in their deaths (Morrow 1991, p. 57).

Making a Live Donor: Bone Marrow Transplants

There is another form of live donation, employed since 1984, that is generating even greater uncertainty and debate about "the permissible limits of one of our most powerful instincts, the one that leads us to fight for the life of our children" (Quindlen 1991). Although there are no complete registry data, major bone marrow transplant centers have reported that between 1984 and 1989 they were involved with more than 40 cases of women who conceived and gave birth to a baby in order to provide a donor for their dying child, including eight infants who actually became donors (Kearney and Caplan 1991, p. 14).

The case that has received the most attention, because of the family's decision to go public, is that of the Ayala family, whose 19-year-old daughter, Anissa, was slowly dying of chronic myelogenous leukemia. Her only possible life-saving treatment was a marrow transplant, but no family members had the correct tissue type, and a subsequent national search did not locate a compatible unrelated donor. Then, in 1990, her parents announced that they had conceived a child on the one-in-four chance that the baby's tissue type would be compatible with Anissa's. A test done when Mrs. Ayala was six months' pregnant showed that there was a tissue match. Marissa was born in April, and at age 14 months was old enough to have the bone marrow withdrawn and infused into her sister.

The Ayalas' story was viewed by many as an act of love as well as of science— all the more so because the parents made it clear that they never considered aborting the fetus if its tissue type did not match Anissa's. Nor should it be assumed, various commentators pointed out, that under supposedly more usual and normal circumstances parents decide to have children for motives that are unquestionable, or that we have the right to restrictively define what these motives ought to be (Kearney and Caplan 1991; Kolata 1991b; Morrow 1991; Quindlen 1991). Nevertheless, a telephone poll conducted for *Time* in June 1991 revealed divided attitudes about the question of whether it is "morally acceptable for parents to conceive a child in order to obtain an organ or tissue to save the life of another one of their children," with 47 percent answering yes, and 37 percent no (Morrow 1991, p. 54). Pervading the discussion evoked by this case was an underlying uneasiness.

> [It was engendered by] the spectacle of a baby being brought into the world not, it seemed, as an end in herself, attended by all the sentiment and sanctity that people supposedly accord a new life. Rather the baby was ordered up to serve as a means, as a biological resupply vehicle.
>
> The baby did not consent to be used. The parents created the new life, then used that life for their own purposes, however noble. Would the baby have agreed to the transplant if she had been able to make the choice? Metaphysics: Would the baby have endorsed her own conception for such a purpose? (Morrow 1991, p. 54)

What was omitted from this and other discussions was a consideration of the heavy obligations and questions of meaning to which having a baby to serve as a tissue donor might subject the family: the "tyranny of the gift" sense of indebtedness that Anissa could feel toward Marissa, who was brought into the world to save her; the doubts that Marissa could eventually experience about her identity and her very reason for being; and the inadequacy, guilt, and pain the whole family may suffer if the transplant that Anissa received from her donor-sister fails to sustain her life.

Efforts to Increase Gifts of Life

Explaining the Organ Shortage

As those involved with the expanding field of transplantation recognized, the "limited organ supply" problem during the 1980s was not due primarily to negative public attitudes toward organ donation. Various surveys demonstrated the same extraordinary level of expressed support for organ donation and transplantation that has been consistently true of the American public for more than 20 years (Prottas 1983, 1988). Up to 90 percent of those polled said that they "strongly approve[d] of organ donation" (Annas 1988, p. 621). Through the Uniform Anatomical Gift Act, provisions to donate one's entire body or specific body parts for transplantation and other forms of treatment, medical research, or education could be arranged simply and directly by signing a witnessed donor card or, in 44 states, through a notation on a person's driver's license. Furthermore, the American organ procurement system had become the largest in the world (Prottas 1985),[2] and facilitated by the establishment of a national registry and donor-recipient matching system in 1986, one that retrieved more organs per capita than any other existing system. As the 1980s revealed, the chief sources of the discrepancy between organ demand and supply in the United States lay elsewhere.

Despite the nationwide adoption of the Uniform Anatomical Gift Act's provisions, and the public's expressed approval of organ donation, fewer than 20 percent of adults in the United States were estimated to have actually filled out donor cards or automobile license donation forms (Task Force on Organ Transplantation 1986).[3] Furthermore, transplant physicians have not relied on such "documents of gift" to legitimate their removal of organs, even though the law permits it. In part because they do not want to give even an appearance of routinely "harvesting" organs, medical staff almost without exception do not take an organ from a newly dead donor who has signed an anatomical gift form without written consent of the next of kin (Peters 1986).

The cadaveric source of most transplantable organs and the tragic circumstances under which they were usually procured impose other basic and powerful restrictions on donation. "Organ donors must be . . . healthy individuals who have suffered sudden and fatal trauma to the central nervous system. In practice, [this means that] most donors are young and have been killed in accidents—usually motor vehicle accidents" (Prottas 1989, p. 43).[4]

> Getting young, healthy adults (the core of the donor pool) to think about death is hard. Getting them to make plans after their death is harder. Getting them to discuss their death with their family yet harder. Getting them to do this based not on their financial responsibilities to their dependents but purely as a consideration to strangers multiplies the problem even further. And finally, to force discussion not merely of death as an inevitable end, but of death of an improbably and particularly tragic type [seems] . . . daunting. (Prottas 1983, pp. 289–290)

Systematically collected attitudinal data repeatedly suggested that reciprocal sentiments of apprehension and distrust in the relations between medical professionals and the American public played a significant role in curtailing the number of organs donated. On the one hand, studies revealed that in the growingly adversarial climate of the 1980s a substantial number of physicians were concerned that their participation in the organ procurement process might increase the likelihood of having a medical malpractice suit brought against them—even though under the Uniform Anatomical Gift Act's provisions they are not in fact legally liable. On the other hand, many respondents to polls on the public's attitudes toward organ donation and transplantation expressed anxiety about the possibility that if they signed a donor card physicians might prematurely take steps to pronounce them dead, to surgically excise their organs, or even to hasten their deaths (Gallup Organization 1985). "The stated willingness to become organ donors is even lower among groups (such as blacks) who perceive themselves to be on the margins of the system and to have even less reason to trust it" (Childress 1989, pp. 91–92).

Throughout the 1980s, medical, legal, ethical, and policy experts on organ donation, procurement, and transplantation continued to be concerned about the relation between the public's attitudes and behavior and the organ donation shortfall. Extensive "donor recruitment" campaigns conducted nationally and on state-by-state bases by groups such as The American Council on Transplantation and the National Kidney Foundation increased awareness of the need for "gifts of life" and in some instances markedly added to the number of people becoming designated donors (Levine 1985; Manninen and Evans 1985).

An example of the increasing effort to enlarge the pool of prospective donors was the Boy Scouts Donor Awareness Program, launched in the fall of 1989 in conjunction with The American Council on Transplantation. Full-page ads accompanied by tear-out donor cards told the American public how Scouts could earn the new Donor Awareness patch.

> Organ donation. It's worth talking about. And the Boy Scouts of America is offering a new patch to families who take the time to discuss it. If you're interested in receiving the Donor Awareness Patch, talk to your family about donation. Keep in mind, we're not looking for a commitment. We just want you to know what organ donation is and how it can benefit the lives of others.
>
> And for just becoming more aware, you'll earn a patch that lets people know your heart is in the right place. (Scouting 1989)

The advertisment campaign escalated in 1990, urging Scouts to tell their families about "the thousands of people who have benefited from transplants" and "the thousands who are waiting," and notifying them that they could purchase the Donor Awareness patch at their local Scout service center. Scouts also were notified that although they did not have to sign up as an organ donor to get the patch, "it's worth doing," so if they wanted to know more about it they could write to Donors Awareness at the National Kidney Foundation (Scouting 1990).

By the mid-1980s emphasis also was being placed on how the knowledge and skills, sentiments, and role behavior of physicians and nurses involved in the procurement process hampered organ donation and what could be done to remedy these problems.

> In recent years, between 70% and 75% of all families asked have granted permission for an organ donation. The willingness of the public to permit donation represents no practical impediment to improvement in the organ-procurement system. It is now widely understood that the cooperation of the medical professionals is the primary factor limiting the supply of transplantable organs. (Prottas 1988, p. 832)

> The transplant community has taken great solace over the years in the view that the public's lack of awareness and understanding of organ and tissue donation is the primary obstacle to broader support for organ procurement. But if opinion surveys are to be believed, the public knows full well about the need for transplants. The public continues to evince a strong interest in organ and tissue donation. . . . It is health care professionals, not the general public, who are in desperate need of education about their duties where organ and tissue procurement is concerned. (Caplan 1988, p. 37)

Required Request

Attention focused particularly on what was viewed as the frequent "failure" of physicians and nurses to approach families of patients potentially qualified to become organ donors, to inform them of the possibility and right they had to donate their relative's organs, and ask them if they were willing to do so. In response to what was now defined as this "main bottleneck" to organ donation, bioethicist Arthur M. Caplan proposed that "required request" procedures be established in hospitals to ensure that the next-of-kin or the legal guardians of every potential donor be notified of the transplantation option and asked to make a donation of their relative's organs for this purpose (Caplan 1984a,b).[5] Caplan's idea was rapidly drafted into law. By the end of the 1980s, required request had been enacted by most state legislatures and mandated in federal leg-islation for all institutions receiving Medicare or Medicaid funds. It also was incorporated into hospital accreditation standards and recommended by the National Conference of Commissioners on Uniform State Laws as a revision in the Uniform Anatomical Gift Act (Martyn et al. 1988).

Despite the almost bandwagon-like conviction and speed with which the required request principle was translated into laws and procedures, preliminary studies of its impact on the attitudes and behavior of doctors and nurses most likely to be involved in organ procurement,[6] and on the number of organs made available for transplants since it became mandatory suggested that its influence was minor at best (Annas 1988; Caplan 1988). One of the notable patterns Caplan and his associates at the University of Minnesota Center for Biomedical Ethics discovered when they conducted a telephone survey of ten states in which required request laws had been in effect for more than 6 months was "resistance by physicians to complying with the new laws. Rates of compliance in many states [did] not exceed 50 percent" (Caplan 1988, p. 35).

Conceptual Confusion and Emotional Unease About Brain Death

The inability of the required request legislation to provide a "legal fix" for the problems of organ procurement and supply and the recalcitrance it engendered in some physicians were associated with one of its most important, though largely unanticipated, consequences. Its enactment helped to surface and under-score the pervasive conceptual confusion over defining and declaring "brain death" and the disquietude about some of its implications for the medical man-agement of the organ donor and for organ retrieval that existed among physi-cians and nurses. In April 1989, for example, the *Journal of the American Med-ical Association* published two articles and an editorial that dealt with physicians' and nurses' knowledge, personal concepts, attitudes, and feelings concerning brain death and with what caring for the brain-dead donor in a hos-pital intensive care unit entailed for the staff. Some of the role conflicts and emo-tional difficulties they underwent while identifying organ donors, making brain death decisions, and approaching families of potential donors were examined (Darby et al. 1989; Wikler and Weisbard 1989; Youngner et al. 1989).

One of the articles was based on an "exploratory-descriptive" study that Stuart J. Youngner and his associates conducted among 195 physicians and nurses "likely to be involved in organ procurement" in four university-affiliated Cleveland hospitals with active transplant programs. In a survey-type interview, respondents were asked the factual question, "What brain functions must be lost for a patient to be declared brain dead?" They also were presented with two cases and asked, first, whether each patient was *legally* dead, and second, whether, aside from legalities, they personally considered these patients to be dead and why. Finally, nurses' and physicians' attitudes toward "required request" were explored through another question: "What is your opinion about a law requiring that hospitals ask families of brain-dead patients who are suitable donors about organ donation?" The Youngner study documented what philosopher Daniel Wikler and jurist Alan J. Weisbard referred to in their editorial commentary as the "conceptual disarray" over the "definition" of death, particularly "brain death," that existed among health professionals (Wikler and Weisbard 1989). "Only 68 respondents (35%) correctly identified the legal and medical criteria for determining death" (Youngner et al. 1989, p. 2205). Those unable to correctly identify the criteria included more than one-third of the physicians "responsible for identifying 'brain dead' patients and declaring them dead . . . [and] nearly three-fourths of another group of medical residents, anesthesiologists, and nurses who work[ed] in the areas of intensive care and transplantation" (Wikler and Weisbard 1989). Furthermore, "personal concepts of death varied widely," and more than half of the respondents "did not use a coherent concept of death consistently" (Youngner et al. 1989, p. 2205). Although these results were "troubling," Wikler and Weisbard cautioned that care should be taken to avoid misunderstanding their import.

> The study . . . does not suggest that brain death is being misdiagnosed; indeed, the diagnosis is as certain as anything in medicine. There is no suggestion that patients are being declared dead, or serving as organ donors who are not brain dead. The problems revealed by the survey lie . . . in the conceptual foundations of the whole-brain definition. Though clinicians can tell which patients have permanent loss of all brain function there is no consensus over whether, and especially why, this means they have died. (Wikler and Weisbard 1989)

There are numerous reasons for the medical profession's confusion about "criteria and concepts of death," "lack of clarity about why brain dead patients are dead," and anxiety and "discomfort" over participating in the processes of acquiring organs, maintaining brain-dead donors, and recovering their organs (Youngner et al. 1989, pp. 2205–06, 2209–10). One set of factors involves the reasons for and ways in which brain death criteria developed, and the fact that these new criteria coexist with the traditional medical and legal standard that persons are dead when they have sustained irreversible cessation of circulatory and respiratory functions.

Some of the persisting confusion about brain death dates from 1968, when an Ad Hoc Harvard Medical School Committee published a landmark report on "the definition of brain death" (Ad Hoc Committee 1968). Although the Committee defined brain death in terms of the abolition of function "at cerebral, brain-stem, and often spinal levels," they also used the term "irreversible coma" as synonymous with brain death. Many people, professionals as well as laypersons, subsequently have been unclear as to whether persons in irreversible coma or persistent vegetative states, such as Karen Ann Quinlan and Nancy Beth Cruzan, are "alive" or "brain dead." Medically and legally they are alive, although they lack those cortical functions that support awareness and cognition, and ethical and legal questions about stopping their treatment are of a completely different nature than that of declaring brain death.

The Harvard Ad Hoc Committee was a response to the growing conviction of medical professionals and legal experts that, for two reasons, new criteria for pronouncing death were needed. First, the Committee cited concerns about the "burdens" on patients, families, and hospital resources caused by "improvements in resuscitative and support measures." These improvements had led to "situations in which lives are saved," but with only "partial success so that the result is an individual whose heart continues to beat but whose brain is irreversibly damaged." Second, "obsolete criteria for the definition of death can lead to controversy in obtaining organs for transplantation" (Ad Hoc Committee 1968, p. 337).

Brain death criteria were progressively developed during the 1970s by the medical community and through a series of court decisions and numerous state statutes on the determination of death. These developments led to the Uniform Determination of Death Act proposed in 1981 by the President's Commission for the Study of Ethical Problems in Medicine and Biomedical and Behavioral Research (President's Commission 1981). The model act, which defined death as either irreversible cessation of cardiopulmonary functions or of the functions of the whole brain, including the brain stem, was endorsed by the American Medical Association, the American Bar Association, and the National Conference of Commissioners on Uniform State Laws, and subsequently enacted by most state legislatures.[7]

However laudable the intent of the new medicolegal definition of death, there have been questions about its necessity and concerns about some of its unintended consequences for organ procurement. In Annas' opinion, for example, "the rush to legislation gave the impression that a new definition of death was being adopted just so organs could be harvested," when in fact, "no new laws were needed for the medical profession to adopt . . . 'brain death' as death," because the law in the United States "has always given physicians the authority to pronounce death, as long as [they] do so in accordance with good and accepted medical standards" (Annas 1988, p. 621).

Whether needed or not, legislation has made irreversible loss of all brain functions widely accepted as a *criterion* for determining death. As Youngner and colleagues pointed out, however, the criterion and its acceptance were not accompanied by "a corresponding, widely accepted *concept* explaining exactly why"— philosophically as well as technically—"brain dead patients are dead" (Youngner et al. 1989, pp. 2205–06).

The reasons physicians, nurses, and families have found it so difficult to comprehend brain death, emotionally and conceptually, have to do partly with the appearance of the brain-dead "patient" and how she or he is medically "managed."

> [A]lthough cadaver organ donors are declared dead, they hardly resemble patients who have died from cardiopulmonary arrest. In fact, they remind us in many ways of living patients. They are warm and retain a healthy color, which is no surprise, because their hearts continue to pump oxygenated blood throughout their bodies. Digestion, metabolism, and elimination continue.
>
> Although it is certainly true that the life processes of these dead could not continue without considerable technologic intervention, the same technologic methods are commonly used to sustain living patients in intensive care units and operating rooms. Maintaining organs for transplantation actually necessitates treating dead patients in many respects as if they were alive. Thus, even health professionals who understand and accept the new criterion for death on an intellectual level may find it difficult to ignore the signs of life that constantly bombard their senses as they provide brain-dead organ donors with intensive and intimate medical care. (Youngner et al. 1985, p. 321)

When the Harvard Committee proposed its definition of "irreversible coma" in 1968, it thought that "if the characteristics [of brain death] can be defined in satisfactory terms, translatable into action . . . several problems will either disappear or will become more readily soluble" (Ad Hoc Committee 1968). More than 30 years later, as our discussion has suggested, numerous problems still confound the acceptance and use of brain death in relation to organ donation. We have yet even to decide what to call those who have been pronounced dead but are being cared for until their organs can be "harvested."

> They are hardly "corpses" in the traditional sense. Although they are "dead patients," they do not resemble our other dead patients. The expression "brain-dead" is accurate but seems to avoid the crucial issues. Most would agree that these donors are no longer "persons." When the patient is admitted to the operating

room, the recorded diagnosis is "beating-heart cadaver"—a term that is offensive to many people. Gaylin coined the term "neomort" 10 years ago, but it has not become popular. Perhaps we will only be able to give these artificially maintained organ donors an appropriate name when we ourselves have made the necessary emotional and cultural adjustments. (Youngner et al. 1985, p. 323)

Youngner is appreciative of what an emotional toll caring for these "dead patients" as if they were alive takes on intensive care nurses and of how difficult it is for operating room nurses to be left to deal with the body of a donor after numerous organs and tissues have been removed from it. As he has suggested, there is a need to develop new nursing rituals that symbolically distinguish caring for the cadaver donor from that of patients and that infuse the macabre nature of what is involved with "gift of life" meaning (personal communication).

"Transplantation Depends on Death"

Advocates of the required request approach to the organ shortage, such as Caplan and Prottas, were not unaware of the added role conflict and stress to which it subjected physicians and nurses. Each responded to its impact on medical professionals in his own fashion. Caplan's reaction was to pugnaciously defend the required request mechanism that he had devised and to severely criticize the "arrogance" of the medical profession in resisting it.

In enacting required request legislation, our society has indicated its collective desire that people routinely be given the option of organ and tissue donation as a last act of respect for the dead and their families and as an expression of concern for those who will die unless more organs and tissues are made available. It has not yet put its money where its ethical concerns are in the form of resources to train health care professionals to feel comfortable rather than angry in discharging their obligations to the dead and those who are dying. . . . [Health care professionals] need to be taught how to make requests, or if they are too discomfited by death, to yield authority over matters pertaining to procurement to others more adept at dealing with this harsh reality. (Caplan 1988, p. 372)

Prottas expressed much more empathy for the predicament of doctors and nurses in the intensive care unit where most organ donors are hospitalized. "[I]n this environment," he wrote, "[i]dentifying and referring the dying are . . . not matters of primary importance." What is more, the intensive care unit staff is asked to "identify . . . donors *proactively* while pursuing their central and most pressing duties" (Prottas 1988, p. 832). As a way to diminish the demands and pressures that the organ procurement process makes on physicians and nurses and to "open the bottleneck . . . constrain[ing] the supply of organs" that these "problems of professional cooperation" created, Prottas proposed that a policy of "routine referral" be instituted that would increase "the organ-procurement system's access to potential donors independently of the behavior of intensive care unit staff."

> This policy would require hospitals routinely to inform organ procurement agencies of *admissions* that are likely to lead to a potential organ-donor situation.... To be sure, everything would not change. The medical staff would still have the final say regarding the donor's suitability. Routine referral would not allow the organ procurement agency to contact a family directly without the permission of those responsible for the care of the patient, nor would this new system eliminate all the reservations that medical professionals have about organ procurement. The need for professional education would continue, but the demands placed on these professionals would be reduced markedly. They would have to respond to a request, much as the family does now, rather than have to initiate a process independently. (Prottas 1988, pp. 832–833)

Prottas was mindful of what he called the "social problems" that routine referral might create for the organ procurement staff, who "would inevitably be contacting intensive care units about patients who are not actually suitable as donors. These encounters could be emotionally demanding and give the impression that the organ procurement agency is waiting for someone to die—that they are 'vultures'" (Prottas 1988, p. 633). Prottas' reflections on the difficulties he foresaw in initiating a routine referral policy were in part philosophical, testifying to his belief in the redeeming importance of organ procurement and transplantation, even though it entailed "waiting for tragedy."

> But if donors are to be located, physicians and nurses must be contacted, and if it appears that the organ procurement agency is "waiting for someone to die," it is because they are. But this is quite different from wanting someone to die, and painful as the thought must be, organ transplantation depends on death. (Prottas 1988, p. 833)

From Gifts of Life to Market Commodities?

The growing imbalance between the demand for transplantable organs and their supply in the United States and other countries has fueled long-simmering concerns about illicit black markets in body parts and debate about the pros and cons of various forms of regulated payment for organ donations. Issues concerning the buying, selling, and brokering of solid organs and tissues have evoked strong responses from many medical groups and from ethicists, lawyers, economists, legislators, and policy analysts; from a variety of local, national, and international political and governmental bodies; and from the mass media. Reactions to the concept of legalized payment for organs and to their illicit brokerage went beyond spirited discussion and debate. On the one hand, it led to the drafting of special guidelines and resolutions by an array of medical societies and health organizations and to the passage of a number of new laws that proscribed buying and selling organs. On the other hand, somewhat paradoxically, a number of individuals concerned with public policy aspects of transplantation began to advocate and develop proposals for the regulated compensation of donors and for dealing with bodily parts as market commodities.

In the United States the 1968 Uniform Anatomical Gift Act was adopted in some form in all states by 1973. In according individuals the right to designate prior to death whether they wished their bodies or organs to be used for transplants or other medical purposes,[8] the Act did not deal explicitly with the sale of organs. Rather, according to the chairman of the drafting committee, it was deliberately neutral on the matter.

> It is possible, of course, that abuses may occur if payment could customarily be demanded, but every payment is not necessarily unethical. . . . Until the matter of payment becomes a problem of some dimensions, the matter should be left to the decency of intelligent human beings. (Stason 1968, p. 928)

Selling the Gift

In 1983 an event occurred suggesting that "the matter of payment" had become an acutely serious issue. Physician H. Barry Jacobs, founder and medical director of International Kidney Exchange, Inc., wrote to 7,500 hospitals asking if they would be interested in participating in his plan to buy and sell human kidneys in a national and international market through his brokerage company. What he proposed was commissioning kidneys from persons living in the Third World or in disadvantaged circumstances in the United States for whatever price would induce them to sell their organs, and then negotiating their acquisition, for a fee, by Americans who could afford to purchase them.

Jacobs' plan aroused consternation in the medical community and in the U.S. Congress. It was denounced as "immoral and unethical" by The National Kidney Foundation, The Transplantation Society, the American Society of Transplant Physicians, and the American Society of Transplant Surgeons, who not only condemned it but resolved to expel any of their members involved in such a commercial scheme. At hearings about Jacobs' brokering enterprise held by the U.S. House of Representatives' Subcommittee on Health and Environment in the summer and fall of 1983, members of Congress expressed their moral repugnance at the specter of exploitation and coercion represented by the buying and selling of kidneys.

Subsequently, some 90 House members cosponsored what became the 1984 National Organ Transplantation Act (Public Law 98-507). The Act authorized federal financial support for local nonprofit organ procurement organizations and for a national organ procurement and transplantation network to assist in matching organ donors and recipients; established a National Task Force on Organ Transplantation to "conduct comprehensive examinations of the medical, legal, ethical, economic, and social issues presented by human organ procurement and transplantation"; and expressly outlawed commercial markets in transplantable organs by making it a federal crime to "knowingly acquire, receive, or otherwise transfer any human organ for valuable consideration for use in human transplantation if the transfer affects interstate commerce."

At a November 1983 Congressional hearing on the proposed Act, philosopher/ethicist Samuel Gorovitz expressed the larger moral and societal reasons for which he fervently believed that the sort of "commercialization of life" represented by Jacobs' plan should be legislatively prohibited.

> I am concerned, of course, with what such a scheme would do to those whose destitution and desperation might move them to sell bodily parts in hope of gaining a foothold for the climb out of poverty. But I am concerned even more about what such behavior would do to the rest of us, and what it would reveal about our compassion, our commitment to equality, our capacity to make voluntary efforts in the public interest, and our willingness to face common problems with collective resolve. (Gorovitz 1984, p. 12)

Gorovitz's convictions were echoed in the "guidelines for the distribution and use of organs" published by The Transplantation Society in 1985, which were reinforced by concrete examples of the "instances of brokerage of kidneys" that had "begun to emerge."

> In a South American country . . . advertisements from desperate individuals have appeared in newspapers offering a kidney or even an eye (for corneal transplantation) for money. In this regard, many of us receive occasional pathetic appeals from people in disadvantaged countries offering to sell a kidney to get money, often for care of an ill relative. Besides being an eloquent comment on the social inequalities of our society in general, such appeals raise unsettling ethical questions of a more specific nature. . . . Furthermore, an active market of living unrelated kidney transplantation with payment to donors is occurring in at least one city in India; some of these donors make their way, with the potential recipient and "proof" of consanguinity, to the West. Thus recently, a major newspaper has described the buying of kidneys from impoverished donors for transplantation in private hospitals in

Western countries. Some donations were coerced, some for meager fees; and allegedly there was no follow-up of the donors after surgery. . . . A similar situation exists in other countries where kidneys are bought from destitute living donors in surrounding regions. It seems clear that when patient care is relegated to the laws of the market place, particularly when the less privileged can be exploited to improve the health of the more privileged, all in society are diminished. (Council of The Transplantation Society, 1985, p. 716)

The Society's guidelines ended with a "special resolution."

No transplant surgeon/team shall be involved directly or indirectly in the buying or selling of organs/tissues or in any transplant activity aimed at commercial gain to himself/herself or an associated hospital or institute. Violation of these guidelines by any member of The Transplantation Society may be cause for expulsion from the Society. (Council of The Transplantation Society 1985, p. 716)

The 1986 final report by the National Task Force on Organ Procurement and Transplantation supported this position taken by the transplant community, reaffirming the ban on commerce in organs that the National Organ Transplant Act had legislated. The report recognized that thus far the voluntary gift-giving on which the American organ procurement system was based had not furnished an adequate supply of suitable organs for transplantation. Nevertheless, the Task Force concluded that it would be "ethically and politically unwise to resort to sales of solid organs until recent and proposed policies to enhance express donation by individuals and family members [had] had sufficient time to work," in part because "transfer of organs by sales would be costly, would probably drive out many donations," and might undermine the simultaneously moral and social principles of "encouraged altruism" (Childress 1989, pp. 100–101, 110). Under the influence of its vice-chairman, James F. Childress, the Task Force also emphasized the seriously adverse effects that allowing organs to be bought and sold could have on "our conception of personhood and embodiment by promoting [their] commodification" (Childress 1989, pp. 101, 110). For Childress, these concerns were not only grounded in basic ethical principles, such as "the dignity of the individual," "respect for persons" and their bodies, and "the obligation to benefit others." They also rested on theological precepts such as the person's "transcendence" and "stewardship" obligations to our bodies and to the community that "set limits on what human beings may do with and to their own bodies, and those of others" (Childress 1989, p. 88; 1986, p. 4).

As various investigative reports have documented, however, the development of national and international commercial markets for "selling the gift" of kidneys and other body parts has not been significantly deterred by these appeals to moral and social values, by professional rules and sanctions, or by laws (Chengappa 1990; Schneider and Flaherty 1985c). By 1989 more than 20 countries had instituted political or legal provisions against commerce in organs. The World Health Organization thought that the practice had become so rampant and problematic that it issued a resolution condemning trafficking in human organs, asking member nations to take appropriate measures against it (Trucco 1989).

The same year, on July 28, 1989, a law was passed by the British Parliament making it a "criminal offense to give or receive money for supplying organs of either a living or dead person," to act as a broker in such a transaction, to advertise for organs for payment, or to transplant an organ from a live, stranger donor. Punishment for breaking the law was either a $3,300 fine or 3 months in prison and, in the case of convicted physicians, the possibility of losing the right to practice medicine. The fact that the British thought it necessary to pass this law, even though their 1961 Human Tissue Act deemed it unethical for medical practitioners to be involved in any way in the buying and selling of human organs, was indicative of the extent to which commerce in organs was considered to be dangerously out of control. Behind it lay a tragic critical incident that had occurred the year before and had received front-page attention from the British media.

> Last summer Colin Benton died after receiving a kidney transplant at a private London hospital. Several months later . . . his case made headlines throughout Britain when his widow disclosed that her husband's kidney transplant had come from a Turkish citizen who was paid $3,300 to fly to Britain to donate the organ. The donor said he had decided to sell his kidney to pay for medical treatment for his daughter. . . .
>
> One investigation led in May to the conviction and imprisonment in Turkey of 55-year-old Tunc Kunter, the kidney broker who recruited the Turkish donor for Mr. Benton's operation. . . .
>
> Two London doctors [also] are being investigated by Britain's Medical Council for their roles in the Benton operation. (Trucco 1989)

By 1990 trafficking in "human spare parts" was a booming business in developing countries such as India, which had no organized systems for procuring cadaveric donor organs, no brain death statute, and no specific laws banning the sale of human organs and tissues. In a story on "the organs bazaar" in *India Today*, Raj Chengappa reported that his country led the world market in buying and selling kidneys from unrelated living "donors," growing from an estimated 50 such transactions in 1983 to more than 2,000 in 1990 (Chengappa 1990, p. 31). In what the International Commission of Health Professionals called a "vile, deplorable, and morally reprehensible development," trade in organs and other body parts was taking on the semblance of marketplace bazaars in large cities and small rural villages across the country, with fixed price ranges for items such as live donor kidneys, live corneas, skin patches, whole cadavers, and skeletons. India's commerce in organs, Chengappa wrote, "is still largely a shadowy business, controlled by an intricate network of touts, donors and hospitals clandestinely performing such operations. . . . A new phrase has even been coined called 'rewarded gifting' to make it sound legal" (Chengappa 1990, pp. 30, 35).

Body Parts as Market Commodities

The resounding concerns about the moral and social dangers regarding the body as a commodity and the attempts to discourage the selling and buying of organs continued throughout the 1980s. However, running parallel to these actions and the convictions on which they were based was a contravening set of trends that gained momentum as the decade unfolded.

To begin with, there were persistent voices, such as that of health policy analyst Jeffrey M. Prottas, arguing that organ donation and procurement was not just "a moral enterprise" and "a mechanism for giving reality to altruism" (Prottas 1989, p. 42). In his view, it should also be defined as a not-for-profit "industry" engaged in "selling altruism" (Prottas and Batten 1991, p. 131). Organ donations, Prottas held, can be maximized and made more efficient by applying more sophisticated business, advertising, and charitable fund-raising strategies, such as "systematically analyzing and planning market strategies, utilizing information technologies, or managing sales forces" (Prottas 1989, pp. 42, 53–54).

Prottas' marketing and business approach remained within the "gift of life" and "encouraged altruism" concept of organ donation endorsed by the National Task Force on Transplantation. From the mid-1980s, however, an increasing number of persons writing about the scarce supply of transplantable organs and about how donation rates might be augmented took leave of such a gift-exchange framework. They argued that many of the problems of obtaining and distributing organs could be ameliorated by the adoption of one or more systems of financial incentives or "regulated compensation" to those providing their organs or to their next of kin. In what physician and medical ethicist Edmund Pellegrino rebutted as a "logically, ethically, and practically flawed" proposal, for example, transplant surgeon Thomas Peters advocated the payment of a $1,000 death benefit payment to "motivate families of potential organ donors" (Pellegrino 1991, p. 1305; Peters 1991, p. 1302). "Our concerns must focus not on some philosophic imperative such as altruism," Peters believed, "but on our collective responsibility for maximizing lifesaving organ recovery" (Peters 1991, p. 1305). As this statement suggests, Peters believes emphatically that payment should not be rendered merely for "goodwill or for consent" but only for the recovery of usable organs. "Unfair? Perhaps, but the focus must remain on saving lives that are now lost because next-of-kin cannot be rewarded in a manner that might increase organ recovery" (Peters 1991, p. 1304).

Other, more far-reaching proposals involved creating a market in organs by methods that are much more sophisticated than simply permitting organs to be bought and sold on the open marketplace. For example, one economist proposed establishing a "futures market" in cadaveric organs through which "the right to harvest a person's organs upon death must be purchased from him while still alive and well" (Hansmann 1989, p. 62).

Elaborating on how such a plan could operate, Hansmann saw health insurance companies as the "natural purchasers of future rights to organs" that could arrange these purchases through provisions in insurance premium statements. Under this market arrangement, it would be assumed that any one who has not "sold a futures contract for their organs" does not want them used for transplantation, eliminating the issue of buying organs postmortem from a person's estate or next of kin.

> The insurance companies would act primarily as intermediaries, purchasing and then reselling rights to harvest organs. Many insurance companies might choose to resell their futures contracts to other firms that would specialize in holding such contracts. . . .
>
> [Under such a system] the price (premium reduction) that insurance companies would pay for the future right to cadaveric organs would depend on the price that they could obtain for those organs at the time of removal. Since the health insurance business is reasonably competitive, presumably insurance companies would be able to take only a market rate of return for their efforts as intermediaries in such transactions. (Hansmann 1989, pp. 63–65)

The chief spokespersons for shifting from a gift to a market model of organ donation and procurement were certain economists, lawyers, and health policy analysts and managers who shared a set of assumptions. They were convinced that an "organ market" would be a more effective mechanism for increasing the supply of organs than "the altruistic 'gift relationship' [which] may be inadequate as a motivator" (Trucco 1989). Although they conceded that markets were driven by the self-interest of buyers and sellers competitively vying with one another, they also saw the market as a social policy instrument that would reduce the "social costs" of transplantation by fostering greater efficiency and coordination in the process of exchange and distribution. Proposals to draft model statutes that would permit regulated sale of human organs for transplantation, rather than prohibit such transactions, were now introduced.

Even if the commercial sales of organs were ethically wrong, these thinkers argued (which they did not believe was the case), "it may nevertheless be preferable to accepting the suffering and death of patients who cannot otherwise obtain transplants" (Trucco 1989). In their view, the main reason people are ethically uneasy about "using markets to handle transactions that were formerly guided in large part by norms mandating a degree of altruism" is that they were "previously socialized to think it immoral to approach [these] transactions from a strongly self-regarding stance." Thus "to see the same transactions now subjected only to the mores of the marketplace" is at first likely to seem "deeply offensive" to them (Hansmann 1989, p. 76). However, those advocating a market approach to organ procurement find it more offensive to argue that "allowing payment for body parts could unduly coerce the poor to donate." In their opinion, "banning payment on ethical grounds to prevent such scenarios overlooks one important fact: to the person who needs money to feed his children or to purchase medical care for her parent, the option of not selling a body part is worse than the option of selling it" (Andrews 1986, p. 32). (Those arguing on these grounds for the right of individuals to sell parts of their bodies do not express concern about ameliorating the impoverished conditions in which such persons and their families live, so they would not feel compelled to resort to this "option.")

Another conviction shared by many proponents of a market in organs is that "people's body parts are their personal property," and they thus have a right to transfer and sell them.

> This is distinguishable from the past characterizations of people as property, which were immoral because they failed to take into account the nonbodily aspects of an individual . . . and they created the rights of ownership by others. . . . I am advocating not that people be treated by others as property, but only that they have the autonomy to treat their own parts as property, particularly their regenerative parts. Such an approach is helpful, rather than harmful, to people's well-being. It offers potential psychological, physical, and economic benefits to individuals and provides a framework for handling evolving issues regarding the control of extracorporeal biological materials. (Andrews 1986, p. 37)[9]

By the end of the 1980s, even medical ethicist and religionist James Childress, a leading exponent of the gift-exchange model of procuring organs, was expressing the opinion that:

> If a system of donation with various modifications proves to be insufficiently effective, then transfer by sales could be tried, even though it would not express the value of altruism that leads many to favor the gift relationship. . . .
> Even if selling some HBPs [human body parts], such as solid organs, would be potentially dehumanizing to the society, there is debate about whether dehumanization results from the sales of all human biological materials, including surplus

tissues and fluids (e.g., hair and urine) and renewable tissue (e.g., blood). It may even be plausible to view the sale of renewable tissues as the provision of a service . . . rather than as a commodity. . . . Furthermore, it would be possible to distinguish types of valuable consideration, such as direct payments and indirect incentives. For example, could the line be drawn between direct payment and coverage of a donor's medical expenses, compensation of a living donor's lost wages, and payment for the burial expenses of a deceased donor? In short, through various distinctions, it may be possible to accommodate some types of transfer of some kinds of tissues for valuable consideration without major ethical costs. (Childress 1989, p. 101)

When giving serious consideration to the admissibility of certain forms of payment for donor tissues and organs, in his role as a transplant policy-maker Childress was pragmatically willing to modify his long-standing commitment to gift-giving as the most ethically preferable basis for organ procurement. The concepts of "stewardship" and "trusteeship" of the body, "altruism," "generosity," "charity," and "community" that he articulated when writing as a moral philosopher were replaced by the language of economics.

Whether human organs will, in fact, become societally legitimated market commodities rather than "gifts of life" is an open question as the 1990s begin. The answer depends as much on social, political, and ideological forces at work on the American scene, as on the magnitude of the organ shortage. For it is more than coincidental that a market approach to organ donation gained momentum during the 1980s, a decade when a certain view of the market has not only become more prominent and "attractive" in the economic sector of American society but in its "moral and social spheres as well" (A. Wolfe 1989, p. 76). This market vision—permeated by supply-side economic and neo-conservative political thinking—is grounded in the conviction that economic and social relations should ideally be organized around and guided by the maximization of rational, self-interested free choices, and that "moral obligations to others can be satisfied [best] . . . by first satisfying obligations to the self" (A. Wolfe 1989, p. 33). In its most extreme laissez-faire form, a market-based outlook is considered to be just as applicable to the procuring of human organs for transplantation, and paying for them, as it is to economically driven decisions about any other "commodity."

Transplantation and the Medical Commons

"The dilemma confronting us," Dr. Howard Hiatt wrote in 1975, "is how we can place additional stress on the medical commons without bringing ourselves closer to ruin" (Hiatt 1975, p. 235). Hiatt's exploration of the nature of the medical commons and who is responsible for protecting its limited resources drew on an earlier paper by Garret Hardin, which used population growth to illustrate the types of human problems that, he argued, are not amenable to technical solutions (Hardin 1968). Both authors addressed the perennial ethical and social policy questions of how we should guard against the depletion of finite resources and how those resources should be most justly distributed. They did so through the analogy of a common pasture, shared by a group of herdsmen who, as their cattle increase, must decide how to balance their self-interests with the need to protect the land from overgrazing and ultimate destruction.

In this chapter, drawing on Hiatt's image of medical care as a common ground that contains a finite amount of resources, we examine three sets of issues posed by the expanding effort to prevent death and hopefully restore health by replacing failing organs. These issues actually involve several "commons." First, within the sphere of transplantation, we look at the ways scarce vital organs are being allocated to potential recipients and the range of policy and human value issues posed by these means of distribution. Second, we consider the question of whether we ought to be committing more and more of our finite material and nonmaterial medical resources to organ replacement; or, as some analysts of health care needs and services have suggested, is organ replacement a pursuit that is forcing us to confront the possibility of protecting the medical commons through nonprice rationing? Third, thinking of medical care in relation to other societal needs and resources, the transplantation endeavor raises, in particularly dramatic and stark form, perhaps the most difficult social values and social policy question we need to confront about the nature and ends of medicine. That question, in the words of philosopher Daniel Callahan, is "What kind of medicine is best for a good society, and what kind of society is best for a good medicine?" (Callahan 1990a, p. 29). How does transplantation speak to what we mean by "medical progress," and is it the type of progress we want to continue to pursue?

The Transplantation Commons

As we discussed in Chapter 1, the 1980s saw an extensive growth in the range, number, and combination of tissues and solid organs that were transplanted, fostered by the introduction of newly developed immunosuppressive drugs and improved surgical techniques and methods for procuring and preserving donor organs. One of the major concomitants of this "boom," which we examined in Chapter 3, has been the way it has exacerbated the imbalance between the supply of transplantable organs and the demand for them.

At least by publicly visible yardsticks such as professional and popular literature and transplant-related policy debates and actions, the transplant community has been far more preoccupied with ways to significantly increase the number of organs available for transplantation than with the thorny distributive justice problem of who, among those in need, should receive these scarce potentially life-saving resources. In Chapters 2 and 3 we examined a variety of strategies employed to reduce the "organ shortfall" within the traditional gift exchange framework of organ donation and proposals to adopt a market framework in which organs and other body parts would be treated like "any other" commodity.

Despite the variety of attempted or proposed strategies to obtain more organs from both the living and the dead, however, the expanding scope and quickening pace of transplantation has meant that the demand far outstrips the supply, forcing transplant teams and organ procurement agencies to grapple with the question of how, in principle and practice, these scarce resources should be distributed. In terms of the principles of equity that, most believe, ideally should govern access to health care resources and their use in the United States (President's Commission 1983), sociomedical policy and value questions permeate two major decision-making stages in allocating organs. First, what criteria do or should determine access to the system; that is, how are patients referred to transplant centers, accepted as transplant candidates, and placed on a waiting list for an organ? Second, once potential recipients are in the system, what criteria do or should govern who receives donor organs?

Social policies concerned with equitable access to vital organs and tissues have been promulgated by the National Transplantation Act of 1984 (Public Law 98-507), the recommendations of the federal Task Force on Organ Transplantation in 1986, and by the policies adopted by the United Network for Organ Sharing (UNOS), our national Organ Procurement and Transplantation Network. To date, the framers of transplantation policies have largely bypassed the question of how access to waiting lists should be handled and focused instead on who receives organs once they have been accepted as transplant candidates (Childress 1987; McDonald 1988; Task Force 1986). James F. Childress, a prominent medical ethicist and religionist, Vice-Chairman of the Task Force, and a member of UNOS' board, holds that concerns about patient access to waiting lists "probably cannot be directly addressed by UNOS and will require attention from other social institutions" (Childress 1989, p. 108). Yet, Childress continued, as the task force, UNOS, and others involved in transplantation have recognized,

> There is evidence that women, minorities, and low-income patients do not receive transplants at the same rate as white men with high incomes. The primary source of the unequal access . . . appear[s] to be . . . in the decisions about who will be admitted to the waiting list. . . . More research will be required to determine the extent to which unequal access to kidney transplantation, for example, hinges on patient choices and legitimate medical factors rather than on physician sequestration of patients in dialysis units, physician failure to inform and refer some groups of patients, or bias in the selection of patients seeking admission to waiting lists. (Childress 1989, p. 108; see also Eggers 1988; Kjellstrand 1988; Task Force 1986; U.S. DHHS 1987)

In addition to particularistic types of selection factors, the major barrier to equitable access at this point of entry into the organ replacement system, as for virtually all other areas of health care in the United States, is the "green screen" of ability to pay. The passage of Public Law 92-603 in 1972, providing Medicare coverage for most of the treatment costs for end-stage renal disease (ESRD), exempted most patients eligible for kidney transplantation or dialysis from the financial criterion for access (Fox and Swazey 1978a, chs. 7, 11; Rettig 1976). However, as detailed in a 1991 report by the Institute of Medicine (IOM) on "kidney failure and the federal government," Medicare funding has not completely removed finances as a significant factor (Levinsky and Rettig 1991a). Transplantation is "unequivocally the best treatment for most patients with chronic renal failure, and over time far less costly to the federal government: excluding copayments and deductibles, it currently costs Medicare approximately $32,000 a year for each dialysis patient, compared to an average of $56,000 for the first year of a kidney transplant and $6,000 a year thereafter"

(Levinsky and Rettig 1991b, pp. 1145, 1144). However, Medicare coverage for kidney transplants has two major restrictions: Eligibility is confined to a 3-year period after a successful transplant, and the costs of the expensive, lifelong immunosuppressive drugs that must be taken to prevent rejection of the transplanted organ are reimbursed for only 1 year.

Dialysis patients eligible for Medicare coverage also encounter costs they must pay themselves, especially for home treatment. Moreover, some 7 percent of ESRD patients—"concentrated disproportionately among the poor and minorities"—are ineligible for any Medicare coverage because of their insurance status under Social Security (Levinsky and Rettig 1991b, p. 1145).

The Institute of Medicine study committee, believing that "access to life-saving therapy should not be limited on any basis other than status as a citizen or resident alien," recommended two major changes in the Medicare "entitlement" for ESRD patients. First, all citizens and resident aliens should receive Medicare coverage for dialysis; second, kidney transplant patients should "be granted a lifetime entitlement comparable to that available to patients on dialysis," including the cost of immunosuppressive drugs (Levinsky and Rettig 1991b, pp. 1145–1146). At the same time, the IOM committee, like many previous analysts, have recognized that the mounting cost of the ESRD program, which now provides Medicare benefits to some 150,000 patients at a price that approaches $4 billion a year, has been a matter of growing concern and controversy in light of efforts to contain the costs of health care. These individual and aggregate costs, generated primarily by dialysis, have escalated far beyond the estimates made when Public Law 92-603 was enacted for two primary reasons: (1) the increasing numbers of persons beginning treatment; and (2) the fact that, in terms of age distribution and severity of illness, there have been marked shifts toward older patients with renal failure secondary to other diseases, particularly diabetes (Cummings 1989; Levinsky and Rettig 1991a,b; Rettig 1980).

Candidates for organs other than kidneys find that the high costs of a transplant and the annual costs of immunosuppressive drugs and medical care thereafter make the green screen an even greater determinant of access to a waiting list. The financing of transplants, as we discuss in the next section, has become a controversial political and policy issue for federal and state policy-makers and third-party payers. Decisions about coverage have been made on organ-by-organ, disease-by-disease, and patient-by-patient bases, resulting in substantial socioeconomic disparities in who gains access to transplant programs and great stress and uncertainty for patients and their families.

Although ability to pay has the greatest impact on transplant candidates who are among the millions of medically indigent or underinsured, it also can be an insuperable barrier to those with normally adequate health insurance, who still may have to pay many thousands of dollars in out-of-pocket expenses. As is attested by frequent stories in local and national media, when patients or their families cannot meet the costs of a transplant, beginning with an initial "down-payment," which for a liver transplant usually is about $100,000, they often resort to desperate fund-raising efforts. Among the newspaper stories in our files, for example, are headlines such as: "Our Towns. Rallying to Help Pay for a Transplant;" "Glen Campbell to Aid Baby in Need of Liver;" "White House Intervenes to Get Mom a Liver;" and "Reagan Call Brings Aid to Boy." As these headlines indicate, attempts to secure funds range from local community efforts spearheaded by families, friends, churches, and civic groups, to special events by celebrities, to engaging the power of the White House.

During the Reagan years the personal involvement of the Presidency was brought to bear not only on federal transplant policy decisions but on interventions for particular individuals, usually children, whose plight caught the attention of the President, his wife, or a special White House aide, Michael Batten. "The involvement of . . . Batten," health policy writer John Iglehart reported in 1983, "has led to an unusual series of federal interventions on behalf of families, including pressuring private health insurers, state Medicaid directors, and the DHHS to pay for organ transplants; making arrangements with the Air Force to ferry organs and patients; and assisting in local fundraising efforts. . . . Batten conceded that his activities amount to 'events in search of a policy'" (Iglehart 1983, pp. 126–127). However humanitarian the motivation for Batten's interventions may have been, the zeal with which he carried them out and the kind of "I represent President Reagan" pressure that he used raised serious questions about his mandate and if he had overstepped it.

Batten's apt characterization of the financing of transplants and other determinants of access to waiting lists as "events in search of a policy" is also applicable to many aspects of the ways that organs are distributed to potential recipients. If transplant candidates do gain access to a donor organ waiting list, they begin an often long period of "many sleepless nights" (Gutkind 1988), playing a waiting game for a suitable organ in which they must "compete" with other candidates who also are hoping for a gift of life. Potential recipients must play this "game," which many of them lose because they die before an organ is procured not only because of the "organ shortfall," but also because of persisting ambiguities and strife about the medical, ethical, and operational criteria for allocating these scarce resources. As a matter of moral principle and social policy, Childress has written,

> The federal Task Force on Organ Transplantation (1986) held that donated organs belong to the community, and this fundamental conviction undergirded all of its "recommendations for assuring equitable access to organ transplantation and for assuring the equitable allocation of donated organs among transplant centers and

among patients medically qualified for an organ transplant." From this perspective, organ procurement and transplant teams receive donated organs as trustees and stewards for the community as a whole, and they should determine who will receive available organs according to public criteria that have been developed by a publicly accountable body with public representation and that reflect principles of justice as well as medical standards. (Childress 1989, p. 102)

In practice, however, there is still a long way to go before these ideals are realized at national, regional, state, or institutional levels. To begin with, at the basic level of medical criteria, the importance of HLA tissue-type matching between a cadaveric organ and a candidate recipient remains, after several decades, a major problem of uncertainty and controversy (Fox and Swazey 1978a, ch. 2; Starzl and Fung 1990). Despite the uncertainty about the relevance of HLA antigen matching for the outcome of cadaveric organ grafts, it is an important element in the use of a "multifactorial point system" for deciding who, on local or national waiting lists, should receive an available organ. This system, initially proposed by Starzl in 1987 for kidney transplants and now used by UNOS for kidney, heart, and liver allocation decisions, assigns a set number of points to a candidate based on factors such as length of time on a waiting list, medical urgency, the logistics (ease and speed) of the transplant, and antigen matching between the donor organ and the patient (Starzl et al. 1987). Although the system's developers saw it as providing a neutral, medically determined way to ensure the equitable distribution of organs, it is not, in fact, value-free. For example, "the vigorous debate about how much weight each criterion should have . . . is to a great extent ethical . . . the points assigned to [the] various factors . . . reflect value judgments about the relative importance of patient [medical and nonmedical] need, probability of success, and time of waiting" (Childress 1989, pp. 104–105).

In addition to the problematic nature of certain medical criteria, as Childress pointed out, distribution based on the concept of donor organs as belonging to "the community" is at best ambiguous. In both principle and practice, it is unclear whether "community ownership" or "stewardship" of a donated organ means it should "belong" to and be used by the local community or region where it was procured, or that it is a national resource that should be assigned according to a country-wide distribution system (Childress 1989, p. 102).

Without clear and agreed-upon normative and medical standards for the equitable distribution of organs, their allocation, like the prior stage of access to waiting lists, has invoked controversy. Dramatic personal appeals for an organ by parents or spouses who can gain the attention of the media or of powerful intermediaries such as the President of the United States, clash with the norms of equity that most people believe should govern the allocation of this or other scarce resources. When identified life appeals are successful, they result in a designated donation, which also undercuts the notion of organs as belonging to "the community." These recurring situations raise questions about whether organ procurers or the family of a cadaver donor should have the "distributional authority" to stipulate who shall receive the gift being made.

The concept of scarce organs as "community property" and a "national resource" also gave rise to a politically and emotionally charged allocative debate during the mid-1980s about "the access of foreign nationals to U.S. cadaver organs" (U.S. DHHS 1986). The controversy and nationalistic demands for an "Americans first" organ distribution policy concerned transplanting organs into foreign nationals at U.S. transplant centers and exporting donor organs to other countries. Somewhat paradoxically, the controversy was rooted in the fact that the organ shortage in the United States is a relative one compared to that in other countries, as Americans donate more organs than persons in any other nation or society and have the world's largest organ procurement system (Prottas 1985).

The nature of the issues and the character of the divisive debate were dramatically publicized in a series of stories in 1985 in the *Pittsburgh Press*. Several of the stories, which themselves generated controversy and acrimony in terms of the accuracy of some of their facts and sources, focused on the policies and practices of the country's largest kidney transplant program, then headed by Dr. Thomas Starzl, at Presbyterian-University Hospital in Pittsburgh (Pierce 1985; Schneider and Flaherty 1985a–c). The tone and substance of the series are captured by the following excerpts from the first two articles in May 1985.

Favoritism Shrouds Presby Transplants

Since January 1984, transplant surgeons at Presbyterian-University Hospital have given some foreign citizens—especially Saudi Arabians—preference over Americans for kidney transplants . . . bypass[ing] . . . the hospital's formal policy of transplanting "locals first, hard-to-match patients second, and then foreign nationals." (Schneider and Flaherty 1985a)

Woman Passed Over After 3-Year Wait

Doctors say that a 60-year-old Pennsylvania woman who has been waiting for a kidney transplant in Pittsburgh for 3 years may be running out of time. . . . The woman was one of three Americans who matched a pair of donor kidneys that became available May 4, but she was bypassed in favor of a foreigner. . . . [H]er case is the latest example of a practice that has been a pattern for 17 months for the kidney transplant team headed by Dr. Thomas Starzl. (Schneider and Flaherty 1985e)

In July 1985, responding in part to the attention generated by the *Pittsburgh Press*, the Presbyterian-University Hospital trustees issued new guidelines for the allocation of organs to U.S. and Canadian citizens and to foreign nationals. The guidelines established an annual quota system, allowing 5 percent of the kidneys and hearts and 10 percent of livers obtained by the hospital's transplant services "to be used for foreign patients" (Pierce 1985).

The newspaper's stories about Pittsburgh's allocation of organs to foreign nationals was followed by a Pulitzer Prize–winning series that detailed various facets of "selling the gift," ranging from the worldwide black market trafficking in organs to another facet of the "Americans first" controversy: the exportation of kidneys from the United States to other countries. In 1984, wrote investigative reporters Andrew Schneider and Mary Pat Flaherty, about 5 percent of the cadaver kidneys donated by families in the United States were exported, "usually to wealthy patients overseas."

> Foreign surgeons say the kidneys, deemed useless by American doctors, were transplanted at success rates that rival or exceed those at the best U.S. centers. Virtually every export broke a covenant made with donor families who had faith that if their gift of organs were usable, it would be used for the sickest patients—not merely the richest or the most influential. (Schneider and Flaherty 1985d)

The ethical, economic, and policy pros and cons of providing foreign nationals with donor organs captured in these and other press accounts were debated at length within the ranks of the federal task force and the directors of UNOS and its Committee on Foreign Relations. Moreover, they became the subject of a DHHS Inspector General's report, a UNOS-commissioned public opinion poll, a Congressional inquiry, and analyses in bioethical publications such as the *Hastings Center Report* (Case studies 1986; Task Force 1986; UNOS 1988a,b; U.S. DHHS 1986).

In the end, at least in terms of the official policies adopted by UNOS, arguments favoring principles of humanitarianism, egalitarianism, and accountability prevailed over those favoring strict quotas for nonresident aliens, "foreigners last," or Americans only for transplants at U.S. centers, as well as a flat prohibition against exporting organs. As summarized by Childress,

> [The policy adopted by UNOS in 1988] establishes some limits and directions but relies mainly on a procedure of accountability in the transplantation of nonresident aliens. The policy requires UNOS members to charge the same fees for [all] patients, to treat all patients accepted on . . . waiting lists according to UNOS policies for the equitable distribution of organs [i.e., the multifactorial point system], and to arrange any exportation of organs . . . only after it has been impossible to find a suitable recipient in the U.S. or Canada. . . . On the local level, UNOS mem-

ber centers that accept nonresident aliens . . . are expected to establish a mechanism for community participation and review. On the national level, the UNOS committee on foreign relations has a right to audit all transplant center activities relating to the transplantation of nonresident aliens and will automatically review any center that has more than 10 percent of its . . . recipients from foreign nationals. (Childress 1989, pp. 106–107)

The mounting scarcity of donor organs has intensified uncertainty and debate about a number of other aspects of organ distribution. As the following four examples suggest, several of these matters reflect broader societal tensions about the relative importance we place on individual liberty and equality as standards governing equitable access to scarce resources. First, the growing number of multiple organ transplants, using two to five organs from one or more donors, has raised the question of "whether a single individual should be allowed to receive several organs while thousands of other dying patients are unable to obtain any" (Altman 1989d). Second, similar questions about "the one versus the many" have been evoked by the estimated one-third of recipients who receive one or more retransplants—in some cases six or more—when their graft is lost due to rejection, infection, or other complications. As transplant nurse-specialist Patricia M. Park pointed out, retransplants also pose questions about "the need and criteria for responsible decisions about when to stop, when to say 'enough is enough' to the transplant process."

> Although noble in its conception, the nonabandonment policy is the root of many of transplantation's problems. . . . Statistically, retransplants have nowhere near the functional success rate of primaries, so each retransplant has a lesser chance of increasing life expectancy.
>
> Retransplants also reduce the number of organs available to patients who are still waiting for their first. . . . While it may make us uncomfortable to think of rationing organs like gasoline, they are, like energy resources, both limited and exceedingly valuable. If the public had a clearer understanding of what can happen when transplantation goes wrong, I suspect they would support . . . legislation [limiting the number of transplants a person can have] without hesitation. (Park 1989, p. 30)

Third, debate about the equity of transplant "multiples" for one person also exists with respect to waiting lists: To wit, is it fair for one candidate to be registered on as many lists as she or he has the knowledge and resources to access? The UNOS Board has switched its policy back and forth in terms of allowing and prohibiting multiple listings by patients. The Board's ambivalence, its Vice-Chairman recollects, "reflect[s] in part . . . uncertainty about whether [UNOS'] underlying philosophy is national or federal." It also reflects the tension between "the dominant argument for permitting [multiple listings, which] stresses maximum freedom of choice and access [and the] main argument against multiple listing [which] centers on the unfair advantage it provides for [those] patients" (Childress 1989, p. 107).

A fourth set of issues, generated by the progressive expansion of eligibility criteria and concomitant decrease in contraindications for transplants, recalls the controversies about the mixture of medical, psychosocial, and behavioral criteria used to select chronic dialysis patients during the 1960s and early 1970s (Fox and Swazey 1978a, chs. 7, 8). During those years, before the Medicare ESRD Program, dialysis facilities such as the Northwest Kidney Center in Seattle formed committees to decide who among the medically qualified dialysis candidates would be chosen to receive one of the limited number of treatment slots available. The Northwest Kidney Center's Committee, dubbed "the God Squad" by its critics, was composed of responsible middle class and upper-middle class members of the community whose selection criteria were, at times, shaped by their largely subliminal views of "social worth," as well as their judgments about a candidate's likely "success" on dialysis given his or her medical, psychological, and behavioral profile.

Today, both the shortage of organs and the human and financial resources that must be committed to a transplant and subsequent care are posing analogous questions and debate. Whether people with end-stage liver disease due to alcoholic cirrhosis (by far the leading cause of such disease) should receive liver transplants is currently a focus of these medical-moral issues in organ replacement. Starzl and colleagues reported that patients with alcohol-related end-stage liver disease (ARESLD) have 1- and 2-year transplant survival rates, comparable to patients with other causes of end-stage liver disease, and seem to have a low recidivism rate (Altman 1990a; Starzl et al. 1988). Based on these data, HCFA recommended in 1990 that patients with alcoholic cirrhosis be included in Medicare coverage for liver transplantation, with the proviso that such patients abstain from drinking; it adopted such coverage as part of its April 1991 ruling that, for purposes of Medicare reimbursement, adult liver transplants are no longer experimental if programs and patients meet a list of specified criteria (Medicare coverage 1991).

Though it may represent a carefully selected patient population, the Pittsburgh data coupled with HCFA's ruling have transformed the question of whether we can obtain "acceptable results" in patients with ARESLD to the question, "Should we?" (Moss and Siegler 1991, p. 1295). Many difficult ethical and sociological questions are involved. For example, is alcoholism a disease, a behavioral deficit that leads people to engage in self-destructive behavior, or a moral failing; and what difference does, or should, the answer make with regard to the alcoholic patient's eligibility for a scarce resource—a liver transplant? Are transplanters justified medically and ethically in requiring that alcoholics stop drinking and pledge not to drink after transplant before they will be accepted as transplant candidates? Does it mean that persons seeking transplants for other diseases, such as smokers who need heart transplants, should be held to the same standards (Altman 1990a)? When allocating scarce organs to persons with alcohol-induced liver failure, are transplanters explicitly or implicitly trying to show that their work is "value free?" As happened with kidney dialysis and transplant decisions of an earlier era, are they assuming that the "gift of life" they are bestowing will cause major, enduring changes in a recipient's behavior—in this case, "converting" him or her to an alcohol-free life (Fox and Swazey 1978a, ch. 9)?

Physicians and bioethicists are beginning to engage in a sharply divided debate as to whether, given the "dire, absolute scarcity of donor livers," patients with ARESLD should be allowed to "compete equally" with other end-stage liver failure patients for a transplant (Moss and Siegler 1991, p. 1298). One position is represented by the Ethics and Social Impact Committee of the Transplant and Health Policy Center in Ann Arbor, Michigan. In terms of principles of fairness and justice, they argued, "there are no good grounds at present—moral or medical—to disqualify a patient with end-stage liver disease from consideration for a liver transplant simply because of a history of heavy drinking" (Cohen and Benjamin 1991, p. 1300). Considering the same types of issues and evidence, Moss and Siegler, from the University of Chicago's Center for Clinical Medical Ethics, come to the opposite conclusion. "Considerations of fairness suggest that a first-come, first-served approach for liver transplantation is not the most just approach. . . . [S]ince not all can live, priorities must be established and . . . patients with ARESLD should be given a lower priority for liver transplantation than others with ESLD" (Moss and Siegler 1991, p. 1298). Both sides in this burgeoning debate agree that their positions may be tempered by further clinical and psychosocial research focusing on alcoholic patients and other candidates for or recipients of liver transplants. Despite such research, however, so long as organs, like dialysis machines in an earlier era, are a scarce resource, we can expect that debate will flourish over assigning them to individuals whose behavioral patterns raise questions about their clinical outcomes and, explicitly or implicitly, invoke questions and judgments about "deservingness" and "social worth."

Transplantation and the Medical Commons

During their deliberations and policy actions relevant to transplantation, members of the transplantation community, the broader medical community, and health policy-makers, with few exceptions, have studiously avoided dealing with the distributive justice question of how the financial and human resources invested in organ replacement endeavors bear on our society's ability and willingness to meet other needs in the medical commons. Rather, as we have indicated, the sociomedical policy thrust has dealt, more narrowly, with how more organs can be procured and, secondarily, how they should be distributed to those who can meet the costs of a transplant. A third major allocative issue, the costs of transplantation and who should or will pay for them, has been avoided as much as possible by federal and state health care policy-makers. They have dealt with the financing of organ replacement when pressured to do so, largely on situational bases, and have only rarely faced it as a matter demanding reasoned policy analysis and action with respect to these procedures per se and their impact on other areas of medical needs and services.

Political scientist Richard Rettig has commented that the ways the intertwined issues of financing, distributive justice, and the rationing of medical resources have been handled in the transplantation "domain" constitute "a parable of our time" (Rettig 1989). Organ transplantation, as we, Rettig, and other of its chroniclers and analysts have shown, has been a parable or paradigmatic case because of the phenomena and issues it embodies, not because of the aggregate size and costs of the enterprise. Because the numbers and thus the overall expenditures for transplants are constrained by the limited supply of donor organs, the total monetary costs of transplantation, which have yet to be calculated, probably represent a relatively small percentage of our total health care expenditures. To date, as Cate and Laudicina pointed out, "available data on transplant costs [are] incomplete and far from perfect"; actual costs are significantly understated by calculating only average hospital charges, not items such as organ procurement charges, physician fees, and post-hospital expenses such as immunosuppressive drugs (Cate and Laudicina 1991, pp. 9, 14–15). Estimates, however, clearly show why the costs of a transplant can be staggering for the individual recipient and a nontrivial item in the increasingly strained Medicare and Medicaid budgets. The median cost of a heart–lung transplant, for example, "is $240,000 for initial care and approximately $47,000 a year for follow-up medications and care" (Theodore and Lewiston 1990, p. 773).

It is these individualized costs of transplants that starkly pose ethical and policy questions about "the trade-offs involved between basic care for the many and expensive, even though [potentially] lifesaving, care for the few" (Rettig 1989, p. 218). These questions are magnified by the oft-raised possibility that the number of transplants could increase dramatically if advances in immunosuppression someday permit the successful use of organs from other species, making it possible, in principle, to offer transplants to all who might benefit medically. Under this scenario, the aggregate costs of transplantation could mount enormously, mirroring, if not exceeding, the fiscal history of chronic dialysis since the government became the chief financer of treatment costs. Thus Rettig observed that one of the factors that has kept the financing of transplantation "off the [federal policy agenda] table has been the dominance of what might be called 'the ESRD metaphor.' The administration and Congress have tended to see transplantation as a fiscal blockbuster due to high unit costs and very high estimates of need" (Rettig 1989, p. 218).

Because policy-makers, particularly at the federal level, have tried to avoid dealing with the individual and aggregate costs of transplantation, it is not surprising that they have shied away from the even more ethically and politically volatile questions about transplantation in relation to other health care needs and costs. Many writers have examined the inevitability of allocation decisions and the temporizing maneuvers we recurrently engage in to avoid the difficult and often "tragic" choices involved in making rationing decisions on ethically and medically explicit grounds (Calabresi and Bobbit 1978). For two decades or more the costs of health care and how to contain them have been a dominant leitmotif in the United States at the levels of individual patients, providers, and institutions and of state and federal policy arenas. By and large, the many cost-containment strategies employed have involved an incrementalist, tinkering approach based on the hope that "quick fixes" might work well enough to avert far more basic decisions about health care needs, how they can be addressed more effectively and equitably, and which theories and principles of social justice should undergird those decisions. As philosopher Norman Daniels pointed out,

> Saying no to [potentially] beneficial treatments or procedures in the United States is morally hard because providers cannot appeal to the justice of their denial. . . . Economic incentives such as those embedded in current cost-containment measures are not a substitute for social decisions about health care priorities and the just design of health care institutions. (Daniels 1986, p. 1383)

The difficulties we have faced in placing fiscal or other limits on transplantation epitomize two of the cardinal, interrelated features of health care in the United States that Daniels addressed. The first is the fragmented and increasingly chaotic nature of what we call our health care "system," whose long-standing signs and symptoms of malaise have been exacerbated by debates over costs and their control. On this point, as Shortell and McNerney have pointedly written, "it would be tempting to suggest that the U.S. health care system is now in disarray were it not for the fact that it has never really been otherwise. There is increasing anger and frustration among employers, consumers, uninsured people, payers, and providers, all of whom are struggling with what are perceived to be competing demands to contain costs while trying to improve productivity, increase quality, and expand access to services" (Shortell and McNerney 1990,

p. 463). Second, as Americans reluctantly face the fact that our society does indeed ration health care based on ability to pay and even more reluctantly begin to consider the possibility of nonprice rationing, our lack of any broad sociopolitical consensus about the values that might provide a foundation for a more just mode of rationing becomes more glaringly apparent.

The fragmented nature of our health care "system" and the sociopolitical and ethical frameworks in which it struggles to function are illustrated by the sagas of the "saying yes" decisions concerning the initiation of heart and liver transplant programs, and reimbursement for these procedures. At a state level, Massachusetts provides a rich case study of the factors that have shaped transplantation policies. These factors include the impact of widely publicized "identified life" cases and the powerful medical-political influences of hospitals and transplant luminaries.

Although the main events in the Massachusetts case transpired during 1983–85, a critical background event had occurred a few years earlier. In 1980 the trustees of Massachusetts General Hospital, to the dismay of their transplant physicians, renewed their 1967 decision that the institution would not initiate a heart transplantation program. The trustees believed that in terms of allocating their institution's resources, such a program would not "produce 'the greatest good for the greatest number'"(Casscells 1986, p. 1365; Leaf 1980). The events and influences that led to a dramatic reversal of this stance and profoundly altered transplantation in Boston as well as nationally began 2 years later. In 1982 hospital administrator Charles Fiske mounted a nationally publicized campaign to obtain a donor liver for his infant daughter, Jamie, dying of biliary atresia, pleading for an organ via television and newspapers and an in-person appeal at the annual meeting of the American Academy of Pediatrics. Mr. Fiske also waged a skilled battle with the state's Blue Cross-Blue Shield company, persuading them to grant his media-celebrated daughter an exception to its policy of not reimbursing the costs of a liver transplant because the procedure was experimental. Jamie Fiske received her new liver, but the procedure was done in Minneapolis because no hospitals in Boston, where clinical transplantation was launched during the 1950s, were performing liver or heart transplants. The 11-month-old girl's transplant and the national coverage it received had a cascade effect on transplantation policies and practices in the state. Boston's premier teaching hospitals, in a rare show of togetherness, formed two powerful consortia that overcame strenuous opposition to their obtaining certificates of need to begin liver and heart transplant programs (Annas 1984, 1985a,b; Fineberg 1983; Knox 1984a,b). Moreover, as these battles raged, Massachusetts Blue Cross-Blue Shield decided in 1984 that their policies would include routine coverage of heart and liver transplants (Knox 1984c).

The same sorts of phenomena involved in the Massachusetts story have played significant roles in the politics of heart and liver transplantation funding decisions at the federal level and thus the consequent growth of transplant programs. Spurred by the skillfully orchestrated publicity to secure organs and insurance coverage for Jamie Fiske and several other critically ill infants and children, liver transplantation "ushered in the contemporary politics of organ transplantation" during the early 1980s "by focusing on children rather than adults" (Rettig 1989, pp. 198–199). In 1982, responding to concerns voiced from the White House and by influential Congressmen such as Representative Albert Gore, Chairman of the Oversight Committee of the House Science and Technology Committee, the NIH agreed to hold a consensus conference in 1983 on the clinical status of pediatric liver transplantation. The key agenda item for that conference and for hearings held by Gore in April 1983 was to deal with what Gore called the "absolutely absurd situation" of the DHHS and CHAMPUS (the health insurance program of the Department of Defense) denying reimbursement for liver transplants on the grounds they were experimental procedures (Rettig 1989, p. 200).

The thrust of Gore's hearings and the agenda arranged for the subsequent NIH conference in June 1983 largely prefigured the content and dynamics of the meeting, the findings and recommendations of the consensus panel, and the funding decision following in its wake. The conference took place in an atmosphere that combined the attributes of a scientific conference with those of a town hall gathering, a revival meeting, and a media circus. In effect, as detailed in Markle and Chubin's anatomy of the conference, it was as much or more "an effort at political lobbying for governmental approval of liver transplantation as it was a scientific assessment" (Markle and Chubin 1987; NIH 1983a,b; Rettig 1989, p. 202). Three of the four liver transplant surgeons who presented data at the conference characterized their overall results as "still medium" and admitted that the preoperative mortality was "unacceptably high." Starzl, however, strongly championed the effectiveness of liver transplants based on the improved 1-year survival rate he was obtaining with cyclosporine; and, as most observers anticipated, his arguments and the testimony of Charles Fiske and other parents prevailed. Although "substantial questions" remain about many aspects of liver transplants, the panel concluded, the procedure is a "therapeutic modality" that "deserves broader application." For, the panel judged, "the operation has been shown to be technically feasible, and interpretable results have been reported. . . . These [results] clearly demonstrate that liver transplantation offers an alternative therapeutic approach which may prolong life in some patients. . . ." (NIH 1983a).

This judgment paved the way for the 1984 decision of the Health Care Finance Administration (HCFA) to cover pediatric liver transplantation for extrahepatic biliary atresia if candidates meet Medicare eligibility criteria for disability or have end-stage renal disease (Lindsey and McGlynn 1988). So few children can meet these criteria that, as of 1988, no liver transplants had been reimbursed under the HCFA provision. As Rettig pointed out, however, the "HCFA decision . . . was very important for state Medicaid agencies, for Blue Cross and Blue Shield plans, and for commercial health insurance firms [because once] HCFA designated the procedure as no longer experimental, these payers would have little choice but to follow" (Rettig 1989, p. 202). More recently, and at a real cost to the federal government as well as to Medicaid and private insurance companies, HCFA agreed to provide Medicare coverage for liver transplants performed for eight conditions that affect adults, including alcoholic cirrhosis. These new financing provisions will cost Medicare an estimated $10 million "in the first year and $120 million by the fifth year, as more hospitals gain approval for reimbursement" (Medicare to Cover Some Liver Transplants 1990).

Federal decision-making concerning funding for heart transplants has a longer history than that for liver transplants but involves much the same mix of events and influences (Casscells 1986; Rettig 1989). In 1979, after the heart transplant bandwagon had faltered, a moratorium phase was in effect among programs other than Dr. Norman Shumway's careful research-based work at Stanford (Fox and Swazey 1978a, chs. 5, 10). In November 1979 the HCFA adopted an interim policy of reimbursing only the procedures done by Shumway's group, but in 1980 the agency was overruled by DHHS Secretary Patricia Harris, who was concerned that the costs of heart transplants might expand to rival those of the ESRD program. Harris signaled DHHS' intention "to require that Medicare coverage decisions," beginning with heart transplants, "be based not just on narrow safety and efficacy considerations but on documentation of cost-effectiveness, ethical implications, and long-term effects on society" (Rettig 1989, p. 197).

To greatly truncate a complex story, Harris' stance led to the DHHS commissioning the National Heart Transplant Study, conducted by the Battelle Memorial Institute under the direction of Roger Evans (Evans and Broida 1985; Evans et al. 1984). The study's central findings were that heart transplants, performed with proper patient selection and by qualified centers, are a clinically effective and cost-effective treatment. Based on these findings and the persuasive advocacy of Evans, by then a member of the national task force on transplantation policy (Evans 1986), HCFA concluded that heart transplants were no longer experimental. Accordingly, in 1986 the agency issued proposed regulations for reimbursing Medicare-eligible patients undergoing heart transplants in facilities that meet HCFA-specified standards of experience and performance.

During the 1980s, in sum, the federal government and many state governments became firmly committed to paying for various organ transplantation procedures. "Because those fiscal commitments generally take the form of entitlement programs for broadly defined, categorically eligible groups," Schuck pointed out, "they entail a large, potentially open-ended claim on public resources. As technological change continues to advance the frontiers of organ transplantation practice, that claim steadily increases. Especially during a period of severe budgetary constraint, the nature and extent of that claim are bound to become divisive political issues" (Schuck 1989, p. 169). The human values as well as the economics involved in these "saying yes" decisions and why we may begin "saying no" were framed evocatively by Havighurst and King. In their conclusion to a paper examining Massachusetts' dealings with liver transplantation, a public policy-making event they likened to a morality play, they wrote:

> Is there any doubt that [a hundred years from now] society will somehow reassess its commitment to saving lives without regard to cost and will come to accept as a matter of course some deaths that could have been prevented by the application of high technology? There are many different ways in which patients can be selected for treatment, not all of which rely on government to act directly or indirectly as the giver or denier of life itself. Without question, our attitudes toward such matters are changing. Ultimately, we must give up some cherished but so far unexamined collective beliefs. The frightening but certain truth is that we are acting out our own morality play—one in which simplistic values, of the kind that flourish most in a political environment, must eventually give way to some hard realities of the human condition. As in any great drama, the central question is whether other, more vital values will be preserved. (Havighurst and King, 1989, p. 257)

Transplantation, Medicine, and the Societal Commons

For both literal and symbolic reasons, we see transplantation as epitomizing many of the issues of what promises to be *the* health policy battle in the United States in the coming years. As Callahan observed: "There is considerable agreement on the outline of the problem: we spend an increasingly insupportable amount of money on health care but get neither good value for our money nor better equity in terms of access to health care" (Callahan 1990b, p. 1811). The growing conflict, then, is not over whether there is a problem but on how to solve it, and the core battle is about rationing.

The State of Oregon has undertaken the first major and highly controversial effort to ration health care services through an open, public process of decision-making that "disavows rationing hidden by the covert workings of a market, or buried in the quiet, professional decisions of providers" (Daniels 1991, p. 2234). Under a bill introduced in 1987 by Senate President Dr. John Kitzhaber, the legislature and a Health Services Commission have been engaged in an arduous effort to design a Basic Health Services Program that, primarily through devising a prioritized list of health services that will be covered by Medicaid, seeks to provide "universal access for the state's citizens to a basic level of health care" (Kitzhaber 1990).

Transplantation was the bellweather case in Oregon's first effort to ration its Medicaid funding through prioritizing services based on a utilitarian cost-effectiveness calculus. In 1987 the legislature voted to eliminate an estimated $1.1 million in discretionary Medicaid expenditures for all soft-tissue transplants except kidneys and corneas, opting instead to accept the recommendation of the state's Division of Adult and Family Services to use those funds to provide prenatal care for an estimated 2,000 medically indigent women (Welch and Larson 1988).

The legislature, in Rettig's words, acted "with a relatively clear understanding" that it was making a "trade-off . . . between basic care for the many and expensive . . . care for the few" (Rettig 1989, p. 218). It was a decision that was premised, in part, on the process and results of the Oregon Health Decisions Project, which provided grassroots input from citizens throughout the state about how they thought scarce health care resources should be allocated (Crawshaw and Garland 1985). As Kitzhaber emphasized, it "was only superficially a transplant issue."

> Rather, it was an economic issue, one which, in Oregon and elsewhere, perhaps can be postponed but not avoided. The question is, can Oregon (or any other state) afford to pay for all the health care now available for anyone who might benefit from it? The transplant issue was a catalyst for a much more far-reaching policy debate, one which has forced us to confront our fiscal limits, our lack of a meaningful health care policy, and the eventual inevitability of explicit health care rationing. (Kitzhaber 1988, p. 22)

Oregon's draft priority list drew vehement criticism partly because it gave higher rankings to relatively minor cost-effective treatments than to potentially lifesaving interventions such as organ transplants (Egan 1990; Oregon rationing plan 1990; Southwick 1990). The Health Services Commission's current list of prioritized services, issued in February 1991, is based on calculations of "net health benefit" tha do not include costs as a factor (Hadorn 1991). A major catalyst for the Commission's rapid retreat from cost-effectiveness criteria and the consequent reappearance of extrarenal transplant procedures on the priority list was the nationally publicized, identified life drama of a young Oregon resident, 7-year-old Coby Howard. Some 6 months after the legislature halted its Medicaid funding for transplants, Coby Howard died of acute lymphocytic leukemia. His mother's efforts to obtain Medicaid funding for a bone marrow transplant or to raise the $100,000 deposit required for her son to be accepted as a transplant candidate had failed. "Amid the glare of cameras, the state and nation watched the little boy die, apparently for want of a medical procedure that would have been available just a few months earlier" (Hadorn 1991, p. 2219).

As Hadorn emphasized in his analysis of Oregon's program, the story of Coby Howard and the changes his death engendered in the state's rationing methods vividly illustrate the difficulties of institutionalizing "saying no" rationing decisions for interventions such as organ transplantation (Hadorn 1991). "Those technologies that do stave off death," ethicist Albert Jonsen reminded us, "pose a particularly daunting problem [for resource allocation] . . . a barrier difficult to climb, a chasm difficult to leap: namely, the imperative to rescue endangered life" (Jonsen 1986).

Whether some explicit system for rationing health care in America is necessary is a topic of heated debate; and if the Oregon experience is any portent, transplantation will continue to figure prominently in the emerging battle. On one side of the battle line are those who, like recently retired editor of the *New England Journal of Medicine* Dr. Arnold Relman, are convinced that we "can improve our health care system sufficiently, and soon enough," through measures to cut costs and improve efficiency, "to avoid either systematic rationing or more restriction of access through pricing" (Relman 1990, p. 1810). The opposing forces are represented by persons such as Kitzhaber and Callahan, who are convinced that some form of *explicit and equitable* rationing is necessary and desirable for the health of health care in the United States.

Among the rationing advocates there are differences regarding whether we should (1) adopt a more open and just system of price rationing that denies "commodities" such as health care to those who cannot pay for them or (2) develop a nonprice rationing system that would place certain limits on medical care even for those who can afford it. The Oregon model, however laudable its goal of providing equitable access to basic medical care may be, is still a form of green screen or price rationing that impacts primarily on "them"—the some 37 million medically indigent people in the United States. There is a vast chasm between this type of rationing and a nonprice rationing that would deny certain treatments or services to "us"—the 85 percent who have insurance or other means to ensure that most of our medical needs and wants are met.

The idea of nonprice rationing is anathema to most Americans because, as Callahan wrote, it seems to violate "several deeply ingrained values" in this society and its health care system. This complex of values includes autonomy and freedom of choice, and a view of "limitless medical progress" in which "every disease should be cured, every disability rehabilitated, every health need met, and every evidence of mortality . . . vigorously challenged. . . . " Concomitantly, we desire "quality" in our medical care, which we define "as the presence of high-class amenities . . . and a level of technology that is constantly improvin*g*, and welcoming innovations" (Callahan 1990b, p. 1811).

Unpalatable as it may be, however, "nonprice rationing" is beginning to be seriously discussed on two grounds. The first, and most familiar, is economic, represented by the thesis of Aaron and Schwartz that we can "arrest or slow the growth of medical cost only temporarily . . . unless we reduce the availability of beneficial services—in short, unless [we] compel nonprice rationing" (Aaron and Schwartz 1990, p. 419). The second and more challenging and unsettling argument for nonprice rationing is a moral one that has been articulated most clearly and compellingly by Callahan. "A consensus to simply limit health care," he argued, "is not enough." Instead of asking the economic question of "how much of what kind of health care we can afford," our society needs to ask (and answer by a consensus-building process) the basic moral question of "how much we *ought* to be willing to afford." The "ultimate problem" behind that question, Callahan asserted, "is our aspiration for unlimited medical progress, which leads us to want more than we can get or can afford. Even if we can better manage our deranged health care system, we will be left with that far more profound issue. We need a change in our perspective, and of a penetrating kind" (Callahan 1990a, p. 32).

We share Callahan's conviction that we need a penetrating change in our collective, societal perspective about the ends of medicine. We have no clear vision of the exact contours of a redefined understanding of the meaning of medical progress and how it would restructure medical care. Like the late René Dubos, however, we believe that our medicine and the society of which it is a part have lost their center in pursuing a "mirage of health"—a belief in "complete and lasting freedom from disease" that "is but a dream remembered from imaginings of a Garden of Eden designed for the welfare of man" (Dubos 1987, p. 2). Our deepening disquietude about the directions of modern medicine, as we explain in the final chapter, is both sociological and moral; and it has been forged, above all, by our views about the nature of the organ replacement endeavor during the past decade.

The Jarvik-7 Artificial Heart Experiment

Desperate Appliance: A Short History of the Jarvik-7 Artificial Heart

Diseases desperate grown
By desperate appliance
  are reliev'd
  Or not at all.

SHAKESPEARE, *Hamlet*, act IV, scene iii

As we stood on the threshold of taking the artificial heart to the clinic, everyone sensed the dilemma that [the device] was not yet ready to support real human existence.... [But] a whole symphony of technology gave us the feeling that maybe the [Jarvik] heart was going to work.

A senior cardiac surgeon, formerly at the University of Utah

Cast of Characters and Their Locales

The Chief Players

The Surgeon-Implanters

William C. DeVries, MD

Chief, Department of Cardiothoracic Surgery, University of Utah Medical Center, Salt Lake City, Utah, and the Humana Heart Institute International at Humana Hospital Audubon, Louisville, Kentucky

Lyle Joyce, MD, PhD

Department of Cardiothoracic Surgery, University of Utah Medical Center

Bjarne Semb, MD

Karolinska Hospital, Stockholm, Sweden

The Jarvik Artificial Heart Developers

Robert Jarvik, MD

> President of Symbion, Inc. (formerly Kolff Medical Associates), Salt Lake City

Willem J. Kolff, MD, PhD

> Inventor of the artificial kidney and a pioneer in the development of artificial hearts; Division of Artificial Organs and Institute of Biomedical Engineering, University of Utah; founder of Kolff Medical Associates/ Symbion, Inc., Salt Lake City

The Patients Implanted with Permanent Jarvik-7 Hearts (Chronological Order)

Barney Clark

> Implanted by DeVries and Joyce at the University of Utah Medical Center on December 2, 1982; died 112 days later on March 23, 1983

William Schroeder

> Implanted by DeVries at Humana Hospital Audubon, Louisville on November 25, 1984; died 620 days later on August 6, 1986

Murray Haydon

> Implanted by DeVries at Humana Hospital Audubon on February 17, 1985; died 488 days later on June 19, 1986

Leif Stenberg

> Implanted by Semb at Karolinska Hospital, Stockholm on April 7, 1985; died 229 days later on November 22, 1985

Jack Burcham

> Implanted by DeVries at Humana Hospital Audubon on April 14, 1985; died 10 days later on April 23, 1985

Featured Roles (Alphabetical Order, by Locale)

Salt Lake City, Utah

Claudia Berenson, MD

> Psychiatrist and member of the artificial heart team

John Bosso, DPharm

> Associate Professor of Clinical Pharmacy and Chairman of the University of Utah Medical Center Institutional Review Board (IRB)

Una Loy Clark

> Wife of Barney Clark

Donald B. Olsen, DVM

Chief surgeon and Director, Artificial Heart Research Laboratory, University of Utah

Chase N. Peterson, MD

Vice President for Health Sciences and university coordinator and media spokesperson for the Artificial Heart Project, University of Utah; became President of the University in June 1983

Ross Woolley, PhD

Department of Family and Community Medicine, University of Utah School of Medicine; Vice Chairman of the IRB and Chairman of its artificial heart subcommittee

Nurses, technicians, physicians, social workers, public relations staff, and other members of the artificial heart group
Louisville, Kentucky

David Jones

Chairman and Chief Executive Officer, Humana Corporation

Allan Lansing, MD, PhD

Chairman, Humana Heart Institute International

Margaret Schroeder

Wife of William Schroeder, and their sons and daughters

George Zenger, MD

Department of Radiology, and Chairman of the IRB, Humana Hospital Audubon

Nurses, technicians, physicians, social workers, and other members of the artificial heart group, and the administrative and public relations staff at Audubon Hospital and the Humana Corporation
At Hospitals in the United States, Great Britain, and Europe

The *patients* who received and *surgeons* who implanted more than 300 artificial hearts, including the Jarvik device and other models, for temporary bridge-to-transplant use from 1985 to 1989

Washington, DC

The *Food and Drug Administration,* Division of Cardiovascular Devices and its Circulatory System Devices Advisory Panel
The *National Institutes of Health,* National Heart, Lung and Blood Institute and its Artificial Heart Program

Prologue

The Night Barney Clark Died

"It was snowing the day he came to the hospital and on the night he died," the nurse said softly, "and I remember the beauty of the mountains and the gently falling snow through the windows of the surgical intensive care unit." It was 112 days earlier, on December 2, 1982, that the 61-year-old Seattle dentist, Barney B. Clark, facing imminent death from chronic congestive heart failure, had been wheeled into an operating room at the University of Utah Medical Center. There two young surgeons, 38-year-old William C. DeVries and 34-year-old Lyle Joyce, the sole members of the center's Division of Cardiothoracic Surgery, removed Dr. Clark's heart. In its place they implanted an experimental device called the Jarvik-7 total artificial heart, which for the first time was intended to function as a permanent replacement for the human heart.

The telemetry equipment that monitored and recorded Dr. Clark's biological life with his Jarvik-7 heart showed that the device beat steadily, 12,912,499 times, for 112 days throughout a series of postoperative complications that gradually and cumulatively caused multiorgan system failure (Berenson and Grosser 1984; DeVries et al. 1984). Then on the night of March 23, 1983, his condition deteriorated rapidly, and his circulatory system began its final collapse. Describing those hours to us, the nurse began to weep quietly.

> The end started about 6:30 p.m. There were very few people around at the time. Bill [DeVries] and Lyle [Joyce] had to decide whether to dialyze Barney or watch him die, and they went to talk to Una Loy [Mrs. Clark] about it. Then three of us went into the anteroom next to the unit to talk to Mrs. Clark. She cried out, "I can't make that decision myself." I can still hear that piercing cry. I went back into the unit to talk to Bill and Lyle, who were with Barney, and told them they couldn't force this woman to make such a decision, that enough was enough, and that they shouldn't start dialyzing Barney just to collect more data. Then I went back to the anteroom to be with Una Loy.
>
> A few minutes later Bill and Lyle came in and told Mrs. Clark she didn't have to make a decision about dialyzing Barney because his blood pressure was going down. By now it was about 8:00, and I sat in the nursing station watching Bill DeVries periodically go into Barney Clark's room, slowly turning the [artificial heart drive] machine down. Nobody was in that room with Dr. DeVries when he finally turned the key [to shut off the drive machine], but about 10:00 he came out and said, "Barney is gone now; I'm going to talk to Una Loy."

Still crying as she recalled that night 3 years earlier, the nurse said sadly, "We all felt we owed Barney something. He gave us a lot, and he was a man who died.

But it wasn't just Barney. He stands for every patient I've ever lost. Barney was a symbol. By now I hardly remember him, but I weep" (Personal interview, August 5, 1986).

Field-Workers in the Land of Oz

Lines from *The Wizard of Oz* about the Tin Woodman's journey to obtain a heart from the Wizard were among the many passages and aphorisms that William DeVries was fond of quoting during the years he was conducting and we were studying the Jarvik-7 artificial heart experiment. As depicted in innumerable media stories, the public persona of the artificial heart implanter was that of the boyish, all-American pioneering surgeon with the physical and personality attributes of a Jimmy Stewart, Gary Cooper, Henry Fonda, and Abraham Lincoln rolled into one. We first met the blond, lanky, 6-foot 5-inch surgeon dressed like a perpetual house officer in a wrinkled green scrub suit on a June day in 1983, less than 3 months after Barney Clark's death. DeVries was carrying a dog-eared copy of our book *The Courage to Fail*, and showed us the marker he had inserted in its underlined chapter on "the experiment–therapy dilemma."

We had followed the intensive dramatic media coverage of Dr. Clark's implant against the background of our earlier study of Dr. Denton Cooley's controversial artificial heart implant in 1969 (Cooley et al. 1969; Fox and Swazey 1978a, ch. 6). Intrigued by what we had seen and read concerning this latest episode in the quest for an artificial heart, and contemplating writing a book of essays that would update some of the topics in *The Courage to Fail*, we had journeyed to Salt Lake City for a week of interviews and discussions with participants in the development and first human use of a permanent artificial heart.

When we met with them, members of the Utah artificial heart team were still in an early phase of "postmortem" stock taking. During those first weeks after Dr. Clark's death, they had difficulty talking with each other about their individual and collective experiences and emotions. Although they were beginning to discuss plans for a second implant, they were ambivalent about whether, on balance, the experiment had been right and good. And they were struggling to understand why, as they repeatedly said, they felt that Barney Clark's case "was the same, but different" from that of the many other gravely ill patients they had cared for and lost (Fox 1984). Most of those with whom we met seemed to welcome the chance to talk to knowledgeable strangers about the events and meaning of Barney Clark's implant and were comfortable with our being introduced by our host, Dr. Chase Peterson, then Vice President for Health Sciences at the University, as social scientists who would be doing an in-depth study of the artificial heart experiment. The thought of doing such a study was not part of our agenda when we planned our trip to Salt Lake City, for the only essay we had drafted for our proposed book was an early version of *Spare Parts'* last chapter, "Leaving the Field." By the end of our visit, though, we were sufficiently captured by what we had observed and heard to decide that some additional exploratory research was warranted.

Two subsequent individual trips to Utah to participate in conferences dealing with the artificial heart enabled us to continue our interviews and observations, and we decided to develop a proposal and seek funding for an ethnographically based study. In August 1984, amidst considerable furor and publicity, DeVries left the University of Utah to continue his artificial heart experiments with the Humana Heart Institute, a group practice loosely affiliated with the Humana Corporation and based at its Audubon Hospital in Louisville, Kentucky. That November he invited us to be participant observers of his second implant, soon to be performed on William Schroeder. We went to Louisville, embarking on what was to become an absorbing, increasingly complex, and ultimately deeply disquieting 5-year study of the "rise and fall" of the Jarvik-7 heart.[1]

Act I: The Development of the Jarvik Heart

In the history of transplantation and artificial organs to date, nothing better exemplifies medicine's relentless efforts to avert death and restore some measure of health to gravely ill patients than the attempts that have been made to replace failing human hearts with man-made substitutes. The development of the Jarvik heart and its experimental use as a surrogate organ is a dramatic and illuminating chapter in the artificial heart story. For many reasons, confined not only to the morbidity and mortality of the five patients, the permanent artificial heart experiment was a small and short-lived one with several quiet and unofficial endings. In terms of the recipients and their survival, one ending came with the death of "Bionic Bill" Schroeder in August 1986—620 grueling days after he became the second recipient in DeVries' permanent implant series. When we learned of Mr. Schroeder's long-anticipated death on August 6, we were in Salt Lake City for a final round of retrospective interviews with participants in the Barney Clark implant. That day we were interviewing Dr. Donald Olsen, a veterinarian, who as chief surgeon and director of the Artificial Heart Research Laboratory at the University of Utah had trained DeVries and other surgeons to implant the Jarvik heart and had been in the operating room as a consultant during Barney Clark's surgery. Dr. Olsen was asked to take an important phone call, and when it had ended he told us somberly that Bill Schroeder was dead. He added reflectively that he was sure there would be no more implants done by Bill DeVries, the only surgeon authorized by the Food and Drug Administration

(FDA) to test the Jarvik heart as a permanent device, so the experiment, to all intents and purposes, was over.

The NIH Artificial Heart Program

Just as there were several endings to the Jarvik heart experiment, so too there were various beginnings. The device that ultimately bore the name of Robert Jarvik, for example, was the product of more than 25 years of work on artificial hearts by an indomitable Dutch-born physician and inventor of the first clinically workable artificial kidney, Dr. Willem Kolff, and the legions of researchers who worked with him in his laboratories in Cleveland and Salt Lake City (Kolff 1983a; Thorwald 1971). The artificial heart work done for so many years under Kolff's aegis, in turn, was part of a longer and larger effort to develop a substitute for the human heart. Some of the first laboratory steps in that effort included the artificial orthotopic (whole heart) pump developed in England by Dale and Shuster in 1928 and the whole-body perfusion device made by Alexis Carrel and aviation pioneer Charles Lindbergh in 1935, which journalists enthusiastically dubbed an "artificial heart" (Hallowell 1985).

Since the 1960s most of the work on total and partial cardiac replacement devices in the United States has gone forward under the imprimatur of and with funding from the National Institutes of Health (NIH) artificial heart program. Several factors contributed to enthusiastic approval by Congress of the establishment of the NIH program in 1963. They included concerns about the high mortality rates associated with cardiovascular disease and the search for various means to reduce them. Partial or total cardiac replacement devices seemed to offer a promising line of attack. Based on work on prototype hearts during the 1950s by prominent physician-researchers such as Michael DeBakey, Adrian Kantrowitz, and Kolff, promoters of an artificial heart program were sure that a workable device could be developed and move into widespread clinical use within a few years. This conviction was based on a widely shared medical and engineering view of the heart as a relatively simple muscular pump whose functions and control systems could be replicated fairly readily through the type of systems development approach used in industry (Altieri et al. 1986; Atsumi 1986; Bernstein 1986; Edson 1979; Szycher 1986).[2] These factors, in turn, meshed with growing industrial interests in developing biomedical capabilities and markets. Lastly, the symbolism of the heart figured prominently in the decision to mount a federal effort to devise a man-made substitute for it. During those years of America's first successful explorations in space, no other organ could have so captured Congressional and public support for launching "with a sense of urgency" an earth-based analogue that would enable us to conquer a leading cause of disability and death[3] (Bernstein 1984; Lubeck 1986; Lubeck and Bunker 1982; Strauss 1984). Although the last several versions of the Jarvik heart were devised and tested with private funds (placing it outside the NIH artificial heart program), it had strong links to that program: A substantial portion of the research and development work on a total artificial heart by Kolff's groups in Cleveland and Salt Lake City had been supported from the mid-1960s to the mid-1970s by contracts and grants from NIH.

"Kolff's Heart"

Willem Kolff is a stubborn, persistent, often embattled pioneer in the field of artificial organs. Described by a colleague as "pure visionary," he has long been staunchly convinced of the desirability and feasibility of creating bionic persons (Wrenn 1982, p. 32). Since the time nearly 50 years ago when he used the artificial kidney machine he had built in Holland during the Nazi occupation and watched his first 16 patients die, he has been willing to incur failure and criticism. In response to doubters or naysayers, he is fond of quoting a much-admired countryman, William of Orange: "Even without hope you shall undertake, and even without success, you shall persevere" (Kolff 1983a). That ideology has supported Kolff's years of work to develop a clinically viable total artificial heart,[4] which he began in 1957 with a team of physicians, engineers, and technicians in his laboratory at the Cleveland Clinic. A decade later Kolff left Cleveland and emigrated to Salt Lake City, where he established the University of Utah's Division of Artificial Organs; soon thereafter he was named director of the new Institute for Biomedical Engineering at the university. The team of artificial heart researchers that assembled in Utah under Kolff's firm and intense direction included Dr. Clifford Kwan-Gett, a cardiovascular surgeon who directed the group's engineering research and animal studies and who later would become embroiled in a priority dispute with Robert Jarvik over credit for the "Jarvik" heart. Between 1967 and 1971 Kwan-Gett designed a simple pneumatically powered (compressed air-driven) artificial heart system that included two "Kwan-Gett heart" models on which the Jarvik versions were based and a pneumatic drive system that was refined into the Utahdrive system that powered Barney Clark's heart (Total artificial heart development at U of U 1982).

One of the first research assistants hired by Kolff when he began his artificial heart program at Utah in 1967 was a first-year medical student, William DeVries. During medical school DeVries worked with Kolff, Kwan-Gett, and the project's veterinarian-surgeon consultant, Dr. Donald Olsen, on the performance of the Kwan-Gett heart models in sheep (DeVries et al. 1970; Kwan-Gett et al. 1969). When he completed medical school in 1970, the Utah native "left the Mormon valley" of Salt Lake City for the first time for 9 years of surgical residency training at Duke University in North Carolina, returning to Kolff's laboratory and the University of Utah Medical Center in 1979.

In 1971, while DeVries was beginning his residency at Duke, Clifford Kwan-Gett left the project to pursue further training in thoracic and cardiovascular surgery, and Donald Olsen joined the laboratory full time, becoming its chief surgeon in 1973 and eventually Kolff's successor as its director. In 1971 Kolff also hired a young man named Robert Jarvik as a design engineer. Uncertain as to what career he wanted to pursue, Jarvik had studied medicine for 2 years in Italy and then dropped out of medical school, ambivalent about where to direct his interests and talents in science, art, sculpture, and engineering. When he was hired by Kolff, Jarvik had just completed a master's degree in biomechanics at New York University. Under Kolff's mentorship, he returned to medical school at the University of Utah from 1972 to 1976, continuing to work part time with the artificial heart project. Medical degree in hand, he became a full-time member of the artificial heart group in 1976.

By the mid-1970s Kolff's laboratory was achieving longer periods of survival for the sheep and calves implanted with successive models of the pneumatically driven artificial heart. At first, survival had been measured in hours, as the project's many specialists struggled with problems of design and functions, materials and their compatibility with human tissue and blood, surgical techniques, and lethal complications such as uncontrolled hemorrhage, infection, and shock. What the team judged as significant temporal milestones were noted and celebrated as hours became days and then weeks and months: the "first 50-hour sheep," the calves that lived for 7 days, then 1 month, and then by late 1974 the calf named Burke who survived for 3 months with his Jarvik-3 model. Further gains in survival times came during late 1975 to 1976 through advances in surgical technique and in the design and fabrication of the ventricles of what, by now, was the Jarvik-5 model. Intimating that human tests were being contemplated, Jarvik and Tom Kessler, a manufacturing technician and mold-maker, reduced the size and stroke volume of the Jarvik-5, which was too large for human use, and produced a smaller version dubbed the Jarvik-7 (Total artificial heart development at U of U 1982).

Another signal to Kolff's group that they were approaching a clinically testable heart, and one that might someday be commercially lucrative, came in 1976. With Jarvik as the prime mover, he, Kolff, and several other investors from the Artificial Heart Laboratory formed Kolff Medical Associates as an independent proprietary company that retained close and subsequently controversial ties to the University of Utah. Five years later, as the artificial heart was on the threshold of its first clinical test, Jarvik convinced his mentor (and, many associates thought, his father-figure), Willem Kolff, that the company was poised for expansion and commercial success, and that he, Jarvik, should become President and raise needed venture capital. That strategy, to those who knew him well, typified the many-faceted character of Robert Jarvik. In person, and as depicted by friends and the media, he was a flamboyant, versatile, intelligent young playboy, artist, inventor, and entrepreneur. His public and professional dress ranged from black leather motorcycle jackets and jeans to pinstripe suits, and his persona from a long interview-based portrait of his "rock'n roll heart" in *Playboy* to his appearance on billboards and in magazine ads as the sophisticated "man in the Hathaway shirt" (Gonzalez 1986). To us, as we knew him during those years of the artificial heart experiment, Jarvik was a man in whom the values of the 1960s and 1980s seemed to be fused in complex ways.

Jarvik succeeded in his efforts to gain control of Kolff's company, duly being named President and raising venture capital. In 1982, the year Barney Clark made history, Jarvik renamed the company Symbion, Inc., reorganized its management structure, and secured Kolff's resignation as board chairman (Carter 1983).

The Move from the Laboratory to the Clinic

In the United States, clinical tests of risky new devices such as artificial hearts have been regulated since 1980 by the FDA's investigational device exemption (IDE) regulations, which are part of a broader set of regulations for the testing and marketing of medical devices. Under the IDE regulations a device such as the Jarvik heart is classified as a "significant risk" investigational device, because it "presents a potential for serious risk to the health, safety, or welfare of a subject" and is of "unproven safety and efficacy." A device manufacturer must obtain permission for "experimental use" from the institutional review board (IRB) at the sites where the device will be tested on human subjects and, contingent on IRB approval, from the FDA's Bureau of Medical Devices (*Federal Register* 1980). Complying with these regulatory requirements, Kolff Associates made their first applications to the University of Utah Medical Center IRB and to the FDA during late 1980, seeking approval to begin testing the Jarvik-7 artificial heart on patients at University Hospital with Dr. William C. DeVries as Principal Investigator.

The decision that "the time is right" to move a new device, procedure, or drug from laboratory and animal testing to human testing is seldom an unambiguous, certain one, either at the time it is made or in retrospect. To a certain extent, given the unknown effects of any innovation on patients, the move from the laboratory to the clinic is always inherently premature, however scientifically and medically warranted it may seem at the time, Not surprisingly, then, the decision to test the Jarvik heart as a permanent replacement for the human heart evoked differences of opinion within and without the Utah artificial heart team, at the time it was made and in retrospect.

Based on data about the Jarvik heart's performance in animals, some members of the Utah group and of the IRB, along with outside experts, had serious doubts about its readiness for human use. In a January 1981 *Scientific American* article by Jarvik, written while he and his associates were drafting their clinical use protocol for the IRB and the FDA, he stated that "neither the Jarvik-7 nor any of the several other total artificial hearts being developed is yet ready to permanently replace a human heart, even on a trial basis, but the pace of improvement in the technology suggests that the day may not be long in coming" (Jarvik 1981, p.74). The judgments by some that it was premature to begin human testing of the pneumatically powered or "tethered" Jarvik heart had several bases. These included long-recognized, persisting problems with biomaterials, the durability of some components, and the pneumatic power supply, all of which were known to cause various types of morbidity and mortality in laboratory animals and in the two previous human recipients of a tethered total artificial heart (Cooley et al. 1981; DeBakey et al. 1969; Fox and Swazey 1978a Ch. 6; Fields et al. 1983; Hastings et al. 1981; Murray and Olsen 1984; Murray et al. 1983; National Institutes of Health 1973).

Since the work initiated by researchers such as DeBakey, Kolff, and Kantrowitz during the 1950s, morbidity problems had been reduced and survival rates substantially improved in test animals. However, the level of success that many artificial heart developers thought was a prerequisite for human use had not been consistently achieved. Researchers from Kolff's former laboratory at the Cleveland Clinic, for example, wrote in 1983 that

> The current goal in artificial heart research is to develop a device which remains functional and viable for a minimum of 2 yrs in a clinical setting. The problem, however, is that to date, not a single animal experiment has achieved this 2 yr status for a variety of reasons, such as overgrowth of animals, calcification, thrombosis, inflow/outflow obstruction or sepsis. (Fields et al. 1983, p. 535)

By the mid-1970s, as we noted, the Utah artificial heart researchers were measuring the survival of their animal recipients in weeks and sometimes months rather than hours and days. Compared to the Cleveland group's clinical goal of a device that functioned for at least 2 years, they defined "long-term" survival in sheep and calves at more than 30 days (Murray et al. 1983).

By 1981, while their protocol was being reviewed and substantially redrafted by the Utah IRB, Kolff's group had achieved a survival record of 5 months or longer in nine calves implanted with Jarvik-5 and Jarvik-7 models, with one animal living for 268 days (Hastings et al. 1981). In these and other animals, a chief cause of morbidity and death was what the researchers called the "dreaded complication of infection." They attributed this often lethal problem to the sanitary conditions in animal barns during chronic experimentation and to the fact that the pneumatically powered artificial heart, with its air hoses penetrating the body's first line of defense, the skin, was proving to be a "particularly susceptible device for the establishment of an infection" from a "wide spectrum of microorganisms" (Fields et al. 1983, p. 532; Murray et al. 1983, pp. 541–42). Other reported causes of death in a series of 35 animals implanted between 1980 and 1982 included broken or malfunctioning mechanical valves, malfunctions in connections between parts of the devices, pneumothorax, respiratory failure, and brain death due to hypotension and acidosis.

As their experiments continued, the team monitored and celebrated what they considered to be their outstanding animal recipients, named by the investigators who had worked with them most closely. These animals included the 268-day record-setting calf Alfred Lord Tennyson; Ted E. Baer, who at the time of Barney Clark's implant was the "world record-holder" sheep, alive for nearly 200 days; and the twin calves used in a series of implant-transplant experiments, who were gleefully named Charles and Diana in honor of Britain's royal romance. Their Diana, members of the Utah group delighted in noting, literally gave her heart to Charles after he had lived for 72 days with a Jarvik device.[5] (The animal names in which the team took the greatest pleasure were those that made some sort of self-mockingly romantic or ironic commentary on the meaning of their experimental work.)

Given the nature of and reasons for complications and death in their calf and sheep recipients, judging the degree of success in animal trials of the Jarvik heart was a matter of deciding whether the proverbial glass was half full or half empty. In part, the Jarvik heart developers assessed their work during the late 1970s to early 1980s by the progress that had been made since the early 1970s, when after more than 15 years of laboratory work the longest animal survival with a total artificial heart was only 1 week. By this comparative yardstick, they thought that the Jarvik-7 had set a "record performance" in terms of durability, functional reliability, and the length of animal survival. In the eyes of its developers, this "level of experimental success rekindled the dream of application . . . in man" (Murray and Olsen 1984, p. 5).

Implementing this dream involved several steps and rationales and was spurred on by several other contributory factors. One step, which we have touched on and will discuss more fully, involved the preparation of human testing protocols and their submission to the Utah IRB and the FDA for review and hoped-for approval. Another preparatory step for the first implant with a patient-subject involved seeing how well the Jarvik-7 model would actually fit inside a human chest and how readily the surgical steps and techniques used in calves translated to clinical use. In Utah and at hospitals in East Germany and Argentina, DeVries and other members of the group used cadavers for "fit" trials to work out the best surgical methods for implanting the Jarvik heart in a human chest. A closer simulation of a clinical implant was undertaken during 1981–82 by Willem Kolff's son, Dr. Jack Kolff, a cardiovascular and thoracic surgeon at Temple University in Philadelphia. Before moving to Philadelphia, the younger Kolff had worked with Olsen and others in the Utah laboratory from 1974 to 1978 on surgical techniques for implanting the artificial heart in calves. At Temple, working both collaboratively and in competition with his father's laboratory in Utah, Jack Kolff continued his research with the Jarvik-7 heart and prepared his surgical team for what each group hoped would be the first clinical implant (J. Kolff 1982, 1984). During 1981 four members of the Utah group—Jarvik, Olsen, engineer Steve Nielsen, and implant coordinator and Utahdrive technician Larry Hastings—traveled to Philadelphia. There they observed and assisted in three practice implants performed by Kolff's cardiac surgical team on brain-dead patients "with the consent of the patients' relatives" (J. Kolff 1982, p. 11).

The Utah group's decision to ready the Jarvik-7 heart and themselves for human use involved several rationales that often play a role in decisions about initiating clinical tests of therapeutic innovations. First, based on "the success of the animal research . . . predictions were made that patients with end-stage heart disease could benefit from the clinical application of artificial heart technology" (Murray and Olsen 1984, p. 11). Second, the Utah group held that lacking a good animal model (that is, an animal with the equivalent of human end-stage cardiac disease), man had now become the "animal of necessity" (Swazey 1978). They had learned all they could about the device by implanting it in healthy animals, this argument ran, and they now needed to study the physiological parameters and the responses of a "sick organism"—a patient—including how being tethered to the Jarvik heart, and the device itself, would affect a recipient's quality of life (Joyce et al. 1983).

Another justification involved a pattern of reasoning discussed in Chapter 1 with respect to the first human heart transplants and the early use of immuno-suppressive drugs such as cyclosporine. What we call *ritualized optimism* blends scientific and clinical knowledge and judgment with a degree of optimism in the face of uncertainty that often seems to involve magicoreligious dimensions. In the case of the Jarvik-7 heart, one hope and expectation was that the human body would be as or more "tolerant" of the device than the bodies of calves and sheep, and that complications accordingly would be less severe (Joyce et al. 1983).

Despite such rationales and the positive interpretations of the animal trials, there was more ambivalence and uncertainty on the part of some of the key players about the success of the animal tests and the device's readiness for human use than is reflected in their published accounts.[6] Not surprisingly, then, a number of other mutually reinforcing factors helped impel the Jarvik heart from the laboratory and animal barns to an operating room at the University of Utah Medical Center. These factors, described to us by various participants in the Jarvik heart's development and the Barney Clark implant, included a strong desire to "win the race" with other artificial heart teams and gain the individual, institutional, and national priority and prestige that would come with the first implant of a permanent replacement for the human heart.[7] In addition, federal support for work on a total artificial heart was waning, as the NIH Artificial Heart Program began to shift its emphasis to partial cardiac assist devices. The prospect of diminishing funds for the development of a total artificial heart, a key member of the Utah laboratory recalled, figured strongly in their decision "to go now with a human experiment, because if successful, it would be a great moral and financial stimulus to the artificial heart program."

The "geist" of Salt Lake City and of many of the principals in the Utah artificial heart program also played a significant, albeit largely implicit, role in moving the Jarvik heart into clinical testing. As we discuss in Chapter 6, the "dream of progress" represented by the device was particularly congruent with the value structure of this dominantly Mormon locale (Fox 1984; O'Dea 1957). Another important element was the conviction and professional and personal drive of a pivotal figure in the decision-making process. In this case it was surgeon William DeVries, who was raised a Mormon and, though no longer a faithful member of the church himself, was married to a devout Mormon who was raising their seven children in the Church of Jesus Christ of Latter-day Saints. Some of those closest to him believed that deep down DeVries saw his work with the Jarvik heart as a surrogate for the traditional Mormon mission he had not fulfilled as a young man (personal interviews). Be that as it may, the young surgeon shared Kolff's belief that "life is always preferable to death"; and in the words of a colleague, he was the one who "championed the research data and had the courage to take it to humans."

As principal investigator for Kolff Medical Associates, DeVries formally initiated their decision to perform a permanent artificial heart implant in June 1980, when he submitted the company's protocol to the Utah IRB. The IRB found the task of dealing with the protocol a difficult and laborious one owing to both the medical nature and ethical complexity of the proposed experiment and to what they judged to be serious deficiencies in the proposal's content and form (Bosso 1984a,b; personal interviews). The IRB formed an artificial heart subcommittee to work with DeVries in order to develop a protocol that, in the words of a subcommittee member, "we [and the FDA] could find scientifically acceptable and approve" (personal interview). After substantial revisions in the body of the protocol and the consent form, initial approval to implant the Jarvik-7 heart was granted by the IRB in February 1981 and then by the FDA in September of that year. The FDA authorized DeVries and Kolff Medical/Symbion to do a series of seven implants—a number chosen, according to an FDA official, more or less at random or perhaps because of a sports analogy to baseball's seventh inning stretch, but not because it had any significance in terms of judging the success of the experiment (personal interview). Rather than giving DeVries permission to perform the entire series of seven implants, however, the FDA stipulated to Symbion that a protocol for each case, including a full report of the previous case, must be reviewed and approved by the IRB.

The protocol first approved by the IRB and FDA restricted the candidate pool to patients who could not be weaned from the heart-lung machine after cardiac surgery. During the next 7 months several possible recipients consented to an implant under such circumstances, but all recovered successfully from their surgery. DeVries and his colleagues then sought IRB and FDA permission, as they had in their original application, to expand the pool of eligible patient-subjects. A second group of candidates for whom the Jarvik heart offered some chance of life, they thought, were patients with severe cardiomyopathy who had been in class IV (end-stage) congestive heart failure for at least 8 weeks and for whom all treatment options except a heart transplant or artificial heart had been exhausted. In May 1982 a protocol was approved for implanting the Jarvik heart in class IV cardiomyopathy patients ineligible for a heart transplant, and the search for a suitable candidate began (Bosso 1984a,b; DeVries, personal interview, June 1983; Eichwald et al. 1981; Woolley, personal interview June 1983; Woolley 1984).

Act II: Barney Clark's Heart

The task of selecting the first recipient of the Jarvik-7 heart was performed by an evaluation committee chaired by DeVries; its other members included two cardiologists, a psychiatrist, a social worker, and a nurse. Additionally, the IRB and the Medical Center took the unusual step of appointing Dr. Ross Woolley, the Board's Vice Chairman and Chair of its artificial heart subcommittee, to monitor the investigators' adherence to aspects of the approved protocol, such as the selection and consent processes (Bosso 1984b). In his increasingly controversial role as a monitor, Woolley served as a de facto part of the committee, and his name was listed on the consent form, along with other members, as a person the recipient could contact if they had questions about the experiment.

The evaluation committee, any of whose members had "absolute veto power" over a candidate (Berenson and Grosser 1984, p. 910), used a number of medical and psychosocial criteria to screen patients, ranking their suitability on a six-point scale. To begin with, the potential candidates, who were referred for eval-uation by their personal physicians, had to meet the basic medical criteria of hav-ing New York Heart Association class IV cardiomyopathy and having been rejected as heart transplant candidates by at least three programs because of their age or other factors. Although patients had to be in a state of "chronic, non-operable, end-stage, progressive congestive heart failure"—essentially, in a "pre-terminal" if not terminal condition—they could not otherwise be "too" ill. Thus they were excluded as candidates if they were known to have "complicating coincidental illnesses, such as chronic renal failure, severe chronic obstructive pulmonary disease . . . cancer with metastases, hepatic disease, or blood dyscra-sia" (Berenson and Grosser 1984, p. 910).

Candidates also underwent a psychiatric evaluation involving the administra-tion of standardized tests and interviews of the patient and his or her "significant others." These assessments were used to weed out patients with "disqualifying major psychiatric illnesses" and to evaluate what the committee thought would be important "specific traits in personality style" that would enable a recipient and his or her family to withstand the rigors of the experiment, the possible com-plications, and the device to which the patient would be permanently tethered. The traits they looked for included "motivation . . . defenses against anxiety . . . adaptability and flexibility . . . mature ego, modulation of affect, and construc-tive use of available support systems." Those support systems, the evaluators thought, must include a family with a great deal of strength and solidarity. The successful candidate, according to the psychiatric evaluators and the selection committee, needed astronaut-like "right stuff" that made him "suitable for a risk-taking venture," and they actually used unpublished criteria for the selec-tion of astronauts as part of their screening procedures (Berenson and Grosser 1984, p. 910).

The candidate who successfully emerged from this selection process, as the world soon learned, was Dr. Barney B. Clark, a retired dentist whom people soon would liken to an "avuncular astronaut" in their letters to him and his wife. Dr. Clark, who was referred to DeVries for evaluation by a cardiologist at the Latter-day Saints Hospital in Salt Lake City, was deemed to be an "ideal candidate" for the first, historic implant. It was only a coincidence, members of the selection committee and implant team later asserted, that Dr. and Mrs. Clark were devout Mormons. And given their patient-subject's stormy postoperative course, the committee and team could not readily explain why, during his medical evalua-tion, they had "missed" identifying the chronic obstructive pulmonary disease that could have medically disqualified him as a candidate (Berenson and Grosser 1984; personal interviews). When Dr. Clark was admitted to the University of Utah Medical Center on November 29, 1982, he was in a deteriorating condition that, in the opinion of consulting physicians, made "death appear imminent within hours to days" (DeVries et al. 1984, p. 274).[8] That night and again the next night, he signed the 11-page consent form approved by the IRB, stating that he "hereby request[ed] and authorize[d] [his] physician to proceed with the implantation of an experimental total artificial heart device" (Shaw 1984, pp. 195–201). Late at night on December 1, as his condition rapidly worsened, Dr. Clark "was taken to the operating room on an emergency basis" (DeVries and Joyce 1983, p. 24). There, during a 9-hour operation that continued into the early morning hours of December 2, he received his new man-made heart.

The details of Barney Clark's 112 days of life with his Jarvik heart were closely scrutinized and chronicled in almost daily reportage by the electronic and print media and subsequently written up by members of the artificial heart team for a number of professional publications. The media coverage of Dr. Clark's implant and that of patients who subsequently received a Jarvik heart proved to be an important aspect of the experiment, with much discussion and debate by journalists and those they reported on about the nature, content, objectives, and effects of such extensive and detailed reportage (Altman 1984a; Blakeslee 1986; King 1986d; Peterson 1984).

As the artificial heart developers contemplated a human test, the public relations dimensions of the venture began to be considered by University officials, especially Dr. Chase Peterson, Vice President for Health Sciences and the institution's coordinator for the program, the public relations staff, and members of the artificial heart team. In the words of Peterson, who would serve as the able media spokesperson for the implant, they decided "that it would be both inappropriate and impossible to conduct the heart experiment in secret" and so began to inform the media about the details of the program and to signal that a historic event was pending (Peterson 1984, p. 130). As *New York Times* reporter Dr. Lawrence K. Altman later said, "The public relations staff did just what it should have done—orchestrated a news-organization march on Salt Lake City to cover the progress of the research that made Dr. Clark's implant possible" (Altman 1984a, p. 113).

Despite their advance planning and the coverage that, as headlined on the cover of one magazine, their "race to have a heart" received (Wrenn 1982), those involved in Barney Clark's implant found they were not fully prepared for the media onslaught that engulfed them: the crowds of reporters and equipment that descended on the Medical Center to cover the event, the number who stayed for the duration of Dr. Clark's hospitalization, and their often intrepid and ingenious strategies for acquiring information not officially released by the hospital. To a veteran reporter such as Lawrence Altman, the fact that people at the University and its medical center were so surprised by the numbers of reporters and the intense interest in the implant was a reaction that "lies somewhere between naiveté and incompetence. . . . [H]ow is it that a medical school can invite the media, get the advance publicity it requested from virtually all major news organizations, and then not expect them to all show up when the real event occurs. Journalists are human and not known for enjoying coitus interruptus" (Altman 1984a, p. 115).

At the time and as they reflected on it afterward, the participants in Dr. Clark's operation and care realized that the media attention was not the only aspect of the experiment they had not realistically anticipated. The nurses and other members of the artificial heart team were aware that their "special patient" was undergoing a novel, uncertain, and potentially perilous venture to save his life and to provide information about the device and its functions and effects in man. At the same time, however, they were largely unprepared for what Dr. Clark, his family, and they themselves underwent during those 112 days. Somehow, the nurses told us later, they had thought Dr. Clark would be "just like any other open heart surgery patient" in terms of his recovery: that he soon would leave the hospital and their care and go home with his new heart. Instead, while the machines recording his vital functions and the device's performance characteristics generated ream after ream of computerized data, Dr. Clark went back to the operating room for three more surgical procedures and suffered a range of complications that gradually diminished both his physical and mental condition.

To the millions who followed the drama of Barney Clark's implant, the quality of his life with a Jarvik heart seemed to be starkly and poignantly captured in a widely televised media event, a videotape of DeVries interviewing his celebrated patient. "To most," Altman later recalled, Dr. Clark "came off looking like a zombie. [He] looked like he was staring off into space, unable to look at Dr. DeVries, his interviewer" (Altman 1984a, p. 121). In fact, as some of those caring for Dr. Clark later told us, and as Altman pointed out in a sharp critique, his zombie-like appearance and halting, stilted speech during that interview was due not only to his flagging mental status: During the interview Dr. Clark was staring fixedly at the event's off-camera stage manager, Dr. Ross Woolley, who unbeknownst to the press or the public was engaged in another of his controversial roles as the IRB monitor (Altman 1984a, pp. 120–121; personal interviews).

Through it all, his psychiatrist later wrote, Barney Clark was a valiant patient who despite "his severe status . . . would consistently reassure the examiner, 'I'm still trying'" (Berenson and Grosser 1984, p. 913). On the final day, March 23, 1983, Dr. Clark was semicomatose most of the time. His death that night "was attributed to peripheral vascular collapse thought to be the result of endotoxin shock from . . . pseudomembranous enterocolitis" (Berenson and Grosser 1984, p. 914). In their first major professional publication about Dr. Clark's case, published in the *New England Journal of Medicine* in February 1984, DeVries and his colleagues judged that the move from the laboratory to the clinic had been warranted, and that the experiment, on balance, was a success. "The initial experience reported here," they wrote, "indicates the feasibility of relatively long-term cardiovascular support with a totally implanted artificial heart in a human being. Despite the relatively complicated postoperative course in our patient, the overall experience of 112 days nonetheless leads to an optimistic appraisal of the future potential for total artificial-heart systems" (DeVries et al. 1984, p. 278).

Postmortem

Some 1,300 friends, colleagues, and admirers, including local and national political figures, joined Barney Clark's family in Seattle for his funeral held at the Federal Way Stake Center of the Mormon Church. The podium was crowded with a large contingent from the University of Utah and Kolff Associates/Symbion. Among those delivering eulogies and tributes to the "medical pioneer" were Neal A. Maxwell, a member of the Mormon Church's governing Council of the Twelve, who praised both Dr. Clark and the research in which he had participated for their at-once scientific and spiritual contributions to the "mortal drive and hunger and quest to know more of what God knows" (Van Leer 1983). In his tribute, Willem Kolff likened Dr. Clark's qualities of dedication, suffering, and persistence to those of William of Orange, who began the Dutch campaign for independence from Spain but did not live to see the success of his efforts. Someday, Kolff said, as many as 50,000 Americans a year may live with artificial hearts, and "their borrowed days, weeks and years will be a precious gift from Barney Clark and Una Loy. He taught us that the artificial heart does not hurt, that its noise is manageable. Most of all, he taught us that it did not destroy his spirit and his ability to love" (Van Leer 1983).

After they returned to Salt Lake City, the participants in Barney Clark's case, each in his or her own way, sought to come to terms with the medical, professional, and personal import of that experience and slowly began to make plans for a second implant. The next months were turbulent ones marked by controversies and tensions about various aspects of Dr. Clark's implant and its sequelae, and about the policies and procedures that should govern the next use of the Jarvik heart. Also there were major dislocations in the membership of the artificial heart group, beginning with the elevation of Chase Peterson to the presidency of the University, which removed him from day-to-day involvement in the program.

In August 1983, as required by the FDA, DeVries submitted Symbion's protocol for a second implant to the IRB. Months passed before that protocol was finally approved by the Board in January 1984 and then by the FDA in June, with charges and countercharges between DeVries and his colleagues and members of the IRB as to who was responsible for the delay. In effect, those months represented the first of several moratoria in the artificial heart experiment (Swazey et al. 1986). An openly frustrated DeVries lamented that he was being contacted by "hundreds" of patients and that these potential recipients were dying while the IRB engaged in "red tape," "foot dragging," internal politics, and poor communications with the principal investigator and his colleagues (Altman 1984b; King 1984b). Members of the IRB in turn acknowledged there were problems and tensions within the committee. Such problems included the difficulties incurred by operating in the unaccustomed glare of the media, including the leakage of privileged committee minutes to the press in September 1983; personality, procedural, and policy differences among members; and operational inefficiency in regard to collecting information about the first implant and communicating questions to DeVries. The Board and others also were in a state of turmoil about the extent to which Vice Chairman Ross Woolley had exceeded the bounds of a monitor's role and acted as the institution's self-appointed medical and moral watchman for the Clark implant; the IRB spent much time redefining the role a monitor should play for the next case (Altman 1984a; Bosso 1984b; Fox 1984; personal interviews). However, as Chairman John Bosso and other members asserted, there were more important reasons for the time it took to approve the second protocol. These reasons centered, first, on the time it took for DeVries and Symbion to prepare a detailed report on Barney Clark's implant and to respond to the IRB's questions about drafts of that report. There were various reasons for the delays, including the team's relative inexperience in analyzing and reporting the results of clinical research and DeVries' well-known disorganization,[9] procrastination, and indifference to schedules. Second, the IRB was continuing to struggle with what they thought were the many serious ethical issues surrounding the Jarvik heart's use with human subjects, including criteria of eligibility, the content of the consent form, the costs of the implant and postoperative care, and commercialization or "paycheck journalism" (Bosso 1984b; Eichwald et al. 1981; Woolley 1984; personal interviews). The fencing that went on over the protocol for a second implant took place in the midst of other problems and concerns that affected the IRB's deliberations and the future of Utah's program more generally. To begin with, the Division of Cardiothoracic Surgery and the surgical duo who had implanted Barney Clark's Jarvik heart were reduced by 50 percent: In the fall of 1983 Dr. Lyle Joyce left Utah for a private practice partnership at the Minneapolis Heart Institute located at Abbott Northwestern Hospital in Minneapolis. Joyce's unexpected move, he said, "was mainly due to a volume problem," for after Barney Clark's implant and death, his and DeVries' referrals from cardiologists in the Salt Lake City area and their surgical caseload had decreased significantly. When Joyce, a research-trained PhD as well as an MD, was "recruited strongly" by a former associate, he decided that the Heart Institute job could "offer . . . everything I had hoped to do at Utah with Bill [DeVries]: a good volume of patients, and the chance to do heart transplants and some clinical research" (personal interview, June 6, 1986).

With Joyce's departure, DeVries was left as the Chief and only member of the Division in a Department of Surgery that, even before the Clark implant, had been without a chairman. In the absence of another physician at the medical center trained in artificial heart surgery, Joyce tentatively agreed to the suggestion that he return to Salt Lake City to assist DeVries when the planned-for second implant occurred. However, as physician-reporter Lawrence K. Altman observed, this plan seemed at best a dubious stop-gap measure to provide the "highly trained surgical team [that] is required to implant an artificial heart. . . . Even if Dr. Joyce returns for the second operation . . . for how long can he stay in Salt Lake City for the postoperative period? . . . If the convalescence took as long as Dr. Clark's, and Dr. Joyce stayed for only part of the period, would that be good care?" (Altman 1984a, p. 128).

Altman raised these questions about the Utah group's readiness and capabilities for a second implant during an October conference in Alta, Utah, attended by some of the key participants in the development and first clinical use of the Jarvik heart and a number of scholars versed in the many issues surrounding the experiment. The conference was arranged by Peterson and others at the university and was co-sponsored by The University of Texas Health Sciences Center at Houston to provide a time for "reflections" on the Utah artificial heart program "after Barney Clark" (Shaw 1984). In addition to IRB-related issues and the vacuum caused by Joyce's departure, the record of the Alta meeting, along with press stories and our own interviews and observations, charted much of the other difficult terrain that the Utah program was encountering on its road toward a second implant. The university and Symbion, for example, found themselves caught up in one of the many acrimonious priority disputes that pepper the history of science, technology, and medicine: In this case it involved claims by Dr. Clifford Kwan-Gett that he had not received appropriate credit for developing the heart implanted into Barney Clark that bore Robert Jarvik's name. Tensions also surfaced over conflicts of interest emanating from the ownership of stock in Symbion by the university and by DeVries. The concerns were twofold: Would it be proper for the university, which had done its research and development work on an artificial heart with public funds, to benefit from the commercial sale of the device? More immediately, could DeVries and the university's interests in the company manufacturing the Jarvik heart affect decisions about its clinical use? Chase Peterson, as the university's new president, acknowledged that there was a conflict of interest for the institution but held that it was minor and by no means unique in the burgeoning world of university-industry relationships. When "Kolff Medical . . . spun off from its university ties," he said, "it [gave] the university a modest amount of stock. I think it is 5 percent, which is a usual figure. . . . Yes, there is a conflict of interest, but it is a very modest one. And it is one that is clearly declared . . . so that people can make their own judgments about the degree of conflict. But it is no different, in my mind, than the conflict between Wisconsin and Vitamin D or between the University of California at San Francisco and genetic engineering" (Peterson 1984, p. 136). To Peterson and other university officials, however, DeVries' ownership of Symbion stock was a more serious matter in terms of perceptions, if not realities. Peterson ordered DeVries, on more than one occasion, to sell his holdings in Symbion before he did a second implant, a directive with which the surgeon, his repeated agreements notwithstanding, failed to comply (Altman 1984b).

A number of other financial matters also beset the program and caused increasing friction among many of its key players and the university community more broadly. One set of problems was finding money to pay for the approximately $250,000 in medical bills incurred by Barney Clark's 112 days of post-operative care and securing an estimated $180,000 needed for a second implant. In his consent form Dr. Clark had agreed to "assume the risk of . . . further hospitalization and treatment [after his implant], including the financial costs thereof." However, neither the Clark family, the artificial heart team, nor the state-funded University of Utah had anticipated just how lengthy, medically complicated, and costly his postoperative care would be, even with all physician fees waived in advance. Recognizing that the Clark family could not pay the bill, the university excused them from any financial obligation. Over several months Peterson, DeVries, and others raised the $250,000 from private donations and sought pledges for the costs of the next implant, a task that DeVries found unduly time-consuming and unpalatable.

Albeit successful, the fund raising efforts had several boomerang effects. One was a wave of protest by Utah faculty members, who because of budgetary cutbacks had accepted a wage freeze, and by medical center staff, who had taken a pay cut. Why, they asked, could the university not have found money for salaries as they had funds for Barney Clark's bills? (King 1984d). The manner in which Dr. Clark's bills were settled also became entangled with unease about the "commercialization" of his historic operation, particularly involving concerns about "paycheck journalism" that excluded journalists and perhaps others from learning about and reporting on various aspects of the case.[10]

William DeVries, lionized by the media as a heroic, pioneering, superstar young surgeon, was at the center of much of the *Sturm und Drang* that swirled around the artificial heart program after Barney Clark's death. In addition to the issues we have already noted, he found himself facing a declining practice and income owing in part to the concern of local physicians that he was too preoccupied with the artificial heart experiment to deal properly with routine surgical referrals, and in part to the fears of some potential patients that they might "wake up after surgery with an artificial heart."[11] Reportedly, he had also received a number of "poison pen" letters, including death threats and threats against his family by people who thought that his implantation of an artificial heart was an unnatural or evil act (King 1984e). To his dismay, DeVries was being criticized by medical peers and expert reporters such as Altman for taking so long to publish scientific reports about the Clark case in medical journals (Altman 1984a).

Despite all the turmoil surrounding the Utah program, most of those involved in it assumed that the FDA approval of a second implant, granted in June 1984, meant that the artificial heart would be deployed again as soon as a suitable candidate was identified (Altman 1984c). It was not to be, however, at least not at the University of Utah Medical Center.

Act III: The Move to Humana

On July 31, 1984, William DeVries was the guest star at a press conference in Louisville, Kentucky held by one of the nation's largest for-profit health care companies, the Humana Corporation,[12] at its Humana Hospital Audubon. Flanked by the company's board chairman and chief executive officer, Mr. David Jones, and Dr. Allan Lansing, chairman of the Humana Heart Institute International, DeVries announced that he and the Jarvik heart experiment had left the University of Utah for greener pastures as a member of the Heart Institute's private group practice.

Feeling harassed by media attention and stressed by many aspects of his personal and professional life, DeVries' trip to Louisville had been unheralded and unnoticed until he appeared at the press conference, for he and his wife had packed their car and left their home to drive to Kentucky in the middle of the night. What Louisville *Courier-Journal* reporter Mike King aptly described as DeVries' "bolting from the University of Utah" surprised many of his friends, colleagues, university officials, and the Salt Lake City community that had taken such pride in the Barney Clark implant (King 1984c). The abrupt departure of the only surgeon authorized by the FDA to implant the Jarvik heart as a permanent device also left the university's artificial heart program in limbo; and university officials, who thought "all the issues" bothering DeVries had been resolved, cautiously said it would take 2 to 3 months to decide if a second implant somehow would be done (Altman 1984d).

At the July 31 press conference and in subsequent newspaper and television coverage, DeVries and his new associates at Humana, Jarvik, and others from Symbion and the University of Utah discussed why he had left the University, the nature of his affiliations in Louisville, and his expectations for the artificial heart experiment under the aegis of Humana. He had decided to leave Utah, DeVries told reporters, primarily because of his frustrations with what he viewed as IRB-caused delays in approving a second implant and because of the chore of raising funds.

The possibility of joining the Humana Heart Institute had been raised earlier that summer by Allan Lansing when he entertained DeVries and his wife at a noted steeplechase race in Kentucky. The DeVries–Lansing connection began in 1983 when, following months of discussions and negotiations with Humana's two principal owners and executives, David Jones and Wendell Cherry, Lansing moved his successful cardiovascular surgery practice from Jewish Hospital to Humana Hospital Audubon, a 484-bed community hospital in suburban Louisville. There he became the founder and chairman/director of the Humana Heart Institute International, a private group practice institute housed by Humana but with no direct financial ties to the corporation. At the time Humana was developing plans to enhance its medical reputation by creating specialized "Centers of Excellence" at certain of its hospitals. These plans meshed well with Lansing's long-cherished dream of building a nationally and internationally prestigious center known for its clinical work in the diagnosis, treatment, and rehabilitation of patients with cardiovascular disease, for its related programs of applied research, and for its medical education efforts (*Centers of Excellence* 1986; Humana Heart Institute International 1985).

One of Lansing's immediate goals for his new institute was to develop a double-barreled capacity to do cardiac replacement surgery—both transplants and artificial heart implants. To this end he and some of his colleagues enrolled in Symbion's training program for surgeons who hoped to do Jarvik heart implants, and beginning in September 1983 he spent time in Salt Lake City performing animal implants under Olsen's tutelage. This training strengthened and personalized Humana's links with Symbion, for the company was one of those that Jarvik had persuaded to invest sizably in Kolff Medical Associates when he became its president.

Given the aspirations of both Lansing and Humana, Lansing met with an enthusiastic reception from David Jones when he broached the idea of DeVries' moving to Louisville. Declaring that "Humana's mission has always been closely allied with the best in research and education in medicine," Jones told reporters he had "jumped at the opportunity" to have DeVries and the artificial heart implant program affiliated with Humana. Although DeVries, like other

Heart Institute staff, would receive no income from Humana, the degree of the company's enthusiasm was signaled by what Jones called a "multimillion-dollar commitment" to underwrite the costs of up to 100 implants (King 1984g).

The "tremendous resources" offered by Humana in terms of money, equipment, facilities, and personnel to support the "growing" artificial heart program, DeVries stated, was the chief reason he had accepted Lansing's offer (King 1984g). There were other reasons too, he told the press. He anticipated encountering less "red tape" and "bureaucracy" in doing implants at Audubon Hospital compared with the Utah Medical Center. Nor did Humana officials, in contrast to the University of Utah, view his stock in Symbion as presenting a conflict of interest problem, thereby removing another of his irritants in Salt Lake City. Additionally, freed from fund-raising duties and with more colleagues and support staff around him, he anticipated having more time to devote to the artificial heart program and to building up his private practice and income (Altman 1984d; Clark 1984; King 1984b–e).

The announcement of DeVries' move to Humana generated a new round of doubts and controversy about the permanent implant series that persisted until the experiment faded away. Doubts about the continuation of the approved series of seven implants at Audubon Hospital under the aegis of Humana quickly were voiced to the media by prominent figures in academic medicine such as Dr. Arnold Relman, editor of the *New England Journal of Medicine*, and philosopher/bioethicist Arthur Caplan, then working with the Hastings Center in New York. Within 24 hours of DeVries' July 31 press conference in Louisville and escalating as he did three implants at Audubon Hospital, six aspects of the experiment's for-profit context were targeted for particular scrutiny (Swazey et al. 1986).

1. Questions were raised about the propriety of for-profit companies assuming control of a device initially developed with federal funds (Carter 1983; Relman 1984).

2. Critics of the Humana Corporation and of the artificial heart experiment—with many overlaps between the two camps—charged that the company's primary motive in agreeing to underwrite the costs of as many as 100 implants was to garner as much publicity as possible in order to increase their market share of patients and increase revenues (King 1984a; Relman 1984).

3. Members of the academic medical research community, such as Relman, promptly questioned whether the level of clinical research demanded by the artificial heart experiment could be carried out in a hospital that was for-profit, community-based, and service-oriented. "I'm not aware," he told a *Newsweek* reporter covering DeVries' move, "that Humana has any experience in basic

medical research. This makes a serious research problem into a public-relations commercial campaign" (Clark 1984; see also Heart of the experiment 1985; Relman 1984; Zenger 1985b).

4. Beginning with comments to reporters and remarks during a MacNeil/ Lehrer Newshour segment on August 1, bioethicist Arthur Caplan led critics of the Audubon Hospital IRB. Caplan and others suggested promptly and continued to assert that the committee would engage in a largely pro-forma review and approval of DeVries' protocols for the second and subsequent implants, acting as a rubber stamp for the interests of the corporation (Caplan 1984c; King 1984g; MacNeil/Lehrer 1984; Preston 1985a,b; Zenger 1985a).

5. Preceeding DeVries' first implant at Audubon, Humana mounted a well-orchestrated, extensive, costly public relations effort that continued with its media facilities and other arrangements for the implants themselves (Irvine 1987). Both Humana and the press were faulted for turning the implants into a "highly publicized media extravaganza," with far too much "emphasis on theatrics and too little on science and ethics" (American Medical Association 1984; Glaser 1985; Korcok 1985).

6. As the implants proceeded, cardiologists and cardiac surgeons complained that they were unable to assess the results because of proprietary constraints imposed by Symbion on access to and dissemination of their data (Buckley 1985; Pennington 1985).

To critics, the Jarvik heart/Symbion/Humana nexus was a case in point of broader alarms about the growth of for-profit medicine during the 1980s and its largely unstudied but presumed negative implications for various aspects of health care (Gray 1983; Relman 1980; Starr 1982). This is not to suggest that concerns about the experiment would not have occurred without the corporate connection. It does seem clear, however, that the debate about the human use of the Jarvik heart would have been less intense and less public had its development and clinical testing taken place *only* in an academic medicine context.

As the experiment and its attendant commentary unfolded, for example, the University of Utah, in contrast to Humana, was not faulted for its desire to "win the race" to perform the first clinical implant and "get on the map" of institutions noted for pioneering medical advances. In contrast to the immediate doubts about the "corporate willingness" of the Audubon Hospital IRB to seriously review the protocol and the degree of experience and expertise they brought to that job, experiment-watchers paid little attention to the "win-the-race" pressures brought on the Utah IRB or to the ability of that or any other committee to handle such a unique and widely publicized human experiment. Similarly, the Humana Heart Institute, Audubon Hospital, and Humana were faulted for their capacities to do "serious" clinical research. Academic physicians, related critics, and the press, however, took little or no note of several comparably relevant aspects of Barney Clark's implant: for example, it was performed by two young surgeons yet to be Board-certified, who constituted the entire staff of the medical center's Division of Cardiothoracic Surgery; they were members of a department of surgery without the organizational structure and lines of senior authority and supervision provided by a chairman; and the "team" involved in the surgery and Dr. Clark's postoperative study and care had little expertise in clinical, in contrast to laboratory and animal, research.

Act IV: The Experiment Continues

William Schroeder: The Second Implant

As we exited from an elevator on the second floor of Audubon Hospital at 8:00 a.m. on November 29, 1984, a tired but ebullient-looking William DeVries strode out of the Coronary Care Unit (CCU), with an entourage of physicians, nurses, and public relations staff. Catching sight of us in the corridor, he stopped, greeted us, and exclaimed, "I want you to see this man," and led us back into the CCU. "This man" was William J. Schroeder, who on November 25 had become the second recipient of a permanent artificial heart.

Preparations for continuing the experiment at the Humana Heart Institute had begun in July as soon as DeVries had accepted Lansing's offer to move there from the University of Utah. The key steps that had to be taken were to secure a new round of approvals from the IRB and the FDA for an implant now that DeVries had shifted the site of his work from Salt Lake City to Louisville. In September the Audubon Hospital IRB approved Symbion's amended protocol for a second implantation, and the document was forwarded to the FDA for review.

The Audubon IRB spent less than 2 months considering and requesting changes in the protocol, which in essence was the same document the Utah IRB and the FDA had respectively approved in January and June of 1984 for a second implant. One new feature of the protocol approved by the Audubon committee included plans to test a portable, battery-powered compressor pack developed for Symbion by Dr. Peter Heimes in West Germany, that would enable a patient to be temporarily "untethered" from the large Utahdrive console that pumped air to the artificial heart. There also were a number of changes in plans for the recipient's medical management and testing based on the experience with Barney Clark. The consent form for the second implant, which DeVries and Symbion released to the public in November 1984, was longer and more detailed than that signed by Dr. Clark, incorporating some of the "lessons learned" from the first implant. The 17-page form included detailed information about Dr. Clark's medical complications, provisions for the recipient to designate a surrogate decision-maker if he became mentally or physically incapacitated, and authority for DeVries to release to the public any information about the implant "within generally accepted bounds of good taste."

The Audubon IRB, which had been established in 1982 and had dealt primarily with protocols for the relatively routine testing of devices such as intraocular lenses and cardiac pacemakers, consulted frequently with the Utah IRB and relied on the latter committee's accumulated experience in dealing with the Jarvik heart protocols. Despite the fact that the Audubon IRB was working with a previously reviewed and approved protocol and that they sought the advice of their more experienced Utah counterparts, their approval of a second implant drew the vigorous criticisms that had begun with the announcement of DeVries' move to Humana. The board was faulted for the speed with which it had approved the protocol and for its members' lack of expertise in reviewing ethically complex research with human subjects. Two further concerns revolved around the private, for-profit status of the hospital and its parent corporation. First, the media and other experiment-watchers found it difficult to garner information about the IRB and its actions because under Kentucky law the hospital was not required to hold open meetings or to disclose information about the committee's membership or its review of the protocol (King 1984c). When the Louisville *Courier-Journal* did obtain details of the Board's membership by filing a Freedom of Information Act (FOIA) request with the FDA, reporter Mike King's story about its composition bolstered the assumption that had been made by "some national medical experts" that it was a physician-and-hospital-dominated committee that needed "more members from the community at large" to guard against its being "too beholden to Humana, Inc." (King 1984f). King also reported that information provided by the FDA in response to the FOIA request raised questions about the IRB's adequacy in handling even the routine device-testing protocols it had dealt with prior to the artificial heart. A 1983 inspection report to Audubon from the FDA's institutional review branch, King wrote, stated that a recent inspection had found the IRB to be "seriously out of compliance with [agency] regulations concerning human subject experimentation" in matters such as record-keeping, follow-up on the results of approved research, and the approval of "completely inappropriate" consent forms (King 1984c).

Despite any FDA concerns about the capabilities of the IRB to handle the artificial heart protocol, Humana announced on November 8 that the agency had approved plans for the second implant. During the fall, in anticipation of FDA approval, DeVries and the other physicians, nurses, technicians, and allied health personnel who would be involved in the implant and postoperative monitoring and care of the patient, along with the public relations staff at the hospital and corporate headquarters, had been readying themselves for the event. Preparations included several exchange visits of personnel from the University of Utah Medical Center and Audubon Hospital, testing of the artificial heart equipment, dry runs for handling various patient care situations, security arrangements, plans for advance publicity about the pending implant and for handling media coverage during and after it, and the formation of a committee to screen candidates.

With FDA approval in hand, DeVries and other members of his selection committee, consisting of two cardiologists and a psychiatrist, nurse, and social worker, began evaluating potential recipients, using criteria similar to those adopted by the Utah committee that had approved Barney Clark. From the time of DeVries' move to Louisville, hospital officials told the press, they had been "receiving dozens of inquiries daily about potential recipients," and several candidates were being considered at the time FDA approval was granted (King 1984b). Discussing the search for a second recipient at a November 8 news conference, DeVries said he expected to be "deluged with candidates" and emphasized that eligible patients must be at least 18 years old, have nonoperable heart disease with no other major medical problems, and have a stable family. "The number to call is 502-636-7135," he told the press. "Operators are waiting" (Surgeon gets federal approval for 2nd artificial heart transplant 1984).

Throughout the month of November, Louisville papers and other media reported on DeVries' search for a second recipient of the Jarvik heart, details of the consent form, and the team's preparations for the implant. On November 19, as part of Humana's extensive public relations work for the event, more than 100 members of the press attended a "sneak preview" at Audubon Hospital, featuring "the first Louisville appearance of Dr. Robert Jarvik," talks by DeVries and Lansing, and a slide presentation of "the Jarvik-7 heart in Dr. Barney Clark" (Barnette 1984). Then on November 23, the Humana Heart Institute issued a news release in which Dr. Allan Lansing announced that "William J. (Bill) Schroeder, 52, of Jasper, Indiana will undergo surgery to implant the JARVIK-7™ artificial heart on Sunday morning, November 25 at 8:00 a.m." (Humana Heart Institute International News Release 1984).

Mr. Schroeder, the news release continued, had been first diagnosed as having coronary artery disease in 1982, and in 1983 he had had a double coronary bypass operation performed by Lansing's team. His congestive heart failure continued to progress, however, and he was referred to the Humana Heart Institute as a candidate for the artificial heart on November 11, having been diagnosed by his physicians in October as having class IV cardiomyopathy. After a review of his medical records, further diagnostic testing, and interviews, Mr. Schroeder had been "unanimously approved" as the second permanent artificial heart recipient by the hospital's evaluation committee.

In this first of what would be many hundreds of press releases about William Schroeder, the media learned that the "Jasper native" was a retired quality assurance specialist at the Crane, Indiana Army Ammunition Activity, had been active in community affairs, and "has been married for 32 years to his wife, Margaret. He has six children, aged 19 to 31 years, and five grandchildren." The press also were informed that a background briefing on the patient and plans for the implantation would be given at 8:00 p.m. on Saturday, November 24, the night before the operation. Due to space limitations at Audubon Hospital, the release stated, this presentation and all subsequent medical briefings and media announcements would not be held at the hospital but at the Commonwealth Convention Center in downtown Louisville, where a briefing area with banks of telephones and "ample working space" for radio and television as well as print media coverage "will operate 24 hours a day."

The November 24 background briefing, carried live on Cable Network News (CNN), and the detailed briefing book and other materials supplied to the media by Humana generated a profusion of press reports the following morning, appearing in newspapers across the country as the implant was in progress. During the day of the operation and for the next several days, television and radio stations presented live coverage of the press conferences held at the Convention Center, with Lansing as the artificial heart team's chief spokesperson. Watching CNN's coverage of the 7:30 a.m. press conference on November 26, the morning after the operation, we saw a tired-looking Dr. Lansing, dressed now in a dark suit rather than the white medical coat he had worn for media announcements the day before, inform the press, "I am happy to tell you the patient is doing extremely well this morning." However, Lansing went on to announce, Mr. Schroeder had been "rushed back to surgery" about 6 hours after the implant to repair "massive bleeding" from his aorta, which necessitated replacement of about one-half his total blood volume. The patient, Lansing added, does not yet know he had additional surgery, and "is in for a rude shock when he wakes up this morning." Promising the reporters they could talk to DeVries the next day and to the Schroeder family that afternoon "if they are willing," Lansing went on to provide medical details about Mr. Schroeder's condition. He framed his report by stating that "his short-term prognosis is good, depending on your definition of short-term," and noted that "basically, we'll be treating him like any other open heart surgery patient, monitoring him and watching for signs of infection, pulmonary embolism, and so on." As promised, William DeVries gave a brief statement at the morning press conference on November 27, reporting that his now-famous patient was "very stable" and might be out of bed by the weekend. In response to questions, he offered some contrasts between the implants done on Dr. Clark and Mr. Schroeder, observing that the second procedure was "much smoother" and that "the most important, impressive thing was that there were no surprises." Invoking a Mormon metaphor, he went on to tell reporters that evaluating the success of Mr. Schroeder's implant would be "a step by step process. There is no point at which we can celebrate and say we've gotten to the top of the mountain."

As we entered the CCU with Dr. DeVries on November 29, four days after the implant, we were introduced to Mrs. Schroeder and then ushered past the security guard and screen blocking access to Mr. Schroeder's room at the end of the unit. Entering a small room crowded with the standard paraphernalia of cardiac intensive care plus the large Utahdrive power console, we saw Mr. Schroeder sitting in a chair, exhausted from being up for the first time. We watched as he was slowly and laboriously helped back to bed by his surgeon and nurses, who in response to his mumbled, anxious queries repeatedly reassured him that he was still "hooked up" to his heart's power supply. Once back in bed, we and a nurse who had not seen him for several days took turns putting our hands on his chest to feel the rhythmic thumping of the Jarvik heart that felt, Mr. Schroeder said hoarsely, "like a threshing machine." During that morning visit, between frequent checking by his nurses and various monitoring tests, Mr. Schroeder periodically sipped a milk shake and water. He also drank part of a can of Coors beer, one of the many gifts that were pouring in to him and his family, leading to a widely publicized picture by the heart team's photographer in which the new medical celebrity, holding his beer, exclaimed with a weak smile, "Coors cures."

During that first morning at Audubon Hospital, we joined various members of the artificial heart team in the small CCU conference room, remote from Mr. Schroeder, where they watched telemetry equipment monitoring the Jarvik heart's functions and studied the data it churned out. We looked at some of the mail arriving by the sackful for DeVries and the Schroeders and talked with the surgeon and several of the nurses and technicians about the implant, the steps leading up to it, and Mr. Schroeder's first postoperative days. "It's been so smooth, like clockwork," said the team's chief technician, Larry Hastings, who had moved from Utah to Louisville with DeVries. "But that first night, when Mr. Schroeder went back to the operating room, it brought back all those memories of Barney [Clark]. Barney did well his first day postop, but I think maybe we had forgotten what it was really like for him. The team here was all riding very high after Mr. Schroeder's implant, and as distressing as his bleed was that night, it did serve the purpose of bringing us all back down to earth and reining us in."

As we saw first hand during the week we spent in Louisville, and as the media chronicled in daily reports based on news briefings and interviews, Mr. Schroeder's first days of life with his Jarvik heart were indeed buoyant ones for him, his family, and his caregivers. Hospital spokespersons and the media spoke of his condition in superlatives, and even the most sophisticated reporters described his implant in terms of a therapeutic success story rather than an experiment. However, as Dr. Allan Lansing had cautioned the press at a briefing we attended on November 29, "at some time in the future I will have to stand up and give you the bad news." That time came when Mr. Schroeder suffered a thrombo-embolic stroke on December 13, nineteen days after his implant.

Many of the medical, technological, and human details of William Schroe-der's remaining 601 days of life have been recorded in professional publications, a book coauthored by his family and reporter Martha Barnette, feature articles in periodicals such as *Life* and *People,* television interviews, and hundreds of newspaper stories (Schroeder 1985; Schroeder Family 1987; Wheelwright et al. 1985). There were intervals when things things went relatively well for Mr. Schroeder and thus for his wife and children and the nurses and other caregivers who became extraordinarily close to and involved with their patient and his fam-ily. Overall, though, as recorded in the sparse medical language of the case report by DeVries, the first stroke marked the onset of a series of "events" that inexo-rably sapped Mr. Schroeder's physical and mental health, culminating in his death on August 6, 1986 (DeVries 1988, p. 851).

Day	19	Stroke—thromboembolic
	68	Neutropenia
	94	Stroke—hypoperfusion
	150–620	Subacute bacterial endocarditis
	163	Stroke—hemorrhagic
	352	Stroke—thromboembolic
	444	Liver biopsy—microabscesses
	590	Feeding gastrostomy
	612	Tracheostomy
	620	Respiratory failure, sepsis, death

Murray Haydon: The Third Implant

After William Schroeder was chosen as the second patient in DeVries' experi-mental series, the selection committee continued to screen additional candi-dates, hoping to perform a third implant as soon as a suitable recipient could be identified. On February 17, 1985, as members of the artificial heart team dealt with Mr. Schroeder's roller coaster postoperative course, DeVries and his sur-gical associates implanted the Jarvik-7 heart for the third time. The patient, Murray P. Haydon, was a 58-year-old retired auto assembly plant worker who lived with his wife Juanita ("Jinx") in Louisville near their son, two daughters, and five grandsons. He was, the press reported, "a tall, white-haired man . . . a fan of history books and puzzles . . . a man known for devotion to his family and his willingness to help neighbors . . . [and] a 'fighter' who won't just lay down and die" (Patient a father, a neighbor, and a 'fighter' 1985). Mr. Haydon was considered as an artificial heart recipient after a 4-year history of "progressive end-stage heart disease secondary to dilated congestive cardiomyopathy (idiopathic)" and exclusion as a heart transplant candidate "on the basis of advanced age" (DeVries 1988, p. 853).

Although Mr. Haydon's evaluation had shown that he, much like Barney Clark, had mild chronic obstructive pulmonary disease (COPD), the initial reports about him and the implant by Lansing, DeVries, and other spokespersons emphasized that he was a far better candidate, medically, than the previous two recipients and that his prospects after a smooth, "record speed" operation appeared to be excellent. On the basis of their briefings, the press recounted that Mr. Haydon was in "good physical condition," was not "on the brink of death when he was wheeled into the operating room," and unlike Barney Clark and William Schroeder did not have "other medical problems, in addition to their heart disease, which complicated their surgery and recovery" (Haydon best hope yet 1985).

Our media files on Mr. Haydon's life as an artificial heart patient are slim ones, primarily containing stories about his implant, his 1-year "anniversary," and his death. As we recognized through conversations with his caregivers and Mrs. Haydon and occasional visits to his room at Audubon Hospital, he was a quiet, intensely private man who insisted adamantly that he and his family be shielded from publicity. He was not, as some of his physicians and nurses at first had hoped, destined to be the first permanent artificial heart recipient to make a "full recovery."

To combat respiratory failure on his 17th postoperative day, Mr. Haydon was intubated and remained respirator-dependent throughout most of his hospitalization, subsequently requiring a tracheostomy and feeding pharyngostomy. His respiratory failure was later attributed to several days of postimplant bleeding into the pleural cavity from a tiny unhealed catheter hole in the remaining auricular portion of his natural heart. The bleeding, exacerbated by the blood-thinning drugs DeVries used immediately after surgery in hopes of preventing the blood clotting problems that had beset William Schroeder, further damaged Mr. Haydon's lungs, already impaired by his COPD. On the first anniversary of his implant, Mr. Haydon's referring cardiologist, Dr. Jeffrey Bracy, described his patient as a "pulmonary cripple" and voiced his judgment that "the bleeding into his chest was the single event that changed the outcome of this experiment. His lungs simply could not expand and in a person who was already debilitated like he was, it was a devastating blow" (King 1986c). In addition to his respiratory problems, Mr. Haydon, like William Schroeder, experienced a series of other "events," including a stroke, subacute bacterial endocarditis, persistent *Pseudomonas* sepsis, and renal failure.

> By day 472, renal failure was evident. . . . A decision was made with the family not to initiate renal dialysis because of poor overall prognosis. By day 482, the patient was totally unresponsive and anuric. . . . On day 487, the patient had no corneal reflexes, and there was no response to iced saline caloric stimulation. On day 488, electroencephalographic tracings were flat, and the patient was declared brain dead by two independent neurologists. (DeVries 1988, p. 854)

Entr'acte: The Artificial Heart as a Bridge to Transplant

On March 6, 1985, as William Schroeder and Murray Haydon lay in their intensive care rooms at Audubon Hospital, Dr. Jack Copeland and his team at the University Medical Center in Tucson, Arizona performed an emergency implantation of a total artificial heart. The device, developed by a Phoenix dentist, Dr. Kevin Cheng, was christened the "Phoenix heart." Copeland explained that he had decided to use the Phoenix heart in a desperate effort to save the life of Mr. Thomas Creighton, who was acutely rejecting his newly transplanted heart, and to sustain him until a second donor heart could be obtained.

Copeland's headline-making implant ushered in a wave of bridge-to-transplant use of artificial hearts. By the end of the decade, more than 300 such implants had been performed by surgeons at various cardiac transplantation centers in the United States and other countries, chiefly using the Jarvik heart and the Penn State heart developed by Dr. William Pierce and his colleagues (Annas 1985a,b; Copeland et al. 1986; Didisheim et al. 1989; Griffith et al. 1987; Joyce et al. 1986; King 1986b; Olsen 1987; Pae and Pierce 1987; Pennock et al. 1986; Swazey et al. 1986).

Bridge use of total artificial hearts rapidly generated a number of concerns and criticisms that by and large were more muted than those surrounding permanent implants. One set of issues involved the allocation of scarce donor hearts. The major allocation question raised by various commentators on bridge implants dealt with equity or fairness: given the likelihood of device-related complications, would temporary implant recipients be given priority for a heart transplant, jumping them to the head of the queue and thus creating even greater inequities in an already problematic system for distributing human hearts? Related concerns included the prospect that the artificial heart's deleterious effects would make a transplant less likely to succeed or that bridge patients might experience complications serious enough to make them ineligible for a heart transplant, thus transmuting them into permanent artificial heart recipients. For these reasons, Senator Albert Gore Jr., a leading figure in federal transplantation policies, officially notified the Commissioner of the FDA in 1986 that he was "deeply troubled by the diversion of donor hearts from use in heart transplants, an accepted medical therapy, to bridge to transplant, an experimental use" (Gore 1986).

In the context of the regulatory definition of total artificial heart models as significant risk *investigational* devices, two other sets of concerns were raised about ways that bridge implants were being performed. One set of issues involved the fact that some surgeons were doing bridge implants as "emergency" procedures without prior review and approval by their IRB and the FDA or by equivalent bodies in other countries. Second, concerns and criticisms were expressed about bridge implants being defined and performed as "rescue therapy" interventions rather than as investigational procedures carried out within a research framework. Limited assessments of the devices' performance and effects in transplant candidates were done by particular implant groups, and some overall information about outcomes was collected retrospectively and reported as "clinical use" registry information. Little in the way of explicitly planned clinical research was carried out, however, and monitoring and data collection were kept to as minimal and noninvasive a level as possible consistent with good clinical care. The medical rationale for this approach to bridge implants was that patients already were closer to death than most other heart transplant candidates and were too "fragile" to withstand implant-related experiments or testing. Rather, the surgeons argued, their recipients had to be clinically nurtured on their artificial hearts, hopefully without suffering from device-related complications that would make them ineligible for a transplant when a suitable donor heart could be procured.

Overall, the FDA accepted the surgeon-implanters' definition of bridge use as noninvestigational therapeutic interventions. As a result, the agency exercised largely *pro forma* regulatory oversight of these procedures until, as we shall discuss, the agency issued a recall of the Jarvik heart in January 1990, partly because of deficiencies in Symbion's conduct of clinical trials with the device.

To many, the laxity with which the FDA treated bridge implants was exemplified by the "emergency use guidance" for unapproved medical devices that was issued in October 1985 (*Federal Register* 1985). The guidelines, which allowed surgeons to perform bridge implants with *post hoc* rather than prior review and approval, were promulgated in response to Copeland's highly controversial use of the Phoenix heart, which had not been tested in animals much less undergone IRB and FDA human use review before it was implanted into Thomas Creighton. "Designed for a calf," Annas wrote in a scathing critique of the implant, "the device was too large, and the chest could not be closed around it. . . . By 3:00 a.m. [the following day] the second human heart transplant was completed. The next day Mr. Creighton died" (Annas 1985b, p. 15).

The press, as Annas wrote, "treated the story like a modern American melodrama," hailing "the implantation of Dr. Cheng's device [as] 'the fulfillment of an American dream,'" proclaiming that the artificial heart "at last has a useful role" and faulting the FDA's investigational device regulations for making "doctors . . . break the law to save a life" (Annas 1985b).

> Melodrama [Annas continued] calls on us to suspend our critical judgment, identify with the protagonists and join emotionally in the drama. This may be an appropriate response to soap operas, but we need to take a rational view of the event in Arizona . . . to decide what transplant policies we should now pursue.
>
> The physicians and their supporters have given three basic justifications for the implant: (1) the "only other option was just to let him die" so "we had nothing to lose"; (2) in an emergency, a physician can do anything to save the patient's life; and (3) FDA regulations do not apply to dying patients. None of these excuses can survive scrutiny. (Annas 1985b, p.15)

In response to such criticisms, which extended beyond the Phoenix heart to subsequent "emergency" implants with the Jarvik heart, an FDA official in 1986 sought to justify the agency's different handling of permanent and bridge implants. He explained that the agency had to act as a "brake pedal" on permanent implants because of the patients' complications but was reluctant to "interfere" with bridge implants because the FDA also had to act as an "accelerator" to increase the development of new technologies. In rebuttal, although he was one of the severest critics of DeVries' permanent implants, Annas declared that "there is a horrible double standard at work now. Dr. DeVries has attempted to provide everything the FDA wants of him, and everybody else gets to do as they please. That is not good public policy, and it's certainly not good science" (King 1986b).

Act IV: Continued

Leif Stenberg: The Fourth Implant

The scene for the fourth permanent artificial heart operation shifted from Louisville to Stockholm, Sweden. There, on April 7, 1985, Dr. Bjarne Semb, a cardiac surgeon at the Karolinska Hospital, implanted a Jarvik-7 heart into Mr. Leif Stenberg, a 53-year-old businessman who had been referred to the hospital's Thoracic Surgical Clinic in March "for severe chronic heart failure and with a history of repeated coronary infarctions" (Gréen et al. 1987, p. 351). For 6 months Mr. Stenberg fared extremely well with his Jarvik heart, experiencing none of the serious complications that had afflicted Barney Clark, William Schroeder, and Murray Haydon. On July 19, dressed in slacks and a sports coat, with the Heimes portable drive unit slung over his shoulder, Mr. Stenberg walked into a lecture hall at the hospital. Flanked by his physicians, a medical engineer, and his wife, he held a 90-minute press conference, telling reporters he had been taking walks in a park near the hospital, had been driven to a restaurant for dinner, and was "living proof" that an artificial heart can extend a person's life and improve its quality. Within a few days, the media learned, the man Dr. Robert Jarvik called his "best patient" was scheduled to move into a nearby specially equipped four-room apartment during the day, returning to the hospital to sleep at night. "I look forward to hopefully getting back to a more normal life," he declared, "and my dream is to be able to work again, maybe contributing more to this cause for future patients" (Heart patient steps forward grateful for extended life 1985).

Despite their patient's excellent recovery, Dr. Semb and his colleagues realized that Mr. Stenberg was at risk for blood clotting and embolic strokes and worked assiduously to devise a regimen of blood-thinning drugs that would prevent clotting without inducing bleeding. Although his Jarvik heart had not been intended as a temporary measure, Dr. Semb placed Mr. Stenberg on Karolinska's heart transplant waiting list after he moved to his daytime apartment. The prospect of a heart transplant, however, was ruled out in early September, 2 weeks after his doctors detected the formation of clots, when Mr. Stenberg suffered a cerebral embolus followed by bleeding into the embolized area. After the stroke he gradually lapsed into a coma and remained comatose until he died of respiratory and vascular failure on November 21, 1985, four days before the first anniversary of William Schroeder's implant. Leif Stenberg's 229 days of life with his Jarvik heart, his surgeon said, provided "grounds for a certain optimism" about such devices, and he affirmed his belief that artificial hearts would be "an acceptable treatment in the future" (Artificial heart recipient dies in Sweden 1985).

Jack Burcham: The Fifth Implant

On April 14, 1985, one week after Mr. Stenberg's surgery in Stockholm, William DeVries and his associates at Audubon Hospital performed another implant. It was DeVries' fourth and the world's fifth such operation, and it proved to be the last time the Jarvik heart was used as a permanent replacement for the human heart. The patient was 62-year-old Jack C. Burcham, a retired railroad engineer from LeRoy, Illinois, who had been in good health until he had a massive heart attack with heart block and cardiopulmonary arrest in October 1984. When Mr. Burcham was referred to DeVries, his medical evaluation confirmed that he had "severe intractable end-stage congestive heart failure secondary to ischemic heart disease and mild chronic obstructive lung disease." When he was admitted to Audubon Hospital after being approved as an artificial heart recipient, Mr. Burcham was undergoing kidney failure, a frequent complication of advanced heart disease; and in the judgment of the Humana Heart Institute physicians "he had an estimated life expectancy of only several days" (DeVries 1988, p. 854).

Jack Burcham, the oldest of the five permanent artificial heart recipients, had the shortest and most medically disastrous span of life with his Jarvik heart. "If you get it in right," he told his surgeon before the implant, "I'll make it work" (Wallis 1985). During the implant, however, DeVries and Lansing discovered to their chagrin that the Jarvik-7 was too large for their patient's chest, even though a preoperative computed tomography scan had indicated his chest's dimensions "to be small [but] adequate for the [device] as determined from cadaver implant data" (DeVries 1988, p. 854). DeVries and Lansing struggled at length to insert the heart, cutting away part of their patient's sternum and twisting the heart's chambers to force it into place. When Mr. Burcham finally left the operating room, his chest, draped with sterile dressings, was only partly closed around the device.

Within hours of his implant, Mr. Burcham began to hemorrhage extensively. In less than 24 hours he lost more than 5 gallons of blood—some four times the volume of an average-sized adult—and received steady transfusions until he was taken back to the operating room for exploratory chest surgery to locate and correct the cause of the hemorrhaging. Mr. Burcham also became anuric immediately after surgery and, in an attempt to restore renal function, underwent 2 days of hemofiltration followed on day 8 by hemodialysis. Because of breathing difficulties he was intubated and placed on a respirator. During his second dialysis treatment on the afternoon of April 24, a nurse checking his chest with a stethoscope heard a diminished flow of air from her patient's left lung. X-rays revealed that a large amount of fluid had collected in his chest, but its true nature and cause were undetected at the time. The heart team physicians, Lansing said later, thought the fluid might be blood from a "diffuse ooze" in the operative area, aggravated by Mr. Burcham's renal failure and the drugs he was receiving as part of his dialysis. The Heart Institute's on-duty surgeon, Dr. Zahi Masri, inserted a drainage tube into his patient's chest and felt large blood clots but retrieved little fluid (Altman 1985a).

As these events transpired, Drs. DeVries and Lansing were attending a Humana Heart Institute conference on heart replacement in downtown Louisville. At a dinner that night, while Lansing was presenting the Humana Heart Foundation award to Dr. Michael DeBakey, DeVries' pager told him to contact

Mr. Burcham's hospital room immediately. When he called, the surgeon learned that his patient's blood pressure was dropping rapidly and that he was hemorrhaging from the endotracheal tube connecting his lungs to the respirator. By the time DeVries reached the hospital, Mr. Burcham's "cardiac outputs and systemic blood pressure [had] dropped to zero, and he rapidly died" (DeVries 1988, p. 855). Some 15 or 20 minutes later, at 9:48 p.m. the key was turned to shut off the Utahdrive system, and the Jarvik heart stopped beating (Altman 1985a). A few hours later, after Mrs. Burcham had given permission for an autopsy, the pathologist and surgeons discovered that Mr. Burcham had died from an acute cardiac tamponade. When his chest was opened, those attending the autopsy could see the large blood clots that had formed outside the artificial heart. The clots had compressed the atria (upper chambers) of his natural heart, to which the ventricles of the Jarvik heart were attached, blocking the flow of blood through the rigid chambers of the plastic heart and causing it to back up into his lungs, where it congealed into a jelly-like mass.

At a postmortem news briefing, Lansing acknowledged that the cardiac surgeons "did not suspect" cardiac tamponade before Mr. Burcham's death. As he explained and as other cardiac surgeons agreed, the "usual early warning signs of cardiac tamponade were not present" because the rigid structure of the Jarvik heart masked the symptoms detectable in a natural heart (Altman 1985a; Saltus 1985). At the same news briefing, a gaunt, serious-looking William DeVries emphasized the experimental nature of the implants and affirmed his intention to continue them despite the deaths of Barney Clark and Jack Burcham and the complications William Schroeder and Murray Haydon were experiencing. At the time, although he described the struggle to implant the Jarvik heart in Mr. Burcham's chest as "like putting a square peg in a round hole," DeVries held that surgical trauma and the device's "tight fit" were not factors in his patient's death (Altman 1985a; Wallis 1985). In the 1988 report on his four implants, however, DeVries recognized that Mr. Burcham's acute cardiac tamponade and renal failure could "be attributed to poor surgical fit of the device with subsequent inflow occlusion (venae cavae and pulmonary veins) and undue stress on the surgical anastomoses with persistent bleeding" (DeVries 1988, p. 855).

Lengthening Shadows: April 1985 to June 1986

Jack Burcham's brief life and death with his Jarvik heart, coupled with the grave complications that Mr. Schroeder and Mr. Haydon were experiencing, cast lengthening shadows over the results of the Jarvik heart experiment and its continuation. Publicly, the Humana Corporation sought to rebut the project's critics and avowed its ongoing commitment to the experiment (Humana Inc. 1985).

In private, however, many persons at Audubon Hospital and corporate head-quarters had grave doubts. They, as well as members of the press and their read-ers, experts in cardiac replacement, and bioethical and legal analysts, wondered if the results of the experiment to date were "worth it" in terms of the knowledge gained and the patients' outcomes and if the project should be allowed to run its allotted course of seven implants.

Duiring press interviews and presentations at professional conferences, DeVries repeatedly affirmed his belief that the experiment should and would continue, arguing that it had been a success as judged by the information it had generated, the survival times of three of his four patients, and the reasonably good quality of life they intermittently had experienced. Overall, however, he and others among the project's principals at the Humana Heart Institute, Sym-bion, and the University of Utah recognized that one of their hopes in initiating human testing had not been realized: the human body did not tolerate the device any better than the calves and sheep who had been its first recipients; patients, moreover, had the devastating problem of strokes which had not been encoun-tered in animals. At an October 1985 conference, for example, DeVries pre-sented a series of slides detailing his patients' major complications: infections, hemolytic anemia, a mysterious severe initial suppression of the immune system that increased susceptibility to infection, acute tubular necrosis and renal failure, respiratory insufficiency, bleeding, and the formation of clots. Because most of these problems seemed to be at least partly device-related, DeVries stated, "at present the use of the artificial heart means giving the patient another disease in place of his original disease" (DeVries 1985).

On December 2, DeVries learned about an impending FDA hearing on the continuation of his permanent implants the same way that we did: He read Mike King's story in the Louisville *Courier-Journal* headlined "FDA panel to discuss artificial heart's future" (King 1985b). King had been told by sources at the agency that the Circulatory System Devices Advisory Panel had scheduled a 1-day hearing in Washington on December 20, with a public morning session for presentations by "interested parties" and a closed afternoon meeting with DeVries, Jarvik, and other representatives from Symbion and the Humana Heart Institute. King learned that the hearing was being convened to provide the panel with perspectives and data on the permanent implants, so they could rec-ommend to the FDA Commissioner whether the agency should allow DeVries' series to continue or restrict the Jarvik heart's use to bridge-to-transplant pro-cedures.

When we arrived at the Heart Institute offices that morning, DeVries was engrossed with a series of phone calls to Jarvik and others at Symbion and to staff at the FDA's Division of Cardiovascular Devices to find out what he could about the hearing's "real agenda" and why he had learned about it from the newspaper rather than from Symbion. The atmosphere at the Heart Institute, the CCU, and the hospital's public relations office was tense and anxious that day. As DeVries and various of his associates told us, they believed the FDA division and its advisory panel had already decided to call a halt to the implants and that the hearing would be a *pro forma* event.

The hearing and the recommendation that the advisory panel issued at its close were an intriguing blend of regulatory process, political exercise, and media event.[13] Nine presentations were made during the open public hearing in an auditorium filled with interested parties, spectators, and the press and their equipment. Strong support for the worth of the implants and pleas for their continuation were voiced by Robert Jarvik, Mrs. Barney Clark, and Mr. Jack Wellman, who had been accepted as an implant recipient but survived bypass surgery and later received a heart transplant. Criticisms and concerns were delivered by health lawyer George Annas from Boston University Schools and Medicine and Public Health, and physician and consumer activist Sidney Wolfe, head of Ralph Nader's Public Citizens Health Group. For the advisory panel members seated at a table on the auditorium's stage, however, the most significant testimony was that offered by physicians representing the American College of Cardiology and the Medical Devices Committee on Circulatory Devices of the Society of Thoracic Surgeons. In their statements these experts in cardiovascular diseases and their treatment made four major points: (1) Decisions about the permanent implants must be based on scientific data rather than press accounts, and DeVries and his colleagues had done a disservice to themselves and their medical communities by not publishing the results of their work. (2) The imposition of a halt or moratorium by the FDA would be premature given the small number of cases to date and the need for a more thorough evaluation of the scientific evidence. (3) The recipients' grave complications are common to Phase I (early clinical) research; and if studies of the artificial heart were stopped, where would the FDA draw the line with other Phase I work? (4) Important information has been gained and can be gained from human testing that cannot be obtained by research with other species. Therefore, each speaker concluded, it would be premature and counterproductive for the FDA to stop the permanent implant series.

At the end of the morning session, DeVries, Jarvik, and their colleagues from Audubon Hospital and Symbion were buoyed up by the unexpectedly positive testimony of the eminent medical society representatives but still apprehensive about their afternoon presentation of data and the panel's subsequent recommendation. For nearly 4 hours that afternoon, the advisory panel and FDA staff met with members of the artificial heart project from Symbion and Audubon Hospital in a crowded conference room, its lights dimmed for the presentation of dozens of slides that reported findings on the Jarvik heart's performance characteristics in humans and the nature and possible causes of the patients' complications. Two outsiders were present at the closed session: one of us (J.P.S.), whom DeVries had invited to attend the hearing as a member of the "team," and a cardiac replacement expert from the Texas Heart Institute, Dr. Howard Frazier, whom the panel had asked to review and comment on the data. To the relieved surprise of DeVries' group, Dr. Frazier's remarks were highly positive, emphasizing the importance of what had been learned thus far, applauding DeVries and his associates for their "courage" in undertaking the experiment, and urging the panel to endorse a continuation of the permanent implants.

When the session ended, the advisory panel remained in the conference room to formulate its recommendation while the Symbion-Audubon Hospital delegation clustered in the corridor and adjacent rooms, anxiously awaiting news of the verdict. Jarvik was summoned back to the conference room to answer some additional "procedural" questions and was joined for a portion of the discussion by DeVries, Symbion's attorneys, and Humana's public relations director. At 6:45 p.m. Jarvik emerged from the conference room, his face wreathed in a huge grin, and summoned DeVries into a vacant room to tell him of the panel's decision. That decision, a relieved DeVries told his associates a few minutes later, was to recommend that the implants continue, contingent on the submission and approval of a revised investigational device exemption protocol by Symbion. Soon thereafter members of the panel and the artificial heart group reconvened for a press conference in the auditorium, at which the panel's chairman, Dr. Charles McIntosh, summarized their recommendations. As he explained at that session and in subsequent testimony at a February 1986 Congressional hearing on the artificial heart, the panel unanimously decided that permanent implants should "proceed, but with caution." Symbion, the panel thought, needed to submit a revised IDE application that included "the experience gained with the last four patients" and specific new patient management and data acquisition plans based on this experience; it also should address those plans and concerns in regard to the range of expertise on the heart team, with "the addition of scientists with needed medical and scientific expertise who will collaborate with Dr. DeVries." If the new protocol was approved, the panel went on to recommend, the FDA should exercise "a more direct oversight role" in any further implants, approving or disapproving them "on a case-by-case basis . . . conditioned upon an analysis of data derived from the preceding implant" (McIntosh 1986).

From the time of the December 20 hearing until the FDA approved Symbion's revised IDE protocol some 2 months later (February 1986), DeVries' work was suspended by what we have termed a "technical moratorium" (Swazey et al. 1986). During the February 5 hearing on the artificial heart program by the U.S. House of Representatives' Subcommittee on Science and Technology,

DeVries angrily charged that the FDA's "bureaucratic over-regulation is becoming a real impediment to further scientific progress" and in particular was stifling his research with the Jarvik heart. In his testimony, wrote reporter Mike King, DeVries "lashed out at the agency for imposing new restrictions simply because it felt pressured by 'uninformed public opinion. Regulatory agencies should evaluate a project based on appropriate scientific reporting and timely publications by the investigator, not by media presentation,' he said" (King 1986e).

DeVries' annoyance with the FDA's tighter regulation of his project notwithstanding, the agency-enforced pause was only one of a number of factors that had stalled the project since his fourth implant in April 1985. "Apart from the many complications that have beset DeVries' patients," King had written in an October 1985 story, "the experiment seems to be stymied by a lack of referrals, by advances in transplantation, and by problems within the program itself" (King 1985a).

During our next round of interviews and observations at Audubon Hospital in April 1986, a determinedly optimistic William DeVries was still discussing plans for a fifth implant. He acknowledged, though, that the referrals of artificial heart candidates had continued to decrease from the several a day at the time of William Schroeder's implant to at most one a week, and no likely recipients had been identified. The mood of most of the other members of the project with whom we talked was far less sanguine than that of DeVries about the likelihood of a fifth implant, and they were less convinced than their principal investigator about whether another procedure was warranted. The nurses and technicians who had now watched over and cared for William Schroeder and Murray Haydon for so many days and nights were stressed, exhausted, deeply worried about their patients' deteriorating conditions, and concerned about their ability to cope with the rigors of another implant patient. Several of them described the troubling, image-filled dreams they had been having about the artificial heart, the patients and their families, and their roles in the experiment. One recurrent image was that of Humana's lavish corporate headquarters: it had been hailed as an architectural masterpiece and as an art deco extravaganza, but in their dreams it was a giant mausoleum in which they were entombed.

We made our next visit to Audubon Hospital 2 months later, playing a participant-observer role that exceeded the usual activities of field workers. At the request of several nurse-members of the artificial heart team and with the approval of the Heart Institute and hospital administration, we had agreed to organize and run two 1-day workshops for staff involved with the artificial heart project, followed by a "debriefing" session with Dr. DeVries and some of the hospital's senior administrators. The workshops, attended principally by nurses, technicians, and allied health personnel were designed to address some of their questions about the nature and conduct of clinical research and to give them a structured opportunity to raise and share concerns, insights, and suggestions about the present and future course of the project and their roles in it. Two of the topics for group discussion, "Team Roles, Relationships, and Stresses in Care Provision" and "Turning the Key: Death with an Artificial Heart," proved to be especially and poignantly germane to the June 19 and 20 dates on which the workshops were held. For at 10:45 a.m. on June 19, while many of his devoted caregivers were attending the workshop's first session, DeVries' third Jarvik heart recipient, Mr. Murray Haydon, was pronounced dead.

Act V: Endings

August 1986

> DeVries took the shiny, silver-colored key from its place inside the Utah's cabinet and leaned over to insert it in the lock on the front of the console. As DeVries held it there, Margaret placed her hand on his, followed by each of the children. In a single, unified act, they turned the key counterclockwise to the OFF position.
>
> The artificial heart, which had clicked inside of Bill's chest more than 68 million times, stopped. (The Schroeder Family 1987, p. 369)

At 1:35 p.m. on August 6, 1986, neurologist Gary Fox determined that William J. Schroeder, after 620 days of life with his Jarvik heart, was brain dead following a final, massive stroke (Gil et al. 1986; King and Gil 1986). Three days later the Schroeder family, relatives and friends, William DeVries, Robert Jarvik, many of those who had cared for Mr. Schroeder during his long hospitalization, and the press gathered in Jasper, Indiana, to pay tribute to the longest survivor of the permanent implant series. After a funeral mass at St. Joseph Catholic Church, graveside ceremonies were held at nearby Fairview Cemetery (King 1986f). The grave is marked by a large black granite tombstone carved into two overlapping hearts. The left-hand heart has a laser-engraved image of the Jarvik-7 heart, and under it are the dates of William Schroeder's birth and death; underneath the right-hand heart Margaret Schroeder's birth date has been engraved, awaiting the time she will be buried next to her husband. Between the apexes of the heart the tomb bears the inscription, "2d Artificial Heart Implant Nov. 25, 1984."

William Schroeder's death received front-page newspaper and prime time television coverage. Many stories during the days after his death not only recounted his long "ordeal" and lauded him as a "medical hero" but also contained reflections by reporters and some of their principal sources about what his experience boded for the future use of the artificial heart. The strokes, respiratory problems, and infections that "plagued" Schroeder's 21 months with an artificial heart, *Philadelphia Inquirer* staff writer Linda Herskowitz wrote on August 8, were a "coda to his life [that] undoubtedly was not what Robert Jarvik . . . had in mind when he declared in 1981: 'If the artificial heart is ever to achieve its objective, it must be . . . reliable and dependable. It must be forgettable'" (Herskowitz 1986). To long-time critics of the permanent implants, such as bioethicist Arthur Caplan and cardiologist Thomas Preston and less-quoted figures such as surgeons Denton Cooley and Norman Shumway, Schroeder's complications with the Jarvik heart and his death were "discouraging" indications that years of further research were needed to develop a clinically safe, "forgettable" device. For now, such commentators opined, use of the Jarvik heart and other total artificial heart models should be restricted to temporary use as a bridge to transplant (Altman 1986; Herskowitz 1986; King 1986f). DeVries, however, staunchly affirmed that despite the outcomes with his first four patients the permanent implants would continue and that he was even now looking for a new recipient. In a page one *USA Today* story on August 7, the day after Mr. Schroeder's death, headlined "DeVries believes in more 'Bionic Bills'," the surgeon was quoted as declaring that "We're very anxious to find another patient. We have a better chance at longer survival and a more useful quality of life" (Mayfield 1986, p. 1).

In retrospect, Mr. Schroeder's death and funeral marked one of several endings to the experimental use of the Jarvik heart as a permanent replacement for the human heart. Another ending, in historical hindsight, was the implant performed on Mr. Jack Burcham on April 14, 1985. Although DeVries and Symbion expected to continue the series, it proved to be the last time a patient received a permanent Jarvik-7 heart (King 1986a). In 1986 it seemed possible that the experimental use of the Jarvik heart was in a moratorium phase and that the implants eventually would be resumed (Swazey et al. 1986). By 1988, however, there were clear signs that the experiment had ended in midcourse, though there had been no explicit or formal decisions to that effect or any official declarations in professional journals or public forums that it was over.

April 1987

For several months we had heard from sources in Salt Lake City and Louisville that the "artificial heart grapevine" had been abuzz with rumors that all was not well at Symbion, Inc. The company's operating losses were said to be mounting, work on the new Jarvik-8 heart was running behind schedule, and relations between Robert Jarvik and other company officials were becoming increasingly strained. On April 27 and 28 newspaper stories confirmed the rumors: Symbion's board had "terminated" Jarvik's employment as chairman and chief executive officer because of "internal company matters" (King 1987b; Symbion board ousts Jarvik 1987).

Those "matters" involved Jarvik's management of the company and the purchase of a controlling interest in Symbion by Warburg, Pincus Capital Co. The venture capital company's earlier buy-out offer had been opposed by Jarvik on the grounds that the price was too low and that Symbion might, for the first time, turn a profit. Shortly thereafter, however, Jarvik quietly sold an estimated $2.1 million of his stock to Warburg Pincus, giving them a controlling interest in the company. Although Symbion's attorney stated to the press that there was no relation between the takeover and Jarvik's departure, associates thought that the inventor-entrepreneur's financial maneuvering had added to already strained corporate relationships (personal interviews).

As part of his severance agreement with Symbion, Jarvik retained his seat on the board but without any administrative duties, and in July he was informed that his faculty appointment with the University of Utah was not being renewed. That summer, after his much publicized engagement and marriage to Marilyn vos Savant, billed as "the world's smartest woman," Jarvik moved from Salt Lake City to New York City (McMurran 1987; Scheier 1987; Vitez 1988). From his new home office Jarvik engaged in a round of media appearances, lectures, and consultations with surgical teams about bridge implants with the Jarvik heart. He also formed a new company, Jarvik Research, and began to seek venture capital to work on a new, electrically powered version of the device that his former company had begun referring to as the "Symbion heart."

May 1987

We made our final research trip to Louisville in May 1987. Though we had kept in touch with many people by phone and letter, it had been 11 months since our last visit, at the time of Murray Haydon's death in June 1986. Over the course of 5 days we talked once more with many of the people who had been involved in the permanent artificial heart experiment: DeVries; his wife Karen; some of the nurses, technicians, and physicians who had cared for Bill Schroeder, Murray Haydon, and Jack Burcham; public relations and administrative staff at Audubon Hospital; and senior executives at Humana's corporate offices. Some of the key members of DeVries' group were no longer affiliated with the project, having taken other jobs at Audubon Hospital or elsewhere. He had recruited a few new people to help him work on his protocols for a hoped-for next implant.

Much like the members of the artificial heart group in Salt Lake City "after Barney Clark," those with whom we talked in Louisville, often for many hours, were in a somber, reflective mood, taking stock of the experiment and their roles in it. With the exception of DeVries and the nurses now helping with his "data management" and protocols, everyone with whom we met thought that the experiment was over. Many by now had strong medical and ethical doubts as to whether, even if another candidate was found, another implant should be done, or if one should be attempted they would be willing to participate in it.

When we had our last interview with William DeVries, it had been more than 2 years since he performed his last implant and almost a year since Mr. Schroeder's death. Portions of our field notes summarize the essence of that meeting:

> The artificial heart group is scattering. Dr. DeVries seems pensive, isolated, and without much to do as a cardiac surgeon or an artificial heart researcher. He is alternately optimistic that his work will continue, uncertain at what the future can hold for him, and angry at those, including ourselves, who question the artificial heart experiment and suggest that he should explicitly call a moratorium. . . . Early the next morning, we stop by his office to see his secretary. In the hours since our interview, a message has been put up on the bulletin board outside his office. We read:
>
>> *It is not the critic who counts; not the man who points out how the strong man stumbled or where the doer of deeds could have done better. The credit belongs to the man who is actually in the arena, whose face is marred by dust and sweat and blood; who strives valiantly; who errs and comes short again and again because there is no effort without error and shortcoming; but he who does actually strive to do the deeds; who knows the great enthusiasm, the great devotion; who spends himself in a worthy cause, who at the best knows in the end the triumph of high achievement and who at the worst, if he fails, at least failed while daring greatly, so that his place shall never be with those cold and timid souls who know neither victory nor defeat.—Theodore Roosevelt*

June 1987

During the winter and spring of 1987 we had heard that relationships were becoming increasingly strained between DeVries and Allan Lansing and the other members of the Humana Heart Institute's surgical group practice. As many of those who talked with us had forecast, DeVries announced on June 1 that he had resigned from the Heart Institute to start his own group practice with two other surgeons in Louisville. In local medical circles the split with Lansing came as no surprise, but it was presented to the public as a relatively smooth one. DeVries explained to reporter Mike King that "now it's time to take the next step. . . . I want to do more surgery. I want to take care of patients, while at the same time explore research and teaching possibilities." Lansing, in turn, expressed regret at DeVries' decision and said, "I certainly understand someone wanting to be his own boss." The Heart Institute's chairman added, "I do think that DeVries has been at loose ends because his work with the artificial heart is stalled," and noted that "we have some differences in the methods of conducting our practice" (King 1987a, p.1).

Even without the Heart Institute's structure and support, including the role that other physicians in the group had played in caring for implant recipients, DeVries maintained that the artificial heart project would continue and indeed would "go forward much smoother and more effectively . . . outside of the current [Heart Institute] environment" (King 1987a). In a meeting with Humana's president, Wendell Cherry, DeVries told reporter Mike King, he asked for "exclusive control over research involving permanent and temporary artificial hearts and ventricular-assist devices," and "came away from the meeting convinced that Humana still supports the project." Publicly Humana officials continued to declare that the company's commitment to the artificial heart experiment was still "as solid as a rock" (King 1987a).[14]

November–December 1987

A number of newspapers, magazines, and professional journals took note of the fifth anniversary of the first permanent implant of a total artificial heart on December 1–2, 1982. More prominent, extensive, and laudatory coverage, however, was given to the fact that December 3 marked the twentieth anniversary of the first human heart transplant, performed in 1967 by Dr. Christiaan Barnard in Capetown, South Africa. The diminished press interest in DeVries' now quiescent work was indicated by the fact that reporters such as Altman, who had chronicled the implants in detail while they were in progress, only mentioned bridge-to-transplant use of the artificial heart in an anniversary story titled "4,000 in U.S. now live with another's heart" (Altman 1987, p.C3). In an interview for a brief story in the *Journal of the American Medical Association (JAMA)*, DeVries again affirmed his and Humana's commitment to continuing with the authorized series of seven implants and said he was still looking for a suitable recipient. In keeping with the heart transplantation anniversary, he recognized that "the best treatment for end-stage heart disease is transplantation," and admitted that "right now the most important use of the artificial heart is as a bridge to transplant." The state of the art of artificial heart technology, DeVries told writer Virginia Cowart, resembled heart transplantation before cyclosporine. "It's still developmental and experimental, but there is a place for another mode of therapy" (Cowart 1987).

In Salt Lake City, which had faded out of the media spotlight after DeVries' move to Louisville, the fifth anniversary of Barney Clark's implant provided an occasion to call local attention to the university's ongoing work on an artificial heart. Stories in the city's two major newspapers, the *Deseret News* and *The Salt Lake Tribune*, recalled the days when Utah had been "tagged as the 'artificial heart of America,'" before "the media circus pitched its tents in Louisville," and then went on to describe how "the heart of the University of Utah's research program is still alive and beating" (Jacobsen-Wells 1987; Mims 1987; VanLeer and Jacobsen-Wells 1987). According to the stories, which updated information we had gathered during our last visit to Salt Lake City in August 1986, the university's artificial heart research group had been quietly moving forward with the development and laboratory and animal testing of a new total artificial heart model, the Utah 100. Members of the Utah 100 team included familiar names from the days of the Jarvik-7, such as Willem Kolff, who had stepped down from his administrative work at the Division for Artificial Organs but was continuing to work on artificial hearts as distinguished professor of surgery and medicine, and Dr. Donald Olsen, now director of the Institute for Biomedical Engineering. New names in the Utah program's lexicon included the calves and sheep being used to test this latest modification of a pneumatically powered heart, such as "Kellog," a sheep who "survived 331 days on the Utah 100" (Jacobsen-Wells 1987). Pending FDA approval, the press went on to report, the Utah group was ready to begin clinical testing of the Utah 100 with a protocol already approved by the IRB for its experimental use as a temporary device, rather than a permanent replacement. For the clinical phase of the project, there was another new name as principal investigator, that of Dr. William A. Gay, Jr., a cardiac surgeon who had become chairman of the medical center's department of surgery in October 1984.

Given the deficits of pneumatically powered artificial hearts, the University of Utah also revealed that its researchers were working on a "totally implantable" electrohydraulic version of the Utah 100, using an external battery pack in place of the air lines that tethered patients such as Barney Clark to the Jarvik heart's power console. Their goal, according to the Institute's associate director, was to produce the new electrohydraulic device by 1992 (Jacobsen-Wells 1987). To meet this 5-year timetable and to deal with the still-worrisome costs of work on artificial hearts, the university had submitted a grant application to the NIH Artificial Heart Program in response to a request for proposals to develop a totally implantable artificial heart system. "The U.," reported the *Deseret News*, was now one of "six finalists" for a $5 million, five-year grant (Jacobsen-Wells 1987).

December 1987

On December 4, when 60-year-old Walton Jones of Louisville, Kentucky began to go into heart failure after coronary bypass surgery, his surgeon, William DeVries, did his first and only "emergency" bridge-to-transplant operation. DeVries first implanted a Jarvik-7 model. Then, because it was too large for the patient's chest, complications developed, and DeVries removed it and implanted the smaller Jarvik-7-70 model in its stead. By December 8 Mr. Jones had recovered sufficiently from his multiple surgical procedures and the hours on the heart-lung bypass machine and the complications they entailed to understand that he now had an artificial heart. After the surgery, DeVries asked Dr. Allan Lansing and Dr. Roland Girardet, his former associates at the Humana Heart Institute, to evaluate Mr. Jones as a transplant candidate. They did so reluctantly, given Mr. Jones's postimplant condition and the fact that a patient normally is designated as a transplant candidate before a bridge implant is performed. On December 19 DeVries explanted the Jarvik-7-70, and a transplant team headed by Girardet replaced it with a donor heart. Mr. Jones died on January 18 of a widespread infection after a series of complications that also included protracted postoperative bleeding, kidney failure necessitating dialysis, breathing problems necessitating a tracheostomy and respirator, and neurological impairments (Gil 1987, 1988; Hazle 1987; King 1987c; personal communications).

February 1988

Two days before St. Valentine's day, *JAMA* published an "artificial heart issue." The doubly symbolic cover illustration for this February 12 volume was Paul Klee's 1920 "An Angel Serving a Small Breakfast," a whimsical lithograph that draws the viewer's eye to the lightly sketched being's bright red heart. By the time this issue was published, its papers and accompanying editorials were, in effect, a tacit memorial to the experimental use of the Jarvik-7 as a permanent replacement for the human heart.

The artificial heart issue, following *JAMA*'s usual format, consisted of four sections. The original contributions provided case reports of the four permanent implants performed in Salt Lake City and Louisville, and three papers analyzed the patients' rampant infectious complications and their causes. A state-of-the-art review by DeVries detailed the surgical technique for implanting the Jarvik heart. Next, the special communications section provided a description of the "clinical management of total artificial heart drive systems," and a paper by DeVries explored the problems "the physician" encountered in dealing with "the media and the 'spectacular' case." Finally, three guest editorials offered perspectives on the experiment and on the future of permanent implants.

A particularly striking feature of the case reports' lead paper, given the numerous medical personnel involved in the four implants and the authorship conventions for scientific publications, is that William C. DeVries was the sole author. In his review he described the patients' preoperative assessments and postoperative courses, including their "neurological, hematological, renal, and infectious complications" (DeVries 1988, p. 849). In the conclusion DeVries implied that his work will continue: "The human permanent TAH study offers several advantages over further animal experimentation and the short-term bridge-to-transplant models for determining clinical applicability. . . . Finally and importantly, fundamental issues concerning the quality of life in artificial heart recipients will continue to be of great concern in this experiment" (DeVries 1988, p. 858). By his reckoning, the results with the "three long-term survivors," Barney Clark, William Schroeder, and Murray Haydon justified the experiment and its continuation both scientifically and because "life of an acceptable quality was realized for significant periods of time, if not the entirety of their postoperative days."

> It is also clear that the TAH is feasible, practical, and durable and offers life to those who would not otherwise be able to continue living. These patients have enjoyed their families, births of grandchildren, marriages of their children, fishing excursions, and even participated in parades, none of which would have been possible without the TAH. It is extremely rare—if ever—that clinical research has been so dramatically successful for the initial subjects. (DeVries 1988, p. 858)

In contrast to DeVries' accentuate-the-positive tone, the *JAMA* reports detailing the recipients' infections, including biomaterial-related sepsis and the accounts of thromboemboli and other complications by DeVries and in previous publications, painted a less sanguine picture of what patients might expect with a permanent artificial heart. To the three experts who wrote editorials for the special issue, the outcomes with DeVries' four implants had been far short of "dramatically successful," and they made it clear that, in their judgment, there were no justifications for continuing the experiment. The first editorial was by Dr. William S. Pierce, who had used the pneumatically powered "Penn State heart" as a bridge device for heart transplant patients and was working on a next-generation electrically powered device in his laboratory at The Pennsylvania State University College of Medicine. To Pierce, "our path [to a permanent heart] seems clear: "the implantable electric hearts . . . when available, will provide an acceptable therapeutic solution for patients with end-stage heart disease who cannot have a transplant. . . . But pneumatic hearts," he stated firmly, "should be used only for bridges to transplantation."

> The articles by DeVries et al. . . . . define the serious problems that have cast a dark shadow on the currently available pneumatic heart: thromboemboli and infections. Unfortunately . . . the suggested solutions to these problems [by DeVries and his coworkers], primarily alterations in patient management, seem unlikely to reduce substantially the incidence of complications. Accordingly, adding patients to this series will serve only to document further the magnitude of the complications rather than to demonstrate an acceptable life-style in the recipient. (Pierce 1988)

In a "clinical perspective" editorial, Dr. Gerald M. Lawrie, from Houston's Baylor College of Medicine and Methodist Hospital, appraised the permanent implantation of the Jarvik-7 against the history of efforts to develop left ventricular assist devices (LVAD) and total artificial hearts (TAH). Like Pierce, he stressed the need of heart transplanters for an "immediately available" fully implantable LVAD or TAH as a bridge device and thought that "despite the obvious limitations of the Jarvik-7 . . . as a permanent . . . substitute . . . [its bridge use] has more than justified its development." Lawrie paid tribute to DeVries' work as a "historical landmark" that "deserves recognition." However, he stated cautiously and equivocally that "the question of whether further use of the Jarvik-7 as a permanent implant should continue is a . . . difficult one" because the problems associated with the device "will not be easily overcome. . . . Pneumatically powered devices," he concluded, "now seem to be outside the mainstream of permanent artificial heart development and their future use in this role will surely remain controversial" (Lawrie 1988, p. 893).

On at least three counts, the final editorial, by Drs. Louis Rice and Adolf Karchmer from the New England Deaconess Hospital and Harvard Medical School, provided the most sobering and critical assessment of the use of total artificial hearts. The authors pointed out that the *JAMA* reports on infections associated with the long-term use of the Jarvik-7 "confirm the experiences derived from studying infection involving other prosthetic devices." Given both "the current limitations of the biomaterials" and the device's "dependence on an external power source and pump," they too thought it "unlikely that the TAH . . . will be useful for prolonged cardiac replacement." Second, because "infection is a dread complication of transplantation," Rice and Karchmer expressed greater concerns than did Pierce or Lawrie about even the temporary use of artificial hearts.

> Use of the TAH as a bridge to transplantation potentially juxtaposes two settings in which the treatment of infection is uniquely difficult: infections of prosthetic devices and infections in immunocompromised individuals. In both situations, eradication of infection is often contingent on removal or amelioration of the predisposing factor. . . . The potential pitfall seems obvious. By using the TAH as a bridge to cardiac transplantation, a setting is created wherein the device, if infected, can only be removed if significant immunosuppressive therapy is instituted. (Rice and Karchmer 1988, p. 894)

The third and most critical part of Rice and Karchmer's editorial assessment, however, was reserved not for total artificial hearts per se but for the caliber of the research and data that had been involved in their use. They directed their comments to temporary use of the Jarvik heart and similar devices, but by indirection they also found deficits in the research associated with the permanent implant series.

> Unfortunately, available data do not allow a meaningful assessment of the risk factors associated with specific infections among TAH recipients or of the impact of each type of infection on subsequent suitability for transplantation. . . . In a 1986 editorial . . . Relman argued in favor of continued clinical experimentation with the TAH as a temporary device, but . . . cautioned [that] "In the absence of protocols and cooperation among institutions, we are likely to see a proliferation of competing and unplanned efforts that will not advance the field and may even set it back." The wisdom of these words persists. (Relman 1986; Rice and Karchmer 1988, p. 895)

May to July 1988

The editorial in the May 16 *New York Times*, vividly headlined "The Dracula of Medical Technology," applauded the news that "the federal project to create an artificial heart is dead." The editorialist granted that "the pursuit of an artificial heart has not been completely chimerical," as such devices "can be of temporary use in patients waiting for a heart transplant" and "mechanisms to assist rather than replace the heart" developed with funds from the NIH Artificial Heart Program "already are proving of value" (Dracula of medical technology 1988). Despite these gains, however, the announcement by Dr. Claude Lenfant, Director of the National Heart, Lung and Blood Institute, that he was canceling contracts to develop a totally implantable artificial heart was welcome news to the *Times* writer.

> During its 24-year life this Dracula of a program sucked $240 million out of the National Heart, Lung and Blood Institute. At long last, the Institute has found the resolve to drive a stake through its voracious creation. "The human body just couldn't seem to tolerate it," explains Claude Lenfant, director of the institute. (Dracula of medical technology 1988)

In January 1988 the NHLBI Artificial Heart Program had awarded a total of $22.6 million in contracts to four centers, to be used over a 5- to 6-year period for work on a "next generation" totally implantable, electric-powered heart. The four centers that won funds to compete in this newest race were the University of Utah; Pennsylvania State University at Hershey; the Nimbus Company in California, working with the Cleveland Clinic; and Abiomed Inc. in Massachusetts, working with the Texas Heart Institute in Houston. Lenfant's decision to terminate these contracts effective September 30 involved a cost-benefit reckoning as to where the institute's limited funds might have their greatest payoff. A new version of the total artificial heart, he and others judged, would probably take at least a decade to develop and might eventually benefit a relatively small number of patients at great expense. Instead he decided it would be more fruitful to redirect funds to accelerate the suddenly promising development of several left ventricular assist devices, which were almost ready for bench testing (Altman 1988; Booth 1988; Browne 1988).

However well-reasoned his decision may have been, Lenfant, in the words of a *Science* magazine story, had not factored in or fully anticipated the "politics of the heart" (Culliton 1988). The reactions to his announcement by those working on total artificial hearts, particularly at the centers whose contracts were to be rescinded, were swift and negative (Altman 1988; Mills 1988). Even though he had no federal funding, DeVries stated, he was "mad as hell" and had felt "wounded" that the *JAMA* reports on his work with the Jarvik-7, noting the "negative as well as positive findings," were now being used "to hurt artificial heart research" (Altman 1988, p. C3). Lenfant's own NHLBI Advisory Council basically endorsed his decision to concentrate funds on the left ventricular assist device; but, in the words of reporter Philip Boffey, quickly "issued a plea for additional funds to rescue the artificial heart program from extinction," seeking to "counter public impressions that, in the words of one member, 'This stuff doesn't work'" (Boffey 1988c).

Soon after Lenfant's announcement, the artificial heart researchers and centers targeted for loss of their multimillion dollar contracts began to mobilize a powerful campaign among senators to restore their funding. The "hardball" assault on Lenfant's position, led by two senators whose constituents had received contracts, Orrin Hatch of Utah and Edward Kennedy of Massachusetts, rapidly paid off. In early July, NIH Director James Wyngaarden ordered Lenfant to restore the total artificial heart program and its contract funds (Boffey 1988a,b). As Barbara Culliton observed in *Science,* "The NIH's struggle for freedom from political interference has been going on for years. For its side, NIH has the power of scientific reasoning; Congress just has plain power. It is not a level playing field" (Culliton 1988).

January 1990

On January 11, 1990, the FDA withdrew its approval for the clinical use of the Jarvik-7 either as permanent device or as a temporary bridge in patients awaiting transplant. In a statement announcing the recall, the agency cited deficiencies in the conduct of clinical trials, manufacturing quality control, and servicing equipment and training personnel by Symbion (Altman 1990c; Merz 1990).

"The decision came like a bolt out the blue," said William C. DeVries. . . . "This is a real blow. The world needs the artificial heart." Dr. DeVries thinks the FDA's action has sounded the death-knell for permanent artificial-heart implantation, and has crippled the use of mechanical pumps as bridges. "I've worked on this project since its inception at the University of Utah. It's like seeing my life's work go down the toilet." (Merz 1990, p. 31)"

Epilogue

January to July 1991

In January 1991, a year after the FDA recall had written the finale to the use of the Jarvik-7, the artificial heart again began to make news. Fueled by the restoration of NHLBI funding for work on a total artificial heart ordered by NIH Director James Wyngaarden in July 1988 in response to Congressional pressures, several developments unfolded during the 7-month period (January to July) when we were completing revisions to this book.

On the research front, testing of a "new generation" of electrically powered devices continued at a number of institutions. In January 1991 the FDA gave permission for Dr. O. H. Frazier at Houston's Texas Heart Institute to perform five experimental implants of the first fully portable, battery-powered LVAD. The "Heart Mate," developed by Thermo Cardiosystems in Massachusetts with contract funding from NIH, was designed for temporary use in patients awaiting a heart transplant. According to the company's chief design engineer and president, Victor Poirier, the device had three features that represented significant advances over the pneumatically powered LVAD the firm had been working on for 25 years: It was completely portable, unlike the Jarvik heart; had "unique textured blood-contacting surfaces" designed to "discourage" the formation of clots; and had a patented access device intended to ward off infection at the point in the body where the electrical leads from the battery to the device penetrate the skin (Goldsmith 1991, p. 2993).

In an enthusiastic report on the FDA's approval to begin human testing of the new LVAD, Lawrence Altman of the *New York Times* wrote that it "offers the potential of reducing the risk of strokes and serious infections that plagued experiments with the permanent Jarvik-7 artificial heart. . . . "Success with Dr. Frazier's five implants," he declared, "would mark an important step toward the eventual goal of a totally implantable artificial heart" (Altman 1991).

The first implant of the "Heart Mate" was performed in Houston on May 2, 1991 in a 52-year-old patient "who was close to death from cardiomyopathy" and remained in critical condition with liver and kidney failure after the operation. Although Mr. Poirier, President of Thermo Cardiosystems, judged that the battery-powered device "worked perfectly in its first clinical trial," the patient died on May 23 from multiple organ failure. "While organ failure is not surprising in patients who are ill enough to require cardiac-assist surgery," Mr. Poirier acknowledged that "the fact that this patient did not respond after having the implanted VAD for two weeks was not encouraging" (Goldsmith 1991, p. 2933).

In addition to the testing of ventricular assist devices for temporary use, work proceeded on devices that would assume the heart's functions on a long-term basis. The dean of cardiac transplant surgeons, Dr. Norman Shumway, revealed that his team at Stanford University Medical Center had obtained FDA approval to test the use of another battery-powered LVAD, manufactured by Novacor in Oakland, California, for long-term use (Scheck 1991). The Novacor has been used since 1984 as a temporary device; but according to the story in which medical writer Anne Scheck reported on her interview with Shumway, "experimentation in animals . . . indicates [the LVAD] could sustain cardiac function over months" (Scheck 1991, p. 1). "It will be tricky selecting these patients" for the first trial of the permanent Novacors, Shumway guardedly commented. The patients probably will be in "pretty bad shape . . . so the initial results may be skewed" (Scheck 1991, p. 17). The FDA also approved clinical tests of the Novacor as a long-term or "permanent" assist device beginning in 1992 at two institutions supported by NHLBI contracts. At the time of this writing, ten patients each at St. Louis University and the University of Pittsburgh are slated to receive Novacor VADs over a 2-year period, with each patient followed "for up to two years" (Hogness and VanAntwerp 1991, p. 1–2).

By spring 1991, the groups in California, Massachusetts, Pennsylvania, and Utah that had funding from NHLBI for work on an electrically driven TAH were midway through their research contracts. As a July 1991 report on the Artificial Heart Program understatedly noted, "the Novacor trial results will have considerable relevance not only for VAD development but also for the future of TAHs. Nevertheless, TAHs are very different devices; replacing a natural heart presents many more challenges than does supporting left ventricular function" (Hogness and VanAntwerp 1991, p. 1–1). The new TAH models were undergoing laboratory and animal testing as a prelude to hoped-for trials with human subjects within the next 5 years. Once again, investigators began to voice their optimism about the increasing success of their "device readiness" testing in animals and its promise for patients. In July 1991, for example, researchers at Pennsylvania State University's Hershey Medical Center announced a new "record" survival time for a calf implanted with their electric total artificial heart. On July 16, according to bioengineer Gerson Rosenberg, "Holly" had lived for 224 days with her "Penn State heart," surpassing the previous record of 222 days set in 1983 by a calf named "E.T." (for "electric total"). Based on the survival of calves and sheep with earlier total artificial hearts, Rosenberg and his colleagues believed that Holly's survival time "is an indication that the devices could potentially last 2 years in patients," and they hoped to begin human testing of their Penn State heart within 5 years (Hostetler 1991).

Meanwhile, on the policy front the National Academy of Sciences' Institute of Medicine (IOM) issued yet another of the periodic studies that have assessed the need for, feasibility of, and issues concerning artificial hearts. The Institute's report, released in July 1991, contained the findings and recommendations of a committee formed in 1989 to conduct an independent evaluation of the NHLBI's Artificial Heart Program. The evaluation was requested by NHLBI Director Claude Lenfant in the wake of the furor over his cancellation of the contracts for work on a TAH. An outside assessment under the prestigious imprimatur of the IOM, Dr. Lenfant thought, would be valuable for the politically and policy-laden decisions he would have to make in 1992 about continued contract support for long-term assist devices and TAHs (personal interview).

Overall, the IOM report strongly supported the continuation of the artificial heart program, as had previous assessments conducted in house by the NHLBI. Focusing their evaluation on long-term mechanical circulatory support through VADs or TAHs, the committee projected that at least one fully implantable VAD "is likely to be approved by the FDA for general use by the late 1990s"; TAHs, which "are being developed on a timetable 5–10 years behind VADs," will probably have a model approved around 2005 (Hogness and VanAntwerp 1991, p. ES-3). At first, the committee believed, "practical "limits" such as insurance coverage and the availability of qualified personnel will "hold the growth of this technology's use." But by 2010 these restrictions should be sufficiently overcome that the devices will be generally available for an estimated pool of 35,000 patients yearly if age 75 is used as an upper limit for candidates, or up to 70,000 patients for age 85. Of that total range, the committee projected that 10,000 to 20,000 people will need a total artificial heart in 2010 (Hogness and VanAntwerp 1991, ES-4).

The IOM report is somewhat more cautious about the prospects for a TAH than for a VAD, in terms of what studies may show about its safety and effectiveness in preclinical and clinical tests, the device's effects on a recipient's quality of life, and its cost-effectiveness compared to assist devices and to cardiac transplantation. In making these assessments, the IOM report utilized previous NHLBI-related studies of the artificial heart and work commissioned for its evaluation. The experience with the Jarvik-7 (conducted outside the Artificial Heart Program) was mentioned only in passing, with only one of DeVries' publications cited in the references, related to a brief discussion of the media's role in "portraying the potential and limitations of these devices realistically" (Hogness and VanAntwerp 1991, pp. 7–12, 7–14).

In this era of preoccupation with the costs of health care, the IOM committee predictably viewed the estimated "cost-effectiveness ratio for TAH use" as the greatest potential barrier to the device's movement into widespread use. The analysis done for the committee, which calculated costs in relation to a less readily quantifiable measure called "quality of life adjusted years" (QALY), compared the TAH with heart transplantation, conventional treatments for end-stage heart disease, and the most widely used organ replacement technology, the artificial kidney. The TAH, presumably to no one's surprise, was by far the most expensive intervention and offered the shortest span of additional "quality adjusted" life: "A TAH yields an average increase of 2.85 years in *quality-adjusted* life expectancy at a net cost of $299,000 for a cost-effectiveness (C/E) ratio of $105,000 per QALY (quality of adjusted life years) gained. Because of transplantation's lower total cost and greater life expectancy, its C/E ratio is $32,000 per added QALY" (Hogness and VanAntwerp 1991, M6–4).

The IOM committee's primary charge was to make a recommendation to the NHLBI and, by implication, Congress about continued federal support for the development of a TAH. Here the committee opted out of squarely confronting the difficult medical, ethical, and economic social policy choices posed by the device, holding that there was no "hard information" on these matters. Instead, in the words of *Science* reporter Eliot Marshall, they fell back on the narrower technocratic posture that "research funding decisions—at least at the agency—should be based purely on technical merit" (Marshall 1991, p. 501). In developing "its main recommendation," the IOM report stated, "the committee is aware . . . that the estimated cost-effectiveness ratio for TAH use . . . is so unfavorable as to be a possible basis for suspending this R&D program." Nonetheless, "the currently estimated C/E ratio is not so extreme that it affects the committee's basic conclusion—namely, that federal support for MCSS [mechanical circulatory support system] development should continue for an interim period. By making possible an earlier approval of TAHs for general use, continuing development for a 2- to 3-year period may benefit patients who would otherwise die by a suspension of funding" (Hogness and VanAntwerp 1991, ES-11, 6, 7).

Some day, Lenfant said plaintively when he received the IOM report, "somebody is going to look at all these [risks and costs], add them up, and see where we are going" (Marshall 1991, p. 502). For now, the IOM committee has tossed the decision-making ball back to Claude Lenfant and his Artificial Heart Program staff, advisors, and contractors.

> Finally, both the committee's recommendations and any NHLBI action consistent with them should be understood by everyone involved *not* to imply a long-term

commitment to TAH development. If clinical performance estimates do not improve as a result of experience during the interim period, NHLBI's proper course in 1994 or 1995 may well be to suspend all support for TAH development until further VAD experience has been gained. (Hogness and VanAntwerp 1991, ES-12)

To those familiar with the history of efforts to create a man-made replacement for the human heart since the 1950s, these most recent events in the artificial heart story have a familiar ring. The developers and testers of the devices, the assorted experts involved in shaping the policy and politics of the heart, and reporters for lay and professional media remain unquenchably optimistic that the barriers to a safe and effective permanent artificial heart soon will be overcome. In a largely unquestioning and unquestioned way, they continue to believe that the perfection and deployment of this "desperate appliance" is a medically and socially necessary and good step in the march of medical progress.

"Made in the U.S.A.": American Features in the Rise and Fall of the Jarvik-7 Artificial Heart

> Unlike so many of our pioneers—most recently the Apollo astronauts who visited the moon and returned from their voyages to reflect upon their experience—the artificial-heart recipients never made it back. And because of the incredible physical suffering they endured along the way . . . we were unable to learn much from them about what it was like to live without a human heart. . . . How it actually felt to be alive with a mono-rhythmic piece of plastic clicking where once the mime—if not the author—of our emotions dwelled is a secret the recipients have taken with them.
>
> (Siebert 1990, pp. 58–59)

> In the fourteen Oz books [Frank Baum] has created a land so rich in palaces, crowns, costume, heraldry, and pomp that he had no grounds for complaining, as James had done, of the poverty of the American environment in supplying the writer with material. Yet Oz remains unmistakably an American fairyland . . . or Utopia. In nothing is this more apparent than in the way Baum transforms magic into a glamorized version of technology and applied science.
>
> (Bewley 1970, p. 261)

The story of the Jarvik-7 artificial heart—its rise and fall in the United States—contains many ingredients of an American morality tale. It takes little sociological and literary imagination to see it as a real-life scenario in which cardinal aspects of the American dream and of American tragedy were publicly enacted allegorically as well as empirically on a nationwide scale. As if scripted by a master author, the settings in which the Jarvik-7 drama took place and the cast of individual and institutional characters it involved called into play values and virtues, as well as vices, that are deeply a part of American culture and its distinctive world view.

American Places, Portraits, and Scenarios

In a way that is congruent with the society's historical reality and the myths and fables it has constructed around it, the development of the Jarvik-7 heart and the experimental attempts to implant it permanently in Barney Clark, William Schroeder, Murray Haydon, and Jack Burcham entailed pioneer journeying over a very American terrain.* The chief sites of these biomedical explorations were the valley-enclosed community of Salt Lake City, Utah, "framed by the snow-clad peaks of the Wasatch Mountains, its skyline pierced by the spires of the Mormon Temple that dominates the dazzling whiteness of Temple Square" (Swazey 1988, p. 45), and Louisville, Kentucky, on the banks of the Ohio River, where "the soaring rose granite and green marble [art deco] tower of the new Humana Building, headquarters for one of the country's leading for-profit hospital corporations" controls the city's horizon (Swazey 1988, p. 46). The artificial heart's American itinerary also included the locales from which the patient-subjects voyaged to receive their implants and to which they returned upon their deaths. In Barney Clark's case, it was Seattle, Washington, the Federal Way Stake Center of the Church of the Latter-day Saints in which his funeral services were held, and his final resting place at the Washington Memorial Cemetery "in a simple polished granite and concrete mausoleum" (Van Leer 1983). For William Schroeder, it was the German-Catholic community in the small Hoosier town of Jasper, Indiana, where he was buried under a large heart-shaped tombstone etched with an image of the Jarvik-7 heart.

The personalities and the character traits of the chief physicians and patients involved in these artificial heart experiments were also imbued with evocative "American story" qualities. Willem J. Kolff, who migrated to the United States from The Netherlands after World War II, brought to this country not only the model of the artificial kidney he had invented and built with his own hands during the Nazi occupation of Holland but also his vision of "bionic man" and his "you shall persevere" philosophy. Here he found a cultural home—a place where his machines, bold innovating, and indomitable spirit were compatible with the technological evangelism, utopianism, and hubris of American social

---

*The analysis in this chapter is confined to the four permanent Jarvik-7 artificial heart implants performed by William DeVries in the United States. It does not include the implant done by Bjarne Semb on Leif Stenberg at Karolinska Hospital in Stockholm, Sweden.

thought and the "we shall overcome" outlook of the American value and belief system (Marx 1964; Rosenberg 1961). Kolff eventually made his physical home in the Mormon American valley of Salt Lake City. He had traveled there, many local inhabitants thought, as a "passionate pilgrim," traversing mountain and desert like Brigham Young himself to come to "this beautiful wilderness, where he was left alone . . . unmolested . . . to develop and strengthen a delicate flower . . . his modern technology" (Fox 1984, p. 87).

As the media quickly recognized and embellished, William C. DeVries had the glamorously folkloric appearance and manner of some of the male movie stars who are viewed as embodiments of the trail-blazing energy and idealism—the dauntlessness, bravery, and missionary zeal Americans associate with their Far West frontiersmen and pioneers. The American aphorisms DeVries collected and delighted in quoting were consistent with this image, sayings such as "I must put my shoulder to the wheel and push on" (a line from an old Mormon song); "If you don't make the first step, you'll never get there"; and the famous dictum of Theodore Roosevelt (which was his farewell message to us) concerning the "credit" that "belongs to the man who is actually in the arena . . . who strives valiantly; who knows the great enthusiasms, the great devotions, and spends himself in a worthy cause; who at best knows the triumph of high achievement; and who, at the worst, if he fails, at least fails while daring greatly."

In these respects DeVries seemed a boyish version of a John Wayne. In other regards he made one think of a Billy Budd, the "Handsome Sailor" created by American author Herman Melville: the golden-haired foretopman, working aloft on the highest sails of a ship, full of "cheery health" and "frank enjoyment of young life," who was the incarnation of innocence (Melville 1924). It was Billy Budd's innocence that made him mortally vulnerable to what Melville described as the evil "monomania" that burned inside Claggart, the ship's master-at-arms. Such "subterranean fire" was not unfamiliar to DeVries, who had what he called "the fever" to implant artificial hearts. "It recharges my batteries," he declared, "to get into the O.R. and play with the knobs and gadgets and learn more about how this device can potentially help people" (Breo 1989, p. 2916). When it became apparent, even to DeVries, that a moratorium had descended on further attempts to implant permanent Jarvik-7 hearts in patients, his figure and the ambience surrounding him took on the contours of another American literary character, Willy Loman, in Arthur Miller's tragic drama *Death of a Salesman*: the "man out there, riding on a shoeshine" and the unrequited dream "to come out number-one," facing the "earthquake" fact that people had started "not smiling back," and that he now had "a couple of spots on [his] hat" (Miller 1949, pp. 138–139).

In the counterculture black leather jacket and executive suite, pin-striped suit phases of Robert Jarvik's evolving public persona, with his *Playboy*-featured antics and his "Man in the Hathaway Shirt" posing, this young physician-inventor-artist-entrepreneur appeared to be the worldly antithesis of William DeVries. Yet the search for his authentic self in which Jarvik swaggeringly engaged and the remaking of himself that he put on view were as American as DeVries' less sophisticated self-presentation. In fact, it could be said that in theatrically different styles both DeVries and Jarvik exhibited the form of American individualism that "represents each person as a virtuoso of his or her self" (Turkle 1987), and that within this common cultural framework each was involved in reconstructing his identity through the artificial heart and his association with it (Turkle 1984, pp. 137–162).[1]

The four American recipients of the Jarvik-7 artificial heart seemed to exemplify an ensemble of family, community, work, athletic, and patriotic values that American culture celebrates. These American virtues were consistently highlighted in the public portraits of the first two recipients, Barney Clark and William Schroeder, who throughout the 112 and 620 days they respectively survived their implants were the foci of intensive media coverage.[2]

Barney Clark was seen as a genial, grandfatherly-looking man, with a "great love for his wife and children" and a "happy, tranquil home." He had been married for a lifetime to his childhood sweetheart, Una Loy, an exceptionally devoted and loving wife and mother, who was a woman of extraordinary "courage," "vision," and "endurance." As a boy, it was said, Clark contributed to the support of his widowed mother by selling hot dogs in ball parks, mowing lawns, and clerking in grocery stores. He had worked his way through university and dental school. The colleague and friend who had shared a successful and respected dental practice with him eulogized Clark as "a practitioner who treated patients like members of his family" (Van Leer 1983). He had a "zest for sports," too, including wrestling, in which he had participated as a "strong, young man," and golf, at which he excelled. "He could drive a ball 200 yards," it was said. Clark's presidency of a local golf club was only one of a number of community activities in which he engaged, among which those associated with the Mormon church and ward[3] to which he belonged figured prominently. He was a man who was thought by many to be genuinely concerned about others, who drew people to him through his sense of humor and his unpretentious, much appreciated qualities as "an honest, warm guy."

Like Barney Clark, William Schroeder was a staunch family man. Married more than 30 years to his wife Margaret, he was the father and grandfather of six children and numerous grandchildren. He reigned over his large, closely knit, extended family with patriarchal German-American and Catholic authority and with fierce love. He was a feisty, tenderly tough, outspoken man with real gusto for life. He also was a sports fan, with special enthusiasm for basketball, baseball, and fishing; and he was an ardent gin rummy player who was determined to win and usually did. Schroeder was proud of his honorable military service record and the fact that he received a congratulatory telephone call from the President of the United States, Ronald Reagan, during the first days after his artificial heart implant. His patriotic sentiments, however, did not deter him from asking President Reagan, while he had him on the phone, to locate an overdue Social Security check the Government still owed him. With the same kind of pluck and small-town earthiness, Schroeder referred to God as "Number One"; requested and downed a Coors beer soon after his implant; and likened the feeling of the Jarvik-7 heart beating inside him to "an old-time threshin' machine."

American Astronaut Imagery

Both Barney Clark and William Schroeder were viewed by the University of Utah Medical Center and the Humana Hospital Audubon staffs involved in their artificial heart implants, by the media, and by the American public as "brave pioneers setting off into unknown territory" (Siebert 1990, p. 57). Some journalists referred to William Schroeder as "Bionic Bill," but it was Barney Clark in particular whose pathmaking "voyage" was equated to the journey of the U.S. Apollo astronauts. With his balding head and bespectacled, pleasant face, this kindly family man and retired dentist in pajamas and bathrobe, tethered to a 230-pound Utahdrive machine with a pneumatically powered artificial heart permanently lodged in the space where his "real" heart was once located, was regarded by many American schoolchildren as a heroic, grandfatherly astronaut who had taken a gigantic "first step for mankind" comparable to landing on the moon. It was in that spirit that great numbers of them wrote to him at the University of Utah Medical Center requesting his photograph, and they continued to do so for quite a while after his death in March 1983. It was not until William Schroeder, the last surviving permanent artificial heart recipient, died in August 1986 that the triumphant astronautical imagery faded completely. It was replaced in some writers' minds by the parallelism they saw between the ill-fated artificial heart explorations and the tragic spaceflight launching of the Challenger.

The American Land of Oz

William DeVries enjoyed referring to the Tin Woodman and the Wonderful Wizard in some of the many Oz stories written by the American author Frank Baum. In those particular tales the Tin Woodman, whose human bodily parts had been severed by an enchanted ax and replaced with tin ones, set out on a journey to the Emerald City, the capital of Oz. It is a pilgrim's voyage to look for his identity, recover his past, and rectify certain sins of omission he committed in his youth. Above all, the Tin Woodman hoped to persuade the Wizard to restore his human heart so he could love again. For DeVries, there was whimsy in the fact that his own mission to substitute plastic and titanium Jarvik-7 hearts for human ones was so closely related—in an inverted, mirror-image way—to the Tin Woodman's quest. DeVries also responded to what he intuitively felt were the American themes in these stories. The correspondence between the Tin Woodman of Oz and the artificial heart implants was noted by journalists too. As one of them ironically commented: "The Tin Man no longer has to settle for a make-believe heart. He can now ask the Wizard of Oz for either a transplant or an artificial heart" ("Heart of Gold" 1983).

What Frank Baum created in Oz was a "specifically American fairyland, or Utopia," in which themes central to American culture and its literature are allegorically expressed (Bewley 1970, p. 255). At the core of the 14 Oz books Baum wrote was the profound American tension between pastoral and spiritual values on the one hand and scientific and technological ones on the other. As Leo Marx contended in his book *The Machine in the Garden* (Marx 1964), the American pastoral dream, which he equated with "the kingdom of love" and the soul, and the American dream of progress through science and technology, which he identified with "the kingdom of power," have "waged war in American literature endlessly since Hawthorne" (Bewley 1970, p. 262). In the enchanted Land of Oz portrayed by Baum, this cultural conflict appears to be successfully and humanely resolved. Here science and technology are magic. The destruction of the pastoral landscape is controlled by Oz's central government, which monitors and curtails irresponsible and unbridled experimentation. Machines exist in Oz, but they are "thoroughly humanized"—even personified—as, for example, in the case of Tik-Tok, the clockwork man (Bewley 1970, p. 265). Once the Tin Woodman has his real heart again, he rules as a benevolent emperor over a country where selflessness and love prevail. He does so with a star engraved on his left breast, marking the spot and covering the patch where his heart was reinserted by the Wizard. In effect, this magical universe, in which a tin heart has been exchanged for a human one, is a land where the morally managed fruits of science and technology have helped to establish a secular Garden of Eden that is quintessentially American.

Factors Shaping the American Features of the Artificial Heart Experiment

What accounts for the fact that the experimental implantation of several permanent artificial hearts conjured up such American tales, themes, images, values, and characters? First, the print and electronic media played a major role in fashioning and conveying these American cultural elements through the massive, continuous, highly organized, thickly descriptive, and theatrically prominent way in which they reported the unfolding story of the Jarvik-7 artificial heart venture from 1982 to 1985. The media did not unilaterally manufacture the amount and type of coverage they produced. To a significant degree it was stimulated by reporters' and editors' professionally trained sense that it was a big story with a great deal of human interest value precisely because it contained such reverberating American material. However, the consistently upbeat accounts of the artificial heart experiment that some of the most prominent journalists wrote seemed to be colored as well by their personal excitement about the endeavor and their enthusiastic belief in its imminent success.

Furthermore, independently of the legendary atmosphere the media helped to weave about them, many of the principal actors in the Jarvik-7 artificial heart implantation events were real-life, and in some ways larger-than-life, American characters. In this connection, the psychological and social criteria used at both the Utah Medical Center and Humana Hospital Audubon to select the "pioneering" recipients of the first permanent artificial heart implants had considerable influence. It was partly as a consequence of the medical teams' efforts to pick individuals with the "right stuff" to cope with all they would have to endure along the way that the four recipients ended up being white Americans of North European origins with traditional American family, community, religious, and patriotic "commonfolk" values and styles of life.[4]

The American aura that surrounded the Jarvik-7 artificial heart experiments was enhanced by the political and ideological atmosphere of the 1980s in which they occurred. This decade was one of almost illusory American optimism and exaltation of self, of belief that individual diligence could solve all human problems, of national confidence, and of patriotic pride incarnated and promoted by the figure of Ronald Reagan. With considerable help from his public relations and video manager, Reagan became the personification of revered, "accentuate-the-positive" American values and virtues—a reassuringly upbeat and humorously gallant "living symbol of nationhood . . . wrapped . . . in the flag," who enacted the leading role in what journalist Hedrick Smith called a "storybook presidency" (Smith 1989, p. 414). In this value climate it seems more than coincidental that a striking overlap existed between the American qualities highlighted by the Reagan administration and those associated with the Jarvik-7 artificial heart implants and their chief participants that received so much attention from the medical profession, the media, and the public. In the mind of at least one senior NIH official whom we interviewed, there was an American "civil religion" connection between the two (Bellah 1970). As he vividly put it: "There's a mystique about the artificial heart. The artificial heart is a bit like a star on the flag, and stopping the artificial heart program would be like picking the star off the flag."

Meanings of the Heart

Underlying these sacredly secular notions about the American connotations of the artificial heart were the powerful symbolic meanings of the human heart for which it was supposed to substitute. According to the most commonly stated medical-scientific conception of the natural biological heart, it is a relatively simple, efficient, long-lasting muscular pump that, like any pump, can be repaired and even duplicated and replaced if necessary. There is a schism, however, between this reductionistic and mechanistic view of the heart and the rich spiritual, emotional, and poetic meanings and mystery with which all cultures—including American culture—endow it (Meslin 1987).

What the permanent implantation of totally artificial hearts in a small group of men made apparent was that older, more vitalistic sentiments and beliefs about the heart and its "deep inner thrum" (Siebert 1990, p. 60) lie below the surface of the scientific and technological view of it that modern-day Americans overtly espouse. The heart, it seems is still regarded and experienced as the locus of the inner self, the home of the soul and the seat of the emotions, the center of knowledgeable wisdom and understanding, the source and repository of love, desire, and courage—a cosmic space where the body, mind, and spirit coexist and penetrate each other.[5] This point was audible, for example, in the statement by Una Loy Clark about how glad she was that her husband Barney "still loved [her], even though he now had an artificial heart." It also was implicit in the commencement address Willem Kolff delivered in 1983 at the University of Utah, when he affirmed that after receiving an artificial heart Barney Clark's "spirit was [still] good, [and] that he never lost his zeal for life, his considerable sense of humor, his desire to serve his fellowman, and his love for his wife and children. Therefore [Kolff concluded], all the qualities of the mind which make life worth living were preserved" (Kolff 1983a).

Perhaps the most eloquent and poignant evocation of the emotional and existential capacities that many believed might have been taken from the Jarvik-7 recipients when their human hearts were removed is contained in an essay on "The Rehumanization of the Heart" by poet Charles Siebert. "I'm looking at an old magazine photo of William Schroeder," he wrote:

> It's April of 1985, five months after his surgery. He's outside in a wheelchair, going on a fishing trip with his family. One son is pushing him up a hill, while a daughter walks alongside with the book-bag size portable heartdriver over her shoulder and, in an upheld hand, the drive lines through which flows the air that powers her father's Jarvik-7 heart. Everyone is smiling eagerly for the camera, while Schroeder, in the foreground, sits slumped forward and tilted to one side, his right hand tugging at his oversize T-shirt near where the drive lines enter through his stomach, his eyes fixed in a downward gaze. It's an unsettled posture, poised somewhere between pro-

test and powerlessness, and his expression in truth can have no "like," no simile: It's the look of a man who has lost his heart. . . .

Schroeder [not only] went on a fishing trip. He also . . . attended a minor league baseball game. If, as a matter of conjecture, his body had completely accepted the Jarvik-7, and no clots had formed to cause strokes, and no infections to bring on high fevers; if there had been no physical suffering to mitigate perception and he had been perfectly lucid, what would his perceptions of and responses to these outings have been like? At the moment a fish is brought to the surface and his new heart does not rise with it, is he aware of that? Or if the team he roots for mounts a late-inning rally and his heart doesn't rally with them, wouldn't that feel different? We know that Schroeder *felt*. He cried at his son's wedding, held at the Humana Hospital chapel, and cried continually over his predicament. But when a man's heart no longer works in concert with his feelings, does he lament that fact and cry more? (Siebert 1990, pp. 57, 59)

Because of these meanings of the heart, Siebert, in common with numerous other writers and many members of the American public (the schoolchildren who wrote to Barney Clark included) saw an analogy between the pioneering journey the artificial heart recipients made to "a realm for which there is no human precedent" and the cosmic voyages of the American astronauts (Siebert 1990, p. 59). In the view of an analyst of science and technology such as medical historian Stanley Reiser, however, building artificial hearts and implanting them in human beings may constitute an even more audacious, hubris-filled attempt to master nature than soaring through space and walking on the moon. "What greater act of domination could we as humans devise," he asked, "than to substitute a machine for the most conspicuous agent of life, the heart?" (Reiser 1984, p. 173).

The Role of Mormonism

Along with the meanings of the heart, the politicized patriotism of the 1980s, the story lines of the media, and the "right stuff" criteria used to select Jarvik-7 recipients, Mormonism played an important part in shaping and accentuating the American cultural features of the artificial heart implants.[6] Salt Lake City, Utah, where the Jarvik-7 heart was developed and was first clinically used, is the geographical and spiritual home of Mormonism and the headquarters and center of The Church of Jesus Christ of Latter-day Saints, commonly called the "Mormon" church. It is an enclave—a "covenant" and a "gathering"—permeated by the values, beliefs, and world view of what sociologist Thomas O'Dea has termed "the most American of religions" (O'Dea 1957, p. 117). Many of those involved with the development of the Jarvik heart and the Barney Clark implant were

Mormons, including William DeVries, the Clarks, Chase Peterson, and Institutional Review Board (IRB) Vice Chairman Ross Woolley; moreover, several were prominent figures in the church's lay-priesthood hierarchy. Even those who were not Mormons felt the strong presence of Mormonism both inside and outside the University of Utah Medical Center. As they noted, Mormonism is so omnipresent in Salt Lake City—politically, economically, and culturally, as well as religiously—that it frames and affects the life of everyone in the area (personal communications). Particularly in the Utah phase of the artificial heart experiment, in largely implicit and unintended ways, Mormonism influenced the heart team's values, vocabulary, and imagery; the team's conception of itself and its purpose; its organization; and the relationships it established with colleagues, its "special patient" Barney Clark and his family, the medical center's IRB, the media, and with the American public.

In more subtle ways Mormonism also colored the implants performed at Humana's Audubon Hospital in Louisville, through the personality of William DeVries and the fervor of his commitment to implanting permanent artificial hearts. DeVries described himself as a "fence-sitting" Mormon. There were ways in which he actively struggled to break through what he called the "life mold" of Mormonism and to liberate himself from the authoritarian structure of the Mormon church, the obedience it demanded, and the powerful social controls it exercised—but he had been raised in Mormon precepts and its way of seeing the world, in Mormon culture, and in the "Zion in the mountains" that Salt Lake City represents. Although moving from Salt Lake City and the University of Utah physically distanced him from a concentrated Mormon world, certain aspects of DeVries' Mormonism traveled with him. It was most notable in his evangelical relationship to the artificial heart experiments. Members of DeVries' family thought that the artificial heart had become his "Mormon mission," an undertaking that made restitution for the fact that he had not gone on a 2-year mission to some part of the United States or to a foreign country when he was in his early twenties, as is customary for young Mormon men (personal communications). DeVries' colleagues at Humana Hospital Audubon also thought that his ardor was special (personal communications).

Some of the Mormon dimensions of the total artificial heart endeavor were verbalized during the days immediately following the death of Barney Clark. "We express our respect and sympathy to Mrs. Clark and her children, and especially to Dr. Clark who was—and I suspect is—a remarkable man, a pioneer to match these Western lands," said Dr. Chase Peterson (then Vice President for Health Sciences at the University of Utah and coordinator and media spokesman for its Artificial Heart Project), when he announced Barney Clark's death on March 24, 1983 (Peterson 1983). One week later, Elder Neal A. Maxwell, a member of the Apostles of the Mormon Church's ruling Council of the Twelve, delivered a eulogy at the funeral service in Seattle. He praised Barney Clark for being a pathfinder who chose to endure the uncertainties of a research project to further knowledge about an untried medical advance. "True scientific research," Elder Maxwell stated, "is but the carefully ordered expression of that mortal drive and hunger and quest to know more of what God knows." Dr. Clark's days with an artificial heart, he affirmed, were "a unique second salute to God in gratitude for the gift of mortal life. . . . To a world increasingly filled with hopelessness and despair, he stood quietly, but resolutely for an entirely different view of life" (Van Leer 1983). Elder Maxwell also extolled Una Loy Clark for the role that she had steadfastly and courageously played as the wife of a medical pioneer, as did Willem Kolff in the remarks he made on this occasion: "Speaking for all of the members of our team," Kolff concluded, "administrators, doctors, nurses, engineers, technicians, physical therapists, dietitians—for all of us who were involved—we thank you, Una Loy, and your wonderful family for your trust and support and wish you Godspeed" (Kolff 1983b).[7]

Mormonism's historical and spiritual identification with the American West—with the manifest destiny of the pioneers who explored and settled it, and their challenges, trials, and achievements —influenced these statements about the trail-blazing significance of the artificial heart project and the roles Barney and Una Loy Clark and their family played in it. Chase Peterson and Neal Maxwell indirectly likened the Jarvik-7 experiments to this American journeying into unknown Western territory: a venture that called for robust optimism and strenuous, faithful effort to master and control the environment and the obstacles it presented.[8] This vision of the American continent and of an energetic, ever-onward pioneering relation to it, fits into the larger Mormon view of an infinite, dynamic universe in which God and man, as superior and subordinate, cooperatively participate in what Mormon theology terms the lawful reality of eternal progression. Rational knowledge and intelligence, along with will, are crucial to this continuous process of increasing mastery, improvement, perfection, and self-deification. It is a process that does not stop with death but continues into the afterlife. "The Glory of God is Intelligence," proclaims the motto of Brigham Young University, which was adopted from the Mormon leader Joseph Smith's teachings.[9] Science and scientific research are viewed as a powerful expression of that intelligence and as an organized way of questing after it. It is to these Mormon concepts and convictions that Elder Maxwell alluded when he praised Barney Clark for his participation in the artificial heart experiment and called his action "a unique second salute to God." Chase Peterson also implicitly referred to the doctrine of eternal progression when he suggested that Barney Clark not only was, but *continued to be*, a "remarkable man." In this way Peterson covertly expressed the Mormon belief that the worthiness of Barney Clark's efforts and the knowledge he had attained and helped to foster during his earthly sojourn had accompanied him into the life hereafter, where they had advanced him in his progress toward perfection.

The tributes that were paid at Barney Clark's funeral to his wife, Una Loy, and to the family that the two of them had created and raised were more than grateful acknowledgments to the Clarks for their role as "co-investigators" (personal communication) or testimonies of the Utah team's profound admiration and affection for Mrs. Clark. Their message took on added significance because of the Mormon contexts in which Barney Clark's artificial heart implant and funeral occurred. In the Mormon religion to which the Clarks devoutly belonged, the nuclear family of husband, wife, and children is defined as the central and most basic unit of human existence, both in this life and in the one that comes after. The family not only links its members to each other but to larger extended kinship groups, to the Church of Jesus Christ of Latter-day Saints, and to the entire Mormon community, including its pioneer ancestors and progenitors. Mormonism teaches that parenthood is next to Godhood; that marriages are everlasting, not just until "death doth you part"; and that children are "sealed" to their parents so that they may rejoin them in eternity. In a Mormon framework, then, the "wonderful family" to which the Utah team wished "Godspeed" is an "eternal family," who because they have lived so worthily can hope to be reunited someday with Barney Clark and live with him in the hereafter.

"Mormonism, in developing a peculiarly American religion," Thomas O'Dea has written, "also established a peculiarly American subculture" (O'Dea 1957, p. 258).

> Freedom, rationality, the universe a world to conquer (a projection of the American continent to infinity), progress, self-improvement, mastery—these are the basic principles of Mormon theology. They are comprehended in terms of the advancement of intelligences toward perfection, an advancement in which one leading intelligence exerts authority over the rest. . . . Secular activity becomes of spiritual significance. In fact, Mormonism obliterates the line between secular and sacred through its theology of utility. But whether Mormonism represents a further secularization of American Protestantism or a sacralization of secular optimism and activism it is difficult to say. It is, in a sense, both. Mormonism has elaborated an American theology of self-deification through effort, an active transcendentalism of achievement (O'Dea 1957, p. 154)

In the ways that we have indicated—pervasively at the University of Utah Medical Center and more restrictedly at Humana Hospital Audubon—what could be described as these exaggeratedly American qualities of the moral and existential outlook of Mormonism made a perceptible contribution to the overall value system and atmosphere in which the permanent Jarvik-7 artificial heart implantations were experimentally conducted.

Corporate Connections

Finally, the institutional frameworks within which the development and manufacture, the animal and human implantations, and the sale and distribution of the Jarvik-7 heart took place involved a skein of structures and a set of patterns and tensions integral to the culture of American medicine and to some of the major social transformations it has been undergoing during the last decades of the twentieth century. Exemplified in the trajectory of the Jarvik-7 from the laboratory to the clinic and the marketplace, and from Salt Lake City to Louisville, is what sociologist Paul Starr has termed "the growth of corporate medicine" (Starr 1982, pp. 420–449). This growth has entailed not only a significant increase in the number and the controlling importance of corporate enterprises in the world of American medicine but also their organization into large-scale conglomerate systems of joint ventures and holding companies. Occurring simultaneously with this "coming of the corporation" (Starr 1982) and the organizational changes accompanying it has been the progressive emergence of what historian Rosemary Stevens described as an "overtly profit-making ethos" in the American hospital system and the national health care enterprise of which it is a part (Stevens 1989, p. 321).

The sort of "new medical–industrial complex" that Arnold S. Relman, editor of the *New England Journal of Medicine* claims has developed as a result of these transformations (Relman 1980) was represented in miniature by the chief institutional actors in the story of the Jarvik heart and their interrelationships. These included the nexus formed by the University of Utah Medical Center, Kolff Medical Associates, an independent proprietary company with close ties to the university that was reorganized as Symbion, Inc., in which the venture capital firm Warburg Pincus acquired controlling interest, and the Humana Corporation (one of the country's largest investor-owned, for-profit health care companies), its affiliated Humana Hospital Audubon, and the Humana Heart Institute International private group practice housed by the corporation. The University of Utah/Kolff Medical/Symbion/Warburg Pincus configuration, and the Humana group were not only linked to one another through the migration of William DeVries from Utah to Humana but also by the substantial amount of money that Humana invested in Symbion and the training in implanting Jarvik-7 hearts that Humana Heart Institute surgeons received in a Symbion program. Internally, and in relation to one another, these Utah and Humana clusters represented an intricate mix of university and industry, public and private, and for-profit and not-for-profit orientations. Their auspices, styles and raison d'être were different, but the two sets of organizations pursued self-promotional goals in combination with both self-interested and disinterested commitments to medical research, technology, medical care, and education. The University of Utah incarnated this very American combination in a characteristically Mormon fashion. It was congruent with the diversified corporate organization that the Church of Jesus Christ of Latter-day Saints has built to support its religious activities and goals, along with the tithing contributions it requires from all members. It also fit the church's pattern of appointing spiritual leaders with the ability to oversee its business and financial as well as religious, educational, and scientific enterprises.

Although the University of Utah is a public institution of higher education, and Humana a privately owned business corporation, there were striking similarities in some of their reasons for becoming so intensively and conspicuously involved in the Jarvik-7 total artificial heart implantations. A major impetus for Humana's decision to recruit William DeVries from Utah and to assume financial responsibilities for up to 100 permanent artificial heart implants appears to have been the corporation's desire to make its name and its health care activities better known and more greatly appreciated throughout the country in a way that might increase their business and profits (Bazell 1985; Cancila 1986). In this connection, corporate headquarters organized and managed the media coverage of the artificial heart implants like a gigantic public relations campaign. When William Schroeder's implant took place, we had a chance to directly observe these activities. As we recorded in our field notes at the time:

> Hundreds of print and electronic media reporters jam a suite of rooms at the Louisville Convention Center, used as Humana's media center for William Schroeder's implant. It is, say some veteran reporters, one of the best organized public relations efforts they have seen since NASA's early space ventures. In the background, against the hubbub of voices and phones, cassette players and radios blare out Louisville's newest hit song, "Plastic Heart."

The University of Utah, being the "homeland" of the invention and development of the Jarvik-7 heart and prominently associated with its pioneering human trials offered a strategic, culturally fitting chance to put itself "on the map" locally and nationally. In the eyes of some of its officers, the artificial heart project had the potential of enhancing the "flagship" status of the University of Utah as the state's oldest and largest public institution of higher education, particularly in relation to Brigham Young University, its private, Mormon church-founded and supported counterpart.[10] At the same time, they saw it as a powerful

"Made in Utah, U.S.A." means of extending the outreach and reputation of the university far beyond the Salt Lake City valley and the Mormon world, while engaging in a trail-blazing, health-connected[11] science and technology endeavor that exemplified core Mormon values and beliefs. In turn, this paralleled a more general process occurring in the Mormon church and community: a concerted attempt to open Mormondom progressively to mainstream American life with the intent of overcoming the persistent image of Mormons as a "peculiar [cultic] people" rooted in polygamy; emphasizing the "typical, uniquely American" characteristics of the Mormon religion and its culture; and strengthening Mormonism's economic, political, intellectual, and moral influence on the larger American scene.

It was against this background, with its own distinctive blend of localism and cosmopolitanism, sophistication and naiveté, that the University of Utah Medical Center set up news coverage arrangements for the reporting of Barney Clark's artificial heart implant that it described as analogous to the NASA model. As *New York Times* journalist Lawrence Altman wrote, the medical center announced the operation before it took place; asked for and received advance publicity from virtually all major American news organizations; invited the media to come to Salt Lake City; and conscientiously reported the complications in Barney Clark's postoperative status as they occurred. Yet, Altman commented, "just about everyone I talked with [at the University of Utah Medical Center] when I covered the Barney Clark story told me that they were flabbergasted at the media turnout as well as the amount of attention the story drew" (Altman 1984a, pp. 114, 125). When this same surprise was expressed to us by members of the Utah team, we found it both ingenuous and disingenuous.

In the end, many of the same American institutional and cultural patterns that catalyzed and shaped the Jarvik-7 artificial heart experiment and infused it with meaning were also responsible for some of its most troubling moral deficiencies and for the way that its downfall and demise happened. As Chapter 7 reveals, nowhere was this point more gravely apparent than in how and why the American multisystem of social controls, designed to govern this kind of human experiment, foundered.

The Rise and Fall of Cold Fusion

Many of the entwined Mormon and American features of the Jarvik heart story in Salt Lake City were replayed in the "rise and fall" of cold fusion at the University of Utah during 1989–1990. In a series of highly publicized and controversial experiments, electrochemists Stanley Pons and Martin Fleischmann claimed to have achieved a dream of nuclear physics: the creation of cheap, limitless energy from a nuclear reaction in a test tube at room temperature (Broad 1991; Close 1991; Mallove 1991; Poole 1989). Some of the same elements that galvanized the Jarvik-7 experiment contributed to the flamboyant manner in which the university used the media to announce and publicize Pons' and Fleischmann's purported discovery, engaged in a dispute with Brigham Young University about priority for the discovery, sought and obtained millions in funding for a National Cold Fusion Research Institute, and dealt with the skepticism and criticism of researchers who could not replicate the experiments. There were overlaps in the "cast of characters" in the two stories, most notably Dr. Chase N. Peterson. His zeal to finance the new cold fusion research institute eventuated in his illicitly transferring $500,000 from a university bank account for the project, presented as a gift from an "anonymous donor," which led to his resignation as president of the university.

Once again, a passionate belief in scientific progress, the energetic desire to promote Mormonism, and an at-once this-worldly and other-worldly vision of entrepreneurship and economics underlay the dynamics of the experiment, its scientific and public presentation, and the excesses committed in its name. While the Mormon dimensions of cold fusion escaped most analysts, some astute commentators, such as Yale physicist Moshe Gai, recognized its "Made in the U.S.A." components.

> My own feeling is that cold fusion represents, more than anything else, the American dream. . . . I think that Thomas Alva Edison would have been proud to design and invent a gadget such as the gadget that is supposed to make this fantastic source of energy. . . . It's the new world, it's a revolution overnight, getting rich overnight, and doing something against the understanding and against the consensus of what our scientific society is. My own feeling is that the American dream turned into an American nightmare. (ConFusion in a jar, 1990)

Who Shall Guard the Guardians?

On an August afternoon in 1986, six members of the University of Utah Medical Center institutional review board (IRB) who had served on the committee during the years that it dealt with the Jarvik-7 heart experiment straggled into a small seminar room. They had gathered, somewhat apprehensively, to talk with us about the IRB's role in the Barney Clark implant and its aftermath and their views of the experiment more generally.[1] It was an occasion that one person likened to a reunion and another to a wake, as it was the first time they had met together since their work on the permanent implant protocols ended with DeVries' move to Louisville.

During their group interview, they recounted to us and talked to each other about the issues with which the IRB and its artificial heart subcommittee had wrestled, the events that had transpired, and the actions they had taken. As their conversation and body language made clear, they were still powerfully affected by their experiences, uneasy, angry, or depressed about some of the roles they and their colleagues had played, and ambivalent about the experiment having gone forward. "The fact that our IRB matured a lot as a by-product of our experiences with the artificial heart experiment was a redeeming feature," one member said pensively near the end of the interview, "but on a personal level it was truly one of the most horrific experiences of my life."

In an individually and collectively personalized way, these painful recollections by the members of the Utah IRB evoked one of the most complex and troubling aspects of the artificial heart experiment: how the systems of social controls that were supposed to govern the work of the researchers engaged in this venture failed to do so in some crucial regards. These social control deficiencies occurred despite the fact that the clinical testing of the Jarvik-7 as a permanent device was conducted in a manner that was highly visible to the medical profession and the lay public, and subject to scrutiny and regulation by such bodies as IRBs and the Food and Drug Administration (FDA).

In the context of the Jarvik-7 heart's development and clinical testing, the term "social controls" encompasses the informal and formal means through which normative standards of scientific, clinical, and moral competence for those engaged in clinical research are established and maintained. When the standards are met, positive sanctions function to endorse, facilitate, and enhance the research endeavor and its continuance. However, significant deviations or departures from these normative standards ideally should elicit processes that help not only to identify and acknowledge the aberrations, but, if appropriate, to deter, delay, or halt the research in question (Bosk 1979; Swazey and Fox 1970; Swazey and Scher 1985).

Who has the obligation and ability to exercise social controls, the types of controls at their disposal, and how effectively the control mechanisms can be wielded are influenced and structured by the social system in which clinical research takes place. Among the individual and institutional "actors" who play key roles in this social system are the therapeutic innovators themselves, their places of work, the wider professional communities of researchers and clinicians of which they are a part, regulatory agencies, the law, and shapers of public opinion such as the media and influential social critics. This social system framework can be visualized as a series of overlapping concentric circles that include within their orbit and loosely link a congery of medical and extramedical persons and organizations on local, regional, and national levels.

Some of the actors in this social system of clinical research, such as the FDA and IRBs, have the specific, designated roles of being "social control agents." The social control responsibilities and functions of most of the other actors, including physician-investigators, are only one part of their total role set. In fact, they may not even define themselves as social control agents or may be reluctant to do so.

When assessing the exercise and effects of social controls on the initiation and continuance of a clinical experiment, at least three questions about the experiment itself need to be addressed. First, is the decision to begin the human experimentation phase warranted by the laboratory and animal data on the safety and efficacy of the new device, drug, or procedure? Second, is the clinical research protocol adequately designed? That is, does it ask scientifically and medically valid and testable questions and use appropriate methods to gather and analyze the clinical data? Third, does the principal clinical investigator and his or her team have the clinical research knowledge, skills, and experience to implement the protocol and to work with, analyze, and interpret the data?

A number of participants in and close observers of the Jarvik heart's development and clinical use had serious reservations about the experiment's initiation and continuance. Both at the time of the experiment and in retrospect they believed that each of the questions about clinical research posed above could or should have been answered "no." Based on their knowledge of the device and its performance in laboratory animals, the content of the protocol for human testing, and the clinical research experience of the investigators, these individuals judged that the initiation of the Jarvik heart's clinical use was premature or that the experiment was not warranted as clinical research.[2] Why, then, did the experimental implantation of the Jarvik heart as a permanent device take place, along with the proliferation of bridge-to-transplant procedures? Why did the individuals and institutions who could have acted as "gatekeepers," on balance, fail to exercise the range of social controls at their disposal?

Initiating Human Testing

Given the inherent ambiguities in deciding that the "time is right" to begin human testing of a therapeutic innovation, it is not surprising that the decision to try the Jarvik-7 heart as a permanent replacement for a human heart evoked differences of opinion inside and outside the Utah artificial heart team, both when the decision was being made and in the wake of the first implant into Dr. Barney Clark. In the view of some of those most intimately involved in this laboratory and animal testing, the decision was prompted by a convergence of personal, professional, and institutional factors that overrode the equivocal bioengineering and biomedical status of the device itself.

When Kolff Medical Associates submitted their first protocol to the University of Utah Medical Center IRB in 1980, a number of potential social control agents had strong doubts about the readiness of the Jarvik-7 heart for human use. From their knowledge of the device's design and its performance in animals, they concurred with Robert Jarvik's judgment that "neither the Jarvik-7 nor any of the several other total artificial hearts being developed is yet ready to permanently replace a human heart, even on a trial basis" (Jarvik 1981, p. 74). Two of the major concerns about the device involved biomaterial–human tissue incompatibilities and problems with the externally driven pneumatic power supply, both of which were known to have caused various types of morbidity and death in laboratory animals and in the two previous human recipients of a tethered total artificial heart model.

Strong reservations about the device's readiness for human use were reinforced by doubts about the caliber of the protocol initially submitted by DeVries and his colleagues: Many members of the IRB believed strongly that it was inadequate for ethical or scientific approval. The IRB was so concerned about the protocol's deficiencies and intent on remedying them that it overstepped its role of reviewing, making comments and recommendations about a research proposal and eventually approving or disapproving it. Over several months, one of the major tasks that the Board's artificial heart subcommittee assumed involved "writing and rewriting the proposal," meeting often with DeVries and his associates until the protocol was transformed "into a scientific document we [the IRB] could accept" (personal interview).

The privately held view of a number of other key players at the University of Utah about the wisdom of testing the Jarvik-7 heart on patients was expressed to us in 1987 by a senior cardiac surgeon who left the Medical Center before Barney Clark's implant. "As we stood on the threshold of taking the artificial heart to the clinic," he reflected, "everyone sensed the dilemma that [the device] was not yet ready to support real human existence . . . but I didn't want to stand in the way of progress. A whole symphony of technology gave us the feeling that maybe the [Jarvik-7] heart was going to work" (personal interview).

During the course of our study we also interviewed a number of distinguished cardiac surgeons who were knowledgeable about the Jarvik-7 heart and its use, but more distantly, as they had no connections with the University of Utah or Humana. Each thought that the Jarvik heart did not embody significant design and performance advances over earlier pneumatically powered devices. "The Jarvik heart," one of these surgeons told us emphatically, "is a cow pump, not a functionally adequate replacement for the human heart" (personal interview).

A number of National Institutes of Health (NIH) officials, including the then-Director Donald Fredrickson and administrators of the National Heart, Lung and Blood Institute's (NHLBI) artificial heart program, also had serious doubts about initiating human testing of the Jarvik heart (personal interviews; Preston 1988). Recalling his reactions when he learned of the Utah group's decision to test the heart on patients, a senior staff member with the artificial heart program said "my perspective was that they should not go forward, and I tried to talk Jarvik and others out of it. . . . We at NIH saw two reasons for developing pneumatic devices: to do research in animals and possibly for temporary or short-term studies in patients. We did not look for the permanent total artificial heart to be a pneumatically driven device. . . . We knew that all the problems the animals had experienced would happen in patients, but I was hoping they would be controllable" (personal interview).

Based on their experience with pneumatic total artificial hearts, several people at NIH attempted to dissuade the University of Utah from initiating what became the Barney Clark implant, advised the FDA not to approve clinical testing, and sought unsuccessfully to at least have an opportunity to examine the protocol and consent form that were under the FDA's purview. Because the Jarvik-7 heart had not been developed with NIH funds, however, and because the device's human testing was under the regulatory control of the FDA, the NIH was effectively cut off from exercising any significant influence or control over the experiment.

Given an at least "reasonable doubt" that the Jarvik heart was ready for human testing, why was such testing launched? The answer, which is not unique to this episode, is that a number of other factors, rationales, and values drove the move to the clinic and helped convince key decision-makers to see the animal data "glass" as half full rather than half empty. There were concerns about declining NIH funding that played into the desires of individual players at Kolff Medical Associates and the University of Utah to "win the race" to implant a permanent artificial heart in man and gain the personal and institutional prestige and presumed funding advantage that would accrue to the winners. Willem Kolff, Robert Jarvik, and many of their associates also had strong convictions about the bioengineering feasibility of building and using artificial hearts, which were reinforced by their strong belief that "life is always preferable to death." These convictions, in turn, were strengthened by the symbolic importance of the heart and its replacement and by the fact that the "dream of progress" represented by the artificial heart was especially congruent with the Mormon values of Salt Lake City.

Jarvik-7 Implants as Clinical Research

Under its 1980 regulations for significant risk investigational devices, the FDA specified the procedures manufacturers must follow when testing and evaluating devices such as the Jarvik heart. These procedures required submission of an investigational plan to the principal investigator's IRB and then, contingent on IRB approval, to the FDA. Components of the investigational plan included a report of previous research with the device and the protocol and consent form for human subjects. In addition, there are stipulations for reporting safety and effectiveness research data to the FDA (Holder 1980). The investigational dimensions of the Jarvik heart's use as a permanent and a bridge device generated a number of questions and concerns about compliance with these regulations and the ethical and scientific research standards on which they are based.

Bridge Use of the Jarvik-7

A major issue about bridge-to-transplant implants of the Jarvik device and other artificial heart models was the extent to which they were being performed as "rescue medicine" interventions, often on an emergency basis, rather than within an investigational framework. In contrast to the largely private ways in which doubts about permanent implants work were handled, the clinical research concerns about bridge use were addressed more openly, in forums such as meetings of those working with cardiac assist and replacement devices, professional journals, and the media. Until the FDA issued its recall of the Jarvik heart in 1990, however, only one strong formal social control action reportedly was exercised with respect to bridge implants, and that action occurred in Sweden rather than the United States.

According to an article in *Le Monde*, Dr. Bjarne Semb, the only surgeon other than DeVries who used the Jarvik heart as a permanent implant, "was removed from his post" in January 1987 as a formal disciplinary sanction by Karolinska Hospital for his bridge-to-transplant implants with the Jarvik-7. He was "accused by his colleagues of using his patients as guinea pigs" and "operating contrary to medical ethics" because, according to Swedish governmental regulations, implantation of the artificial heart should have been considered experimental and subject to review and approval by the hospital's ethics committee. The case that led some of Semb's colleagues to request an inquiry by hospital officials involved a 49-year-old German woman admitted to Karolinska in the fall of 1986 as a heart transplant candidate. The patient underwent three operations in 2 weeks: A temporary Jarvik heart was implanted on an "emergency" basis, followed 9 days later by a heart transplant and then, when the transplant failed, a second Jarvik heart implant. Some of the specialists on Semb's service contended that the first implant was not warranted by the patient's condition, and that a "classic transplantation" should have been performed. Defending his decisions to perform bridge implants, Semb stated: "It is evident that we are not doing experiments but rather we are caring for patients. It is research insofar as we are at the beginning of the development of a technique. But we are saving human lives" (Un pionnier du coeur artificiel est suspendu de ses fonctions 1987). It is interesting that, given the discussion and debate about emergency bridge use of artificial hearts in the United States and what some viewed as the laxity of controls by the FDA and IRBs, we saw no mention of this action in the American press or professional journals.

Permanent Implants

In contrast to the more public discussion about the investigational aspects of bridge implants, clinical research issues concerning DeVries' permanent implants were raised largely *sub rosa*. They were voiced within the confines of the artificial heart teams in Salt Lake City and Louisville, discussed internally by other administrative and professional staff at the institutions, and critiqued in private by experts in cardiac replacement and research who were knowledgeable about the implants.

Unlike bridge use, permanent implants were consistently defined and treated by the Utah and Audubon Hospital IRBs and by the FDA as human experimentation. Thus they were subject to the scientific, medical, and ethical norms and regulatory requirements governing clinical research. As the consent form for permanent implantation of the Jarvik-7 heart stated, it was being used experimentally, with two objectives: "to determine if it will help other people with [the recipient's] condition, and for the possible beneficial affects [sic] that [the recipient] may obtain from the experiment" (DeVries and Symbion, Inc. 1983).

In practice, no matter how clearly and how often the experimental nature of a new drug, procedure, or device and the primacy of research objectives are affirmed, the boundaries between experiment and therapy blur and shift, and therapeutic hopes and judgments are virtually inevitable on the part of both physician-investigators and their colleagues and patient-subjects and their kin. As he discussed with us on many occasions, DeVries, not atypically, swung back and forth between viewing and dealing with his permanent implants as an experiment and as a "desperate remedies" treatment (Moore 1989). When Barney Clark, William Schroeder, and Murray Haydon seemed to be doing well, DeVries recognized that he was particularly prone to let therapeutic hopes and goals override the experimental dimensions of doing research on as well as caring for his patient-subjects (personal interviews). In fact, in the face of his patients' complications and eventual deaths, he maintained that the artificial heart had been successful as a therapeutic intervention. "I believe the artificial heart is therapeutic," DeVries stated in response to reports and comments about Dr. Clark's poor physical and mental status after his implant. "I believe it helped Barney Clark and that it gave him a good quality of life. And I think he appreciated the life he lived on the pump" (King 1984h).

From a clinical research perspective, however, investigators do not answer the question, "was the experiment worth it?" by redefining an experiment as a treatment. Rather, they base their determinations about the merits and results of clinical experimentation primarily on the knowledge gained about the modality's benefits and risks assessed by the investigators and informed peers according to professional standards for competently designed and executed clinical research. To some members of the artificial heart teams at Utah and Humana, members of the Utah IRB, and some knowledgeable outsiders, the adequacy of the clinical research involved in the permanent implants, and therefore their ethical and medical justifiability, were the most disturbing aspects of the Jarvik heart's use.

The implants had many familiar characteristics of early clinical research with a risky innovation that is being tested on gravely ill persons, such as problems of uncertainty, experiment–therapy tensions, and grim outcomes for patient-subjects. On close scrutiny, however, even to social scientists such as ourselves, DeVries' implants also differed in significant ways from other features of "experiment perilous" clinical research (Fox 1959). As we conducted interviews, made observations, and studied the protocols and other primary source materials bearing on the clinical research aspects of the implants, we progressively felt as though we were in an Alice-in-Wonderland state. Were we, we asked each other, the only ones in the world of the Jarvik-7 who thought that the experiment we were studying had few of the attributes we associate with clinical research? Over time, many participants in the experiment voiced similar doubts as we talked with them. Toward the end of our study, we asked Dr. Alvin R. Feinstein at Yale University School of Medicine, a leading authority on the epistemology and methodology of medical research, a basic question: As the permanent implants were planned and conducted, did they constitute clinical research; and if so, what kind? They can be called "research," Dr. Feinstein replied, because Dr. DeVries and his associates were doing something "which has received little exploration . . . The research may be good or bad in its quality, but it is surely research. . . . and I would be willing to call it experimental, in the sense that the intervention is still relatively unexplored and has unproven efficacy." The artificial heart experiment, Dr. Feinstein continued, was "highly empirical, trial-and-error research, which is usually the case whenever any major new innovation is introduced and tried out in people" (personal communication).

Although granting the empirical nature of much first-phase clinical research, members of DeVries' teams at Utah and Humana and others who had an opportunity to study the implants and the information collected by the investigators thought that the research had serious flaws. The postoperative monitoring and testing of the artificial heart recipients, they told us, involved a more than usual amount of inchoate data gathering that was not set within a well thought out, well designed research protocol (personal interviews). The nurse-members of the artificial heart teams in Utah and Louisville, who had little training or experience in clinical research, were uncertain and often anxious about the research aspects of the cases and how it might be affecting their patients. Having received sparse if any instruction or edification from the physicians about the clinical research involved in the implants, they resorted to asking us questions such as "What is clinical research?" "What is a clinical research protocol?" "Are we doing clinical research?" Some of DeVries' more technically sophisticated associates sarcastically described their computerized monitoring, data gathering, and occasional analyses of raw data as "garbage-in/garbage-out,"[3] DeVries himself characterized his research as "shotgun" and "wandering around in the field" (personal interview). Members of the Utah IRB, in turn, depicted the artificial heart group's research perspective and protocol as "put the thing in and see if it works" (personal interviews).

Prior to the December 1985 FDA hearing on the permanent implants, the agency sent Symbion a list of questions about the performance of the Jarvik heart and the recipients' courses after their implants, requesting that the company and its principal investigator, William DeVries, prepare analyses of some of the raw data they had collected. The presentations of their findings by Jarvik, DeVries, and others at the hearing led the Circulatory System Devices Advisory Panel to recommend continuation of the implants. Concerns about the research caliber of the experiment however, were, reflected in the panel's recommendations that more persons with scientific expertise be added to DeVries' team and that the FDA should approve further implants on a case-by-case basis, contingent on the submission of more regular and detailed reports by Symbion. The panel's chairman, heart surgeon Charles McIntosh, also recognized that the lack of published data by DeVries and his colleagues made it difficult, if not impossible, for researchers and clinicians to evaluate the experiment and its results. Perhaps most tellingly with respect to canons for sound clinical research, McIntosh remarked in a press interview that DeVries' recipients, in the words of a reporter, "would undoubtedly have benefitted if the scientific data had been analyzed systematically along the way" (Herskowitz 1986).

The Gatekeepers

A varied range of social control agents, sometimes referred to as gatekeepers, were involved in the initiation and continuation of the permanent implants with the Jarvik-7 heart. There were significant differences among the statuses and roles of the gatekeepers, which in turn helped to determine the controls they could have used or did exercise to affect the course of the experiment. Analytically, we can distinguish three groups of social control agents within the social system framework of the experiment.

The *primary gatekeepers* were those who had the most immediate and direct ability to determine whether the clinical experiment would begin and continue. The *secondary gatekeepers* were not in direct decision-making roles; but by virtue of their statuses and the positions they occupied they could attempt to strongly influence the views and actions of primary gatekeepers. Finally, there was a group of actors we classify as *tertiary gatekeepers*. They helped to shape the opinions of professional groups and the public about the nature of the experiment; but because of their sociological distance from both the primary and secondary gatekeepers and the nature of their authority they were not in a position to exert a major, immediate influence on the course of the experiment. The chief gatekeepers in each of these three categories included the following:

Primary gatekeepers

- Scientists, bioengineers, and physicians directly involved in the Jarvik heart's laboratory development and animal testing, and the decision to move that testing to human use
- Institutional review boards at the University of Utah Medical Center and Humana Hospital Audubon
- The FDA's Division of Cardiovascular Devices and its advisory panel
- Patients and their families who consented to an artificial heart implant and their referring physicians
- The chief surgeon-principal investigator for the clinical implants and other members of the artificial heart teams (e.g., physicians, nurses, technicians)

Secondary gatekeepers

- Senior administrative officials and senior physicians at the University of Utah and its medical center, and at Humana Hospital Audubon and its parent corporation
- Senior officials at the NIH, the NHLBI, and the Institute's artificial heart program
- The wider professional community of cardiovascular and cardiac surgeons and cardiologists, especially those involved in cardiac replacement

Tertiary gatekeepers

- Professional journals and their editors and peer reviewers
- Expert analysts and commentators in areas such as health law, medical ethics, and health policy
- Print and electronic media
- Social scientists who were studying the experiment

The Primary Gatekeepers

Throughout the entire trajectory of the permanent artificial heart experiment, three of the key members of its "inner circle"—Willem Kolff, Robert Jarvik, and William DeVries—remained its staunchest, most unwavering champions. Some of the other important figures in the device's development had reservations about its readiness for human use, but for various of the professional and personal reasons we have identified they did not try to deter its implantation in patients.

In the face of the innovators' determination to move the Jarvik heart from the laboratory to the clinic and to continue the permanent implants after Barney Clark, the social control responsibilities of the IRBs and the FDA to critically appraise the experiment took on added importance.

As the Utah IRB engaged in its reviews of the artificial heart protocols, they were buffeted from within and without by pressures from the heart's proponents, their medical center and university, and the Salt Lake City community to approve and support the experiment. They also were unsettled by the extensive publicity given to the experiment and their role as its reviewers, as the media eagerly responded to the university's public relations work.

DeVries' protocol for the first implant generated a gamut of issues and problems for the IRB as a whole and the subcommittee it formed to deal with them. Two concerns that "caused a lot of emotional battles during meetings" were the ways patient selection and consent for the implant would be handled and the quality of life of the artificial heart recipient. Other aspects of the protocol that preoccupied them, members of the IRB told us, were its overall scientific quality and the information they were given about the results of the implants in animals. Their unease about these matters and how they should handle them was exacerbated by having to interact with a "galaxy of people and institutions" rather than, as is usually the case when reviewing protocols, only with the principal investigator. This "galaxy," members said, included "some very vocal forces" urging them not to delay the experiment, which made them feel that "we had to have a protocol we could accept."

Because the IRB was dealing with a proposal for the first clinical implant of the Jarvik heart, the results of the test implants in animals were a particularly important part of the protocol and of their review. "Most of us were fairly accepting of the animal data at that point," one IRB member recalled, "and the main issue for us was how the complications seen in animals would be dealt with in patients." "Dr. DeVries assured me," said another member, "that the problems with the device, including thromboembolism, had been ironed out and it was ready for human testing." After Dr. Clark's implant, however, according to some of our interviewees, they began to get a different picture of the results with animals. "A lot was ignored in the original protocol. We learned that the investigators had seen complications in the animals like those Dr. Clark had. They knew the valve in Dr. Clark's device that broke just after his operation had broken in animals. They knew the valve was faulty, but they insisted it was important to get the heart into a human being to see what would happen."

The protocol that DeVries first submitted in 1980, members of the IRB thought, "had the mask or aura of science, but it was not a scientific protocol. . . . It basically said that the investigators want to implant the heart and see if it works, and that kind of protocol offended a lot of us on the committee." "When we looked at it," another IRB member recalled, "the heart was pretty much presented to us as 'this is it . . . this will do it . . . if I was dying I'd want the device in my chest.'" Said another member, growing increasingly irate and emphatic as he spoke, "the protocol entered with trumpets and medieval trappings. It was like the entrance of Macbeth. It included a quote from Theodore Roosevelt, and we told Dr. DeVries we wanted that page removed or we would not deal with the protocol."

As they worked with the principal investigator and gradually modified the protocol into an acceptable document, a key member of the committee said, "we realized that Dr. DeVries was not experienced with protocol design. In fact, no one on the team, including Dr. Kolff, had much experience with protocol design. There was even an initial push to have the IRB exempt the device from review on the grounds that it was innovative therapy. But as we worked on the protocol the ethical issues were so great that we tended to defer to the investigators on the science. There were scientific issues or points that we wanted to have defined better, but when an IRB looks at the scientific merits of a proposal the investigator has a leg up. The IRB has to depend on the investigator's integrity."

After Barney Clark's implant and death, the IRB found itself struggling with several more concerns as they considered DeVries' application to perform a second implant. One issue, which we touched on in Chapters 5 and 6, was the appropriate role of the IRB monitor in terms of determining how faithfully the approved protocol was being followed by the team. Another was the type of direct and supervisory care and testing by physicians the first patient-subject had received. In the words of an IRB member, "Barney Clark was handled very differently than patients are usually handled in this hospital, and that was a big mistake." Committee members cited two examples of the "importantly worse ways" that Dr. Clark's care was not like "the way we usually take care of patients in a teaching hospital." First, they said, "house staff were only involved in Dr. Clark's care in a peripheral way." Second, "there was input into the protocol and the selection and consent phases from many specialists, which we assumed would continue after the implant. But that cadre of specialists weren't there after Dr. Clark had his implant." Another person explained, "The rationale we were given for handling Dr. Clark's case like this had to do with security . . . and avoiding leaks to the media by having a small, tight loop of people directly taking care of the patient. . . . The whole thing created a situation that was destined to be an aberration, and I think it thwarted some of the usual clinical care processes."

IRB members attributed the time it took them to review the protocol for a second implant to several factors. They described difficulties in obtaining the kind of data about Dr. Clark that they wanted to examine in relation to plans for the next patient-subject's selection, consent, and care. Other time-consuming matters included (1) revisions of the protocol by DeVries and colleagues in response to the committee's questions and recommendations, and (2) resolving heated differences of opinion within the group as to whether they should approve a second case, and if so, with what changes from Dr. Clark's protocol. In the end, although several members of the IRB had serious reservations about continuing the experiment, only one person voted against approving the protocol for a second implant. "I thought it was fair to allow the benefit of doubt with the first case," that individual told us. "But how in good faith anyone could go on after

Dr. Clark I do not know." "We should have stopped it right after Dr. Clark," another IRB member said regretfully, "but we didn't." Agreeing with this hindsight judgment, another person reflected that "by approving human implantations of the heart, we opened the door to legitimizing the device."

When DeVries moved to Louisville, the protocol for a second implant had to be considered anew by the Humana Hospital Audubon IRB. As we described in Chapter 5, Audubon was predominantly a community hospital, and its IRB was relatively new and inexperienced. Although they had corrected some of the deficiencies for which they had been cited after an FDA inspection, the committee operated with far less rigor, expertise, and sophistication than did most IRBs in a teaching hospital. Nor, as an IRB member said, had they had any prior scientific or clinical experience with cardiac replacement via heart transplants, much less an artificial heart. It was largely for these reasons that the Audubon IRB relied heavily on the more experienced Utah IRB and its reviews and approvals of the protocols for the first and the anticipated second implant. To the Audubon IRB, the prior reviews and approvals of the protocols in Salt Lake City did seem to legitimize the Jarvik heart's clinical testing. Thus the Louisville IRB decided that they "did not need to delve very deeply into the protocol." Their review, handled by various subcommittees, concentrated primarily on what they thought were ethical aspects of the consent form and process, the wording of the consent form, and arrangements for in-service training for nurses and others who would be involved in the care of recipients and their equipment.

The Audubon IRB members did not describe the pressures to approve the Jarvik-7 protocol related to us by the members of the Utah IRB, but the Louisville committee had a number of reasons for supporting the experiment that transcended the protocol itself. To our knowledge they were not overtly pushed to approve the protocol, but they were aware of the importance that the hospital's owners, the Humana Corporation, attached to work on the Jarvik heart going forward under their aegis and of the money that had been pledged to support Dr. DeVries' work. Additionally, they felt enormous personal, institutional, and community pride at the presence of the celebrated surgeon and his work in "little old Louisville" and that they were "privileged" to be at the "forefront" of "such a great humanitarian effort." Moreover, the committee was impressed by the qualities they perceived in the surgeon-investigator. "We have excellent rapport with Dr. DeVries," a committee member told us in 1985. "We recognize more and more that he's a man with high moral standards, a religious man, and the IRB admires those traits. He's not like one of the good old boys."

Ultimately, members of the Audubon IRB thought, the FDA would be the body that decided if the data on the permanent implants warranted their continuation. In response to their critics, the IRB's members argued vehemently that they "had never rubber-stamped anything." They did recognize, however, that in common with most IRBs they lacked the technical expertise to thoroughly evaluate the investigators' reports of the Jarvik heart's performance and its effects on the patient-subjects in whom it had been implanted. In the final analysis, they believed, no matter how well they dealt with the experiment, "the FDA has the bat, the ball, the glove, and the rule book."

It is difficult for us to assess how adequately the FDA exercised its ethical and technical regulatory responsibilities when reviewing the various protocols and interim reports from DeVries and Symbion. We were not granted interviews with relevant agency staff from the Bureau of Medical Devices or its Division of Cardiovascular Devices, and the records of their reviews and decision-making are considered to be confidential information because manufacturers have proprietary interests in their products. In the opinion of several "Washington insiders" knowledgeable about the FDA's actions whom we did interview, however, the FDA too felt pressure to support the initial and subsequent clinical testing of the Jarvik-7. Among the pressures these individuals cited were the "extraordinary visibility and symbolism" of the artificial heart and political worries about the reactions of Congress and the public if the agency disapproved the experiment after the federal government had invested millions of dollars in research on similar devices. "I think the FDA saw the overall artificial heart program as one that had a positive goal for the country," said an NIH official, "and even though the Jarvik heart wasn't developed with NIH funds, my sense is that [the agency] thought it wouldn't be a bad strategy to let DeVries' work go on in a very slow, cautious manner."

There also are questions about the thoroughness with which the Circulatory Systems Devices Panel performed its task as expert advisers to FDA staff concerning the experiment with the Jarvik-7. One panel member, for example, felt strongly that the advisory committee exercised a largely *pro forma* role, meeting only once prior to the December 1985 hearing they held in Washington. Moreover, this panel member had never seen Symbion's protocol for the permanent implants.

That there were deficiencies in the material submitted to the FDA by DeVries and Symbion about the four implants performed in Salt Lake City and Louisville is indicated by the fact that the panel requested additional data and analyses for its 1985 hearing. At least one panelist, Rebecca Lake, a nurse and healthcare consultant who was serving as the consumer member, felt strongly that the material they received for the hearing was inadequate in its scientific content and organization. After the hearing, she submitted a report to the FDA's Office of Consumer Affairs that received media coverage when it was leaked to the Public Citizen Health Research Group. In her report, Lake characterized the information submitted to the panel by DeVries et al. as "hurriedly thrown together, disjointed ... with little substance, organization and conclusions [and as] definitely not representative of academic research by any stretch of the imagination" (King 1985b). The panel's post-hearing recommendations that Symbion be required to submit a substantially revised protocol and that DeVries' team acquire additional scientific expertise suggest that the panel shared some of Lake's concerns about the quality of the data that had just been presented to them. When the panel met in private to formulate their recommendations, a source told us, one member proposed that DeVries be required to add a "well-qualified clinical researcher" to the team. This recommendation, however, was viewed "as inappropriate" by the majority of the group "because they felt that it might embarrass Dr. DeVries."

Once the IRBs and FDA had given the green light for the implants, their realization depended on the readiness of physicians to refer patients to DeVries' group and the willingness of the candidates selected and their families to participate in the experiment. As is clear in the accounts of why the gravely ill men who became the pioneer recipients of the Jarvik heart consented to do so with the support of their wives and children, they viewed this venture as the last best hope for their survival. Even if the experiment did not forestall their deaths, they thought, it was still a meaningful way to contribute to medical science and to the care of future patients like themselves.

It was perhaps the nurses involved in the clinical aftermath of the implants who suffered the most acutely from their growing doubts about the undertaking on the one hand and their anguished loyalty to the physicians under whose aegis they worked on the other. As the primary hands-on caretakers of the patients, they were the most continuously exposed to their physical and psychic ordeals. The nurses also developed close relations with the families of the Jarvik-7 recipients and had intimate knowledge of the painful experiences the family members underwent as a consequence of the media attention to which they were subjected and the catastrophic strokes, infections, and other complications that overtook their husbands and fathers.

In common with several of the technicians on the artificial heart team, some of the nurses became increasingly uncertain about whether the implanted devices and their patients' reactions to them were being studied in a way that met the scientific and moral criteria of good clinical research. The nurses and technicians, however, were reluctant to express their doubts, principally because they were unsure about their competence to pass judgment on the quality of the research, an uncertainty reinforced by their subordinate roles in the team hierarchy. Despite their uneasiness about the experiment, they were inclined to assume that they did not have enough scientific training and experience to challenge the investigators' conception and execution of the research or its approval by the IRBs and the FDA.

The Secondary Gatekeepers

The major groups of what we have roughly classified as secondary gatekeepers for the artificial heart experiment consisted of senior administrative officials and physicians at the institutions where the implants took place, a wider professional community of physicians esteemed by their colleagues for their expertise in cardiac replacement, and senior personnel at the NIH and its NHLBI. Had the NIH been involved in funding the Jarvik heart's development, it would have been a primary gatekeeper by virtue of its authority to review a principal investigator's protocol and the results of his or her experiment. Because the Jarvik heart's final stages of development did not take place with NIH funding, however, the NIH had no official role to play in approving or disapproving the experiment. Thus, the NIH was relegated to the domain of secondary gatekeepers. In this capacity several senior NIH personnel did try, to no avail, to persuade the University of Utah not to initiate human testing and attempted to interact informally with FDA staff when the agency reviewed the first protocol and consent form.

A number of senior administrators and physicians at the University of Utah, and later at Audubon Hospital and Humana's corporate headquarters, also thought that either the experiment should not begin or, after the first implants, it should stop. Some of them publicly supported the experiment despite their reservations, whereas others chose not to express any judgment, either pro or con. During the period that DeVries and his associates were seeking approval for the first implant, for example, a number of influential persons at the University of Utah were privately concerned about the composition of the artificial heart team and their ability to design and carry out clinical research. They also worried that the department of surgery, then without a chairman, could not provide the organizational structure and lines of authority and support in which clinical ventures such as the artificial heart implants usually are embedded. In the judgment of a senior surgeon who left the university before Barney Clark's implant, "Bill DeVries was technically good at putting the artificial heart in calves, but he didn't have much training in scientific methods and clinical research. . . . I think [he continued] that if Bill had been a good scientist like Tom Starzl he would have done one or two implants and then stopped, because a surgeon and researcher like Tom wouldn't have kept the carnage going." After a long, reflective pause the surgeon added, "I guess now that I should have said something about my concerns, but once I had decided to leave Utah I just stuck my head in the sand and ignored the artificial heart" (personal interview).

Without exception, the senior surgeons we interviewed from the wider professional community of physicians expert in cardiac replacement thought that the experiment, at best, was a dubious undertaking. One of these surgeons recounted a conversation he had with DeVries and Jarvik after Dr. Clark's implant. "I told them [he said] that I didn't see much difference between the Jarvik heart and the models we were using in animals years ago." The surgeon continued, "In my judgment there has never been good experimental evidence that there is a reasonable chance of success with the human use of a [pneumatic] total artificial heart. A few calves living 9 months or more do not warrant human trials. In the end, we've been killing healthy animals by giving them total artificial hearts, and we've just been repeating the same mistakes because there have been no really new thoughts on how to prevent problems like infections and clots" (personal interview).

Another senior surgeon, who had known William DeVries for many years, said that he shared the concerns of some of the senior medical and administrative staff at the University of Utah about DeVries' maturity as a surgeon and the extent of his clinical research experience. "Bill has talent and has been almost religiously dedicated to bringing the artificial heart to proper usage for people with cardiac disease," this surgeon stated. "It's been his quest, and I have great respect for his dedication to that cause. But he does not have experienced judgment. For one glistening moment in the sun, Bill DeVries may have to spend the rest of his life in darkness" (personal interview).

With few exceptions, the secondary gatekeepers who doubted the wisdom or medical and ethical propriety of the experiment and were in a position to most strongly affect it found countervailing personal, professional, or political reasons for not publicly expressing their concerns. Some senior NIH officials did try to intervene in plans to initiate human testing. According to the content analysis of our extensive media files, Dr. Norman Shumway, the dean of heart transplantation, became the only senior cardiac surgeon to publicly oppose the use of the Jarvik-7 heart because of the morbidity and mortality it caused and the type of "tethered" existence it necessitated (Langone 1986). Others dissuaded themselves from taking any steps that might preclude or later halt clinical testing.

The Tertiary Gatekeepers

Among the more distant agents that exercise social control influence over clinical research, medical journals play a doubly significant role. As the principal vehicles for the publications of medical researchers and an important source of information for stories carried by the media, they straddle and interconnect the medical profession and the lay public.

The chief social control authority and power of medical journals reside in their prerogative to decide whether articles submitted to them merit publication. The slow and relatively sparse output of manuscripts by DeVries and his asso-

ciates did not give journal editors and peer reviewers much opportunity to critically evaluate the quality of the team's scientific and clinical work. In one
instance where a major report on the experiment was submitted to a leading
journal, however, the editors, much like members of the Utah IRB, apparently
crossed over the line from critical reviewers to helpful collaborators. Partly out
of their competitive desire to publish the results of such a celebrated medical
happening, they devoted an unusual amount of editorial time, energy, and skill
to reshaping the manuscript they received into a scientifically and literarily
acceptable professional communication.

The most explicit criticisms and concerns about the experiment were voiced
by individuals with expertise in areas such as health law, medical ethics, and
health policy and by a few physicians who spoke from outside the professional
communities involved with cardiac replacement. From the first announcements
that permission would be sought to test the Jarvik heart in patients, these experts
engaged in a public point–counterpoint debate with supporters of the experiment about whether the implants should take place (Swazey et al. 1986, pp. 397–
404). Only two critics, health lawyer George Annas and physician and consumer
activist Sidney Wolfe, persistently called for a halt to permanent implants and,
later, bridge use; and they worked to influence the FDA and Congress to impose
a moratorium (Annas 1986a,b; Wolfe 1985). Although both men are highly
knowledgeable and respected in their professional domains, their arguments and
political strategies did not prevail. This was chiefly due to the fact that they are
viewed in medical circles as persistent opponents of many aspects of medical
research and practice and because they did not speak with the authority of
experts in the study and treatment of cardiac disease.

A somewhat larger but still relatively small group criticized various aspects of
the artificial heart's clinical use, writing and lecturing about their misgivings for
lay and professional audiences and being regularly quoted by the media when
stories were written about problems with the device. Prominent members of this
group included cardiologist Thomas Preston, Arnold Relman (physician-editor
of *The New England Journal of Medicine*), historian Barton Bernstein, and bioethicist Arthur Caplan (Bernstein 1981, 1983, 1984, 1985; Caplan 1982; Preston
1983, 1986, 1987, 1988; Relman 1984, 1986). These critics, however, were not
as actively and uniformly opposed to the experiment as were Annas and Wolfe,
nor did they have the same direct interactions with agencies such as the FDA.

The media, one of American society's most powerful shapers of public opinion and social policy, played mixed roles as social control agents. When the most
renowned of the patient-subjects, Barney Clark and William Schroeder, were
doing well, even the best medical journalists tended to be swept away by the
drama of the device and its therapeutic promise. They portrayed the implants as
heroic life-against-death interventions and down-played or ignored their risks,

experimental nature, and research objectives. In many ways, as journalists later recognized and discussed, the way media reported the artificial heart story helped to generate a crisis of failed expectations about what the Jarvik heart would accomplish for its first recipients. The detailed coverage also framed recurring questions about the rights and responsibilities of journalists in obtaining, reporting, and shaping news (Altman 1984a, 1985b; Blakeslee 1986; King 1986d; Winsten 1985).

The reportage patterns, intensified by the "identified life" drama of each case, the daily recounting of as many medical and human details as journalists could obtain from hospital spokespersons or their private sources, and the impact of live coverage on television led the public and some medical professionals to judge the success or failure of the experiment according to the day-to-day therapeutic status of the patients. Predictably, as complications such as infections and strokes mounted and as the patients, one by one, died, the artificial heart story was reported in a more negative and pessimistic fashion.

One result of the dramatically changed perceptions about the outcomes of the experiment, according to DeVries, was that his once numerous referrals from physicians and from patients themselves about candidacy for an implant slowed to a trickle and then essentially stopped (personal communication). This "drying up" of candidates, which also was partly attributable to expanded criteria for heart transplantation eligibility, was a principal cause of the experiment's end.

During the post-Jarvik-7 era of work on a next generation of artificial hearts, the media continue to influence significantly the attitudes of the public and the medical profession toward these devices. The initial media accounts of the research leading to clinical tests of electrically powered ventricular assist and total replacement devices are so comparable to the optimistic and uncritical reportage about the preclinical and early clinical use of the Jarvik-7 that there is cause for concern about whether the risks and limitations, as well as possible benefits, of these devices will be realistically portrayed. Much of the present press coverage makes no reference to the lessons that should have been learned from the prematurity of the Jarvik-7 experiment, its questionable competence, and the human suffering it caused, or from the crisis of risen expectations that was created in large measure by the media.

Our analysis of the tiers of social control actors in the artificial heart story would be incomplete without commenting on the gatekeeping role that we inadvertently came to play. As field workers we had privileged access to the spectrum of participants and gatekeepers in the experiment and to primary materials such as protocols, patient charts, and research data and reports that gave us detailed and comprehensive insiders' knowledge of both the achievements and shortcomings of the Jarvik-7 endeavor. Over time, as some of the experiment's troubling features became more apparent, our distress mounted. It was enhanced by the fact that persons on every level of involvement in the permanent implants were confiding their concerns and disquietude about them to us. Implicitly and on occasion explicitly, some of these individuals expressed their hope that we would find an appropriate way to "blow the whistle" on the experiment.

By virtue of the intensive, long-term relations that field workers characteristically develop with those they study, especially through participant observation, they not only become repositories of private thoughts and sensitive information but may also obtain first-hand knowledge of ethically dubious behavior and practices. As a consequence, field workers may be confronted with the question of whether their own professional ethics and personal morality obligate them to disclose what they have learned or to treat it as confidential information.

This situation was the quandary we faced as our study progressed. Although we were familiar with what sociologist Charles Bosk has called the "watcher and witness" dimensions of field work (Bosk 1985), we were shaken by the choices we believed we had to make. On the one hand, we were not sure that we were qualified to set into motion a process that might discredit or possibly end the experiment, or that it would be appropriate for us to write a muck-raking exposé. On the other hand, we considered it unacceptable to remain silent witnesses, although at one point we seriously considered calling a halt to our study and to any further publications based on it.

What helped us to resolve this field workers' crisis was the recognition that the deficiencies accompanying the rise and fall of the Jarvik-7 artificial heart were not unique to it. Rather, we concluded, they were special and in some ways magnified instances of patterns that can and do occur in other clinical experiments. With the hope that this insight was more than a sociological rationalization, we decided that we would "go public" through our professional lectures, the final report that we would write to the study's funders, the National Science Foundation and the NHLBI, and through this book.

Moratoria and Endings

As we recounted in Chapter 5, the implantation of a permanent total artificial heart had several moratorium phases and, in retrospect, several endings. One major endpoint came in April 1985, when DeVries performed the fourth and what proved to be his final implant in the series of seven that had been authorized by the FDA. By the time William Schroeder, the second recipient, died in August 1986, most of those involved in the experiment acknowledged privately that it was, and should be, finished. The ending of the experiment in midcourse, with no explicit or formal decisions to that effect, much less any declaration in professional or public forums, is one of the more interesting and problematic sociological features of the ways social controls operated and did not operate in the case of the artificial heart.

There were three moratoria in the use of the Jarvik-7 heart as a permanent device, each of which occurred for different reasons (Swazey et al. 1986). The first moratorium period began in August 1983 when DeVries submitted a protocol to the University of Utah Medical Center IRB for the required case-by-case approval to perform a second implant. That pause ended in November 1984, when DeVries, now in Louisville, operated on William Schroeder. The chief cause of this first moratorium was the time it took for DeVries and Symbion to gain the needed approvals for a second implant. The Utah IRB and the FDA, respectively, approved a revised protocol in January and June 1984. Then DeVries' move to the Humana Heart Institute necessitated a new round of regulatory reviews by the Audubon Hospital IRB and the FDA. Permissions to proceed with an implant were granted in September and November 1984, respectively, paving the way for William Schroeder to become the second permanent artificial heart recipient.

A second, brief halt was imposed by the FDA from late December 1985 to late February 1986. This suspension was called by the FDA so Symbion could prepare and file a revised protocol after the agency's advisory panel hearing in Washington. Many, including members of the artificial heart group, had expected that the hearings would result in the implants being halted by the FDA based on the outcomes with the first four recipients and a barrage of negative publicity about the program. However, because of supportive testimony given by representatives of professional societies at the hearing's public session, the data presented by Symbion during the closed session, and political concerns about the consequences of stopping the experiment, the panel recommended to the FDA that the implants be allowed to "proceed, but with caution" (McIntosh 1986, pp. 10–11).

At the time that the FDA called its brief moratorium, 9 months had elapsed since DeVries had done his fourth implant. He and his team were still screening a few candidates and working on changes in their patient management protocols, and they were outwardly optimistic that more implants would occur. As time would show, however, the FDA moratorium was superimposed on what in fact was an enduring halt. But until January 1990, when the FDA ended the use of the Jarvik heart, DeVries officially still had FDA permission to perform three more implants. Because neither he, the Humana Corporation, nor Symbion had explicitly stated that no more permanent implants would be done, or acknowledged that, with or without their input and consent, the experiment had stalled and then stopped, this moratorium was what we would term a de facto one.[4]

Other than DeVries' obstinate belief that permanent implants with the Jarvik heart would continue—and indeed that they had never really halted—only one other artificial heart surgeon, Dr. Jack Copeland, publicly called for a resumption of their use. Copeland's argument, much like the one he advanced for his use of the "Phoenix heart" in 1985, was that the device was available and could be used to prolong the lives of patients who were not eligible for a heart transplant because of other health problems or age. Dr. Robert Jarvik agreed with this viewpoint but was less sanguine that the pneumatically powered heart would again be used as a permanent replacement. In an Associated Press story in July 1989, Copeland and Jarvik were quoted as follows.

> "I think in small terms about individual lives, one at a time. . . . " says Copeland. . . . "I know there's something I can do [for somebody dying of heart disease]. I just don't have the money, I don't have the support. . . ."
> The biggest obstacles to anyone resuming implanting artificial hearts, [Copeland] says, are money, the pressure of life in a fishbowl, and the public's inability to view such procedures as experimental and "allow us to fail." . . . "If I could get somebody to come up with enough bucks to do it, I would do it," he says.
> "If Dr. Copeland has resources and the availability to work on it, that's fine, it's ethically justified," Jarvik says. "But I think in general most people want to work on electric powered systems." (Doctor says its time to resume using permanent artificial hearts 1989)

As the decade ended, DeVries and Copeland seemed to be the only cardiac replacement surgeons who thought the Jarvik heart might be used again as a permanent device. The prospect of such implants being resumed became even more improbable in January 1990, when the FDA issued a recall notice to Symbion, withdrawing the agency's approvals for investigational use of the Jarvik-7 heart, the smaller Jarvik-7-70 model, and the company's ventricular assist device. In its recall notification the FDA cited various ways in which the company had violated requirements for the production of an experimental device and its use by investigators. They included "deficiencies in manufacturing quality control, monitoring of research sites [by the company], training of personnel and reporting of adverse reactions to the FDA." According to an agency spokesman, "the FDA believe[d] that, on balance, the deficiencies in the Symbion studies were great enough that the risks to patients were outweighing benefits" (Gladwell 1990).

Although the FDA recall was described by the press as "an action that stunned heart researchers," reporters pointed out that it was not expected to have a major impact on "medical practice." Because many heart transplant surgeons had started using ventricular assist devices to support a candidate's own heart until a donor heart was available, and because other total artificial heart models were available for temporary procedures, there had been a "downturn" in the Jarvik heart's use, with only five implants done in the United States and 15 in other countries during 1989 (Altman 1990c). Not surprisingly, Symbion, which had moved from Salt Lake City to Tempe, Arizona, disputed the validity of the FDA's charges. The company's chief financial officer declared that Symbion "stood by its products" and, because FDA regulations apply only to devices used in the United States, "would continue to sell them [abroad]" (Altman 1990c).

News of the recall prompted various eulogistic comments about the Jarvik heart from the press and those who had been directly or indirectly involved with its use. The reporter who broke the recall story in the *Washington Post*, for example, began his article by describing the Jarvik heart as "the medical device that captured the imagination of the world when it was implanted 8 years ago in a dying Seattle dentist named Barney Clark" (Gladwell 1990). French surgeon Christian Cabrol, who had used the Jarvik heart for 47 bridge implants—and could continue to buy the device from Symbion—proclaimed that "he was shocked by the FDA's action against the device that he termed 'one of the most wonderful tools in medicine'" (Altman 1990c). Dr. Jack Copeland, who only a few months previously had called for a resumption of permanent implants with the Jarvik heart, noted that he had stopped using the device for bridge implants about a year ago, favoring ventricular assist devices instead. "The Jarvik heart," he affirmed in January 1990, "was the Model T. Now we have to go on to other ideas" (Altman 1990c; Gladwell 1990). From his position as director of the National Heart, Lung, and Blood Institute, Dr. Claude Lenfant—who personally had many reservations about the Jarvik heart and its clinical use—declared that "in a way, the Jarvik heart was a failure. But it was a step that needed to be taken so we could see where we were going. The first experiments paved the way for much of the work that is going on now" (Gladwell 1990).

As Lenfant indicated, the FDA recall of the Jarvik heart and the earlier halt of DeVries' implants did not signal an end to artificial hearts. Research and development efforts with a new generation of devices and timetables for their clinical testing are going forward with unquenched convictions about the feasibility and desirability of a man-made replacement for the human heart.

The clinical experiment with the Jarvik-7 heart as a permanent replacement for the human heart proved to be a relatively brief one. It ended not with a bang but a whimper. That the experiment came to a halt, however, had little to do with the exercise of professional governance by those most closely involved with the experiment and their wider professional community or, the FDA recall notwithstanding, the application of formal regulatory controls. The fact that most of those with grave doubts about the artificial heart experiment, who might have altered its course, remained silent and inactive despite their concerns is a familiar, recurrent, socially predictable pattern in medicine, as well as other professions. Integral to this pattern is the shared belief that individuals will regulate themselves regarding standards of professional competence and conduct, as well as the norms of loyalty to the group that foster a collective self-protectiveness. As a result, physicians and other professionals are reluctant to criticize, confront, or "blow the whistle" on colleagues they identify as incompetent, impaired, or engaging in various forms of misconduct. They also are disinclined to openly challenge, much less try to stop, research they find scientifically and ethically dubious, either by taking action within the confines of their institution or professional community or in a more public fashion (Bosk 1979; Freidson 1975; Swazey 1980; Swazey and Scher 1982, 1985).

We are not contending that social control mechanisms did not work at all in the case of the Jarvik-7 artificial heart. In our judgment, however, they were weakened and compromised by the zeal with which the quest for a viable mechanical heart was pursued, as well as by the various forms of individual and institutional self-protectiveness and self-interest that came into play. To a chastening degree (as we have documented in Chapter 6), some of the most valued characteristics of American society and culture contributed to the dangerous excesses and forms of misconduct associated with the Jarvik-7 experiment.

Recognizing and understanding these patterns, however, does little to resolve the disturbing issues of moral agency they raise. The experiment ended, and we left the field, with the unanswered question, "Who shall guard the guardians?"

The Participant
Observers:
Final Journeys

Leaving the Field

"Well, imagine you had a great-great-grandson . . . and he lived to see the end of the state. No injustice, no inequality—how would he spend his life, Sancho?"

"Working for the common good."

"You certainly have faith, Sancho, great faith in the future. But *he* would have no faith. The future would be there before his eyes. Can a man live without faith?"

"I don't know what you mean—without faith. There will always be things for a man to do. The discovery of new energy. And disease—there will always be disease to fight."

"Are you sure? Medicine is making great strides. I feel sorry for your great-great-grandson, Sancho. It seems to me that he may have nothing to hope for except death."

The mayor smiled. "Perhaps we may even conquer death with transplants."

"God forbid," Father Quixote said. "Then he would be living in a desert without end. No doubt. No faith. I would prefer him to have what we call a happy death."

"What do you mean by a happy death?"

"I mean the hope of something further."

(Greene 1983, pp. 72–73)

As journeyers into the field, participant observers, and chroniclers, we have been involved in the development of organ transplantation, the artificial kidney, and the artificial heart throughout most of their contemporaneous medical and social history and for many years of our working lives. Since 1951 (RCF) and 1968 (JPS) we have had the privileged opportunity to watch, from the inside, how dialysis and kidney, heart, and liver transplantation, which began as "desperate remedies for desperate patients," with certain "desperate[ly] hopeless" conditions (Moore 1989, p. 1483), evolved into "nonexperimental," though far from ordinary, interventions to treat a wide gamut of end-stage diseases. During those years we have seen the range and combinations of different organs transplanted, the numbers performed, and the array of artificial organs designed increase dramatically, and we have charted at firsthand the early phases of the drive to replace the human heart with a man-made device.

Our intensive, long-term relationship with these therapeutic innovations and their clinical unfolding has had many of the characteristics anthropologist Margaret Mead identified as inherent to field research, no matter where it is located or what its subject matter may be. Field work, as she described it, entails not just the unique

> but also cumulative experience of immersing oneself [*sic*] in the ongoing life of another people, suspending for the time both one's beliefs and disbeliefs, and of simultaneously attempting to understand mentally and physically this other version of reality. . . .
>
> Immersing oneself [*sic*] in the field is good, but one must be careful not to drown. One must somehow maintain the delicate balance between empathic participation and self-awareness, on which the whole research process depends. . . .
>
> Only very slowly did we [field workers] begin to take into account that we ourselves change with each step of the journey, with each new image presented to us . . . and with each day in the field. . . . (Mead 1977, pp. 1, 7, 15).

Our research did not transport us to geographically and culturally isolated primitive villages, where we lived and worked day after day for months without the respite of returning to our home-world. Yet, in many crucial respects, our field experiences parallel those of Mead. We have journeyed far, horizontally and vertically, in our questing after transplantation, dialysis, and the artificial heart—coast to coast in this country, and to Europe, Hawaii, Majuro, and China; down long corridors into the high technology surgical and intensive care chambers of the modern hospital; and ever more deeply into the corridors and chambers of ourselves. The people we have studied have been our "teachers" as well as our "subjects," helping us to learn their language and their ways. We have risen "at cock crow" to accompany transplant teams, donors, and recipients into operating rooms, and we have stayed up all night to "listen for some slight change" in a patient's or prospective donor's condition and "revel or mourn" with medical professionals, patients, and families. We have "used ourselves as instruments," striving to attain and reattain the "kind of reflexive objectivity that calls for continuous self-scrutiny and self-analysis, along with observing and interpreting the actions and interactions of others." For years, as participating observers and observing participants, we have walked the thin line between detachment and concern and between "belief and disbelief." And like Mead, "only very slowly did we realize" that, as a consequence of our "immersion" in the field, deep and enduring changes were taking place in us (Mead 1977, pp. 1–16).

Foremost among the people whose "reality" we have been allowed to share are the physicians and nurses, patients and families who have been the chief actors in the "experiments perilous" through which organ transplants, dialysis, and the efforts to fashion a viable artificial heart have been advanced. It has kept us in close contact with the grave illnesses and frequent deaths they have mutually faced, with the hope and renewal, the "breakthroughs," and the despair and disappointments they have experienced, and with the ways of navigating and coping they have forged. We often have been enriched and energized by the many transplantation- and artificial organ-centered communities we entered and by the professional and personal relationships we have established within them. Our association with the human story of these therapeutic innovations, their scientific and clinical significance, and their social and moral import has never been academically detached. In fact, the process of disengaging ourselves from this field has made us feel at times as though we were getting a divorce, departing from a religious order, or forsaking comrades in crisis.

Our decision to leave the field has been a complex one and a long time in the making. Over the past decade or so, we gradually recognized in ourselves the signs and symptoms of what we diagnosed as "participant-observer burnout"— akin to what we have witnessed over the years in some of the medical professionals immersed in the world of organ replacement efforts. Our burnout has its roots in the fact that there have been aspects of these efforts that we always have found especially troubling. Prominent among them have been some components of the "courage to fail" value system prevalent among transplantation and artificial organ pioneers. This ethos includes a classically American frontier outlook: heroic, pioneering, adventurous, optimistic, and determined. It also involves, however, a bellicose, "death is the enemy" perspective; a rescue-oriented and often zealous determination to maintain life at any cost; and a relentless, hubris-ridden refusal to accept limits. It is disturbing to witness, over and over, the travail and distress to which this outlook can subject patients:

I have often seen transplant surgeons, confronted with a clinical dilemma, begin to invoke a litany of names, like a litany of Roman Catholic saints [a transplant service chaplain reflects]: "It may be a real long shot," they say, "but remember Vernie and remember Toni and remember Carl and remember . . . and remember . . . and remember. . . . " (The litany, which always consists of patients who survived against seemingly impossible odds, is used as an argument for pressing on. There does not seem to be a parallel list that would argue for giving up.) (Reimer 1989, p. 41).

It is sometimes hard to meet the eyes of patients who have improved enough to have been moved to the regular postop floor and finally become alert enough to communicate their despair and disappointment.... Often, after entering the experience with such great hope, patients for whom transplantation has been a series of setbacks clearly articulate their feelings of betrayal: "No one ever told me it could be like this." ...

Certainly they were told that there would be no guarantees, and that it would be hard, and that there would be setbacks—but probably not how hard, or what some of the worst-case scenarios could be. When they were told, "You have to have a transplant or you're going to die," they were left a very slim margin for decision making. These people need to know not only what it will be like not to be dying any more, but what it may be like to not live so well. (Park 1989, p. 31)

Another early source of unease was our conviction that if our society is to engage in such endeavors, we have a moral obligation to ensure equitable access to organ replacement. In the absence of such equity, we have observed again and again how specifically designated individuals have been privileged to obtain needed organs and funding for transplantation by wielding special emotional, media, political, and economic resources available to them, including, during the Reagan years, the power and resources of the presidency.

Rather than focusing on conditions that ultimately are defensible in terms of equality and justice, ... designated ... person-specific ... organ donation ... ties access to an organ to the emotional appeal (or lack thereof) of the prospective recipient, the public relations skills of the physician[s] involved, of the next-of-kin, and of those who orchestrate the media campaign, and the financial abilities of everyone concerned to mount such a campaign in the first place. ... [I]n effect [it] ... singles out a specific individual and characterizes him or her as someone to whom an organ may be given independently of the established means of access. The assumption is that this person is ethically special; that he or she has some particular quality or characteristic that permits an exemption from the criteria that would otherwise apply to all. (Kluge 1989, pp. 11–12)

Our decision to leave the field actually occurred in two phases. Our first attempt to do so turned out to be no more than a brief moratorium. During 1979–82, partly under the aegis of the James Picker Foundation Program on the Human Qualities of Medicine, we conducted targeted field research for a book of essays that would be a sequel to *The Courage to Fail*. It was during the course of this work, as we immersed ourselves once more in the "lived-in reality" of the world of organ replacement endeavors, that we first seriously discussed leaving this field.

Many people and experiences from those years remain indelibly etched in our minds. It was the identified cases, relationships, and advances we were privileged to study first-hand that both powerfully bound us to the field for so long and, cumulatively, led us to withdraw from it. Among those still vivid images are the vista of an empty thoracic cavity awaiting the implantation of a heart and lungs from a brain-dead donor at Stanford; the sight of desperate parents and their tiny, dying children with huge eyes, bloated bellies, pale, lifeless hair, and ochre-colored skin, who had made pilgrimages to Dr. Thomas Starzl in Pittsburgh to plead for a liver transplant; and, in both of these settings, the first exuberant discussions about the miracles that were being wrought by the discovery of cyclosporine.

Above all, it was the "identified lives"—the patients and families we came to know, some only slightly and others more intimately—that made us feel sadder and more anxious than we had in the past and filled us with painfully unanswerable questions of "why?" Though we had met him only briefly when he was a heart transplant patient at Stanford Medical Center, for example, we felt true human ties to Talcott (Sam) Poole and real sorrow when we read of his death from renal failure in December 1982 at age 24. We thought also of his family and of his caregivers at Stanford, who were portrayed so vividly in an extraordinarily moving book by Sam's mother, *Thursday's Child*, which chronicled the onset of his incurable heart disease, his transplant and life thereafter, and his at-once joyous and stoical spirit through it all.

Another such experience was with Doris, a close, kin-like friend whose "case" we had both studied and participated in personally and professionally for many years. We had talked many times with her and, after her death, with her family about trying to capture in a written "portrait" all that her story entailed about the worst and best of being a chronic dialysis patient. For she, more than any other person we have known, exemplified the finest elements of the "courage to fail" ethos in her life with progressive renal failure, several humanly and medically difficult years of dialysis, and then a death that represented some of the worst features of a "House of God" teaching hospital (Shem 1978). There is a sense in which we have vicariously experienced what Thomas Starzl has described as "the sense of personal loss" and "the cumulative weight of grief" that transplant surgeons like himself have undergone in response to the deaths of the "desperately ill" persons for whom they have cared, particularly the deaths of individuals who have come to personify for them the suffering of all their patients and the embodiment of their "determination to make things better" for them through transplantation. "The burn-out rate," Starzl has observed, was especially "high in the early days of transplantation. Because of this, and because aging spares no one [he added], only a handful of workers in transplantation have stayed in the field continuously throughout its 30-year modern history" (Starzl 1990).

Six weeks of field research during the summer of 1981 in the People's Republic of China also had a powerful impact on us (Fox and Swazey 1982, 1984). During that era of the "four modernizations," China's medical workers had a collective commitment to "serving the patient" by progressively "scaling the heights" of modern medicine. It was part of a larger "golden dream" they shared with their compatriots about what science and technology might achieve for their country and its people. As part of this drive for medical modernization, hospitals in Tianjin were making their first forays into organ transplantation and chronic dialysis. As we watched these beginnings, we were vividly reminded of what Dr. Francis D. Moore termed the "black years" of renal transplantation in the United States—complete with the high mortality rate of patients and organs and what would now be considered in our country and in Western Europe excessive doses of corticosteroid immunosuppressive drugs, with all their side effects. Absorbed though we were by many features of our Chinese field experience, we were reluctant to "go through again" what RCF observed 40 years ago on the metabolic research ward of the Peter Bent Brigham Hospital in Boston, where renal transplantation and dialysis were pioneered (Fox 1959). We also found ourselves in the peculiar cultural and ideological position of being more preoccupied than our hosts with the allocation of scarce resources dilemma that their dawning interest in transplantation, dialysis, intensive care medicine, and other advanced forms of Western medicine would pose for a country as poor as China, with a population of more than one billion persons and massive public health and primary care needs.

China also provided us with a societal telescope through which, from a great historical, cultural, and physical distance, we were able to connect our thoughts about transplantation and dialysis with our growing sociological and moral concern about the state of American ideas, values, and beliefs, as epitomized by the predominant themes of bioethics a decade ago. In a comparative analysis of "medical morality" in China and bioethics in the United States, we wrote that

> if . . . bioethics is not just bioethics and is more than medical—if it is an indicator of the general state of American ideas, values and beliefs, of our collective self-knowledge, and our understanding of other societies' cultures—then there is every reason to be worried about who we are, what we have become, what we know, and where we are going in a greatly changed and changing society and world. (Fox and Swazey 1984, p. 360)

Although we gathered a great deal of material between 1979 and 1982, we kept postponing the task of turning it into a book. Our problem, we finally admitted to ourselves, was that we had lost much of the detached concern that had enabled us to study and write about this field for so many years. Tellingly, by the end of 1982 we had drafted only the final essay in our unborn volume. It was called, as is this chapter, "Leaving the Field," for we had decided that all the signs and symptoms of our self-diagnosed field worker and writerly malaise indicated that we should withdraw from our work on organ replacement.

In December 1982, as we were completing a draft of "Leaving the Field," newspapers headlined the first implantation of a permanent total artificial heart by Dr. William DeVries and his colleagues at the University of Utah Medical Center. For the next 112 days, we and millions of others followed the drama of Dr. Barney Clark's life and death with a Jarvik-7 heart. However, because of the extensive case study we had made of the total artificial heart implant Dr. Denton Cooley attempted in 1969, the Barney Clark/William DeVries story had a magnetic effect on us, drawing us back into the field despite our resolve to leave it (Fox and Swazey 1978a, ch. 6). And so, in June 1983 we found ourselves en route to Salt Lake City, for what we defined as a brief, one-time period of interviews and observations. However, more than 5 years passed before, in the fall of 1988, we completed what became a detailed and profoundly disquieting study of the development and use of the Jarvik heart. It was that research project and some of the participant observation experiences associated with it that brought our journeying into this field of medical research and therapeutic innovation to a definitive end.

During the 1980s we also continued to monitor developments and issues in transplantation and dialysis, and our uneasiness about the attributes and side effects of organ replacement endeavors continued to grow. It has become increasingly difficult for us to "suspend [our] beliefs and disbeliefs" and "maintain the delicate balance" between "immersion" and detachment that field work optimally requires (Mead 1977). Through the ongoing process of self-scrutiny and self-analysis that participant observation also entails, we have recognized that our years in the field have made us more, rather than less, emotionally and morally perturbable. For example, we found ourselves responding with stronger negative sentiments than in the past to such *déjà-vu* experiences as hearing some of the same transplanters who proclaimed the "cosmic" significance of cyclosporine now hail the newly discovered experimental immunosuppresive agent FK-506 as a once-in-a-lifetime miracle drug and learning that the Boy Scouts of America are offering a Donor Awareness Patch to induce Scouts to talk to their families about organ donation. We reacted with concern to a proposal by Paul I. Terasaki, a pioneer of transplantation tissue-typing methods, that organ recipients "who are now enjoying a second chance at life, thanks to the compassionate generosity of the families of donors" be organized into "a trained . . . volunteer . . . self-perpetuating advocacy group" that could "take turns being on call to ask grieving families to consider organ donations, . . . visit hospital personnel . . . who . . . have limited personal contact with . . . a person who has been given life and health with someone else's heart, liver, or kidney," and "promote awareness" of the mounting . . . need" for donations of cadaveric organs (Terasaki 1989). When we read about multiple organ transplants, live-donor liver and lung transplants, conceiving children to serve as bone marrow donors, the temporary use of diseased donor hearts, and about the merits of markets in "HBPs," we wondered, as did philosopher Daniel Callahan, "what kind of life" our values are driving us to seek, and if we can accept "limits to medical progress" (Callahan 1989).

We are not therapeutic nihilists, nor do we lack appreciation for the impressive medical, surgical, and technological progress that has been made with transplants and artificial organs over the course of the past three decades, or just in the past 10 years. If anything, our in vivo historical relationship to their development has heightened our recognition of just how far they have advanced. Nor have we lost our capacity to respond with empathy to the "stories with happy endings" (Park 1989) and to those that tragically never came to pass:

> For my family and me [a friend wrote us], the pain and grief of losing John was complicated by the bitter disappointment that we did not receive a heart in time to sustain his life. Intellectually, I know this is an incontrovertible fact. Emotionally, I know that we, his family, were his life and all of you are helping to sustain us. Perhaps, John did receive a heart. Although few of you knew him, you gave him yours.

But we have come to believe that the missionary-like ardor about organ replacement that now exists, the overidealization of the quality and duration of life that can ensue, and the seemingly limitless attempts to procure and implant organs that are currently taking place have gotten out of hand. In the words of a transplant nurse-specialist, "perhaps the most important issue in a critical examination of transplantation involves the need and criteria for responsible decisions about when to stop, when to say 'enough is enough' to the transplant process" (Park 1989, p. 30).

In our view, the field of organ replacement now epitomizes a very different and powerful tendency in the American health care system and in the value and belief system of our society's culture: our pervasive reluctance to accept the biological and human condition limits imposed by the aging process to which we are all subject and our ultimate mortality. It seems to us that much of the current replacement endeavors represent an obdurate, publicly theatricalized refusal to accept these limitations. Physicians are morally guided by what the late Protestant theologian and ethicist Paul Ramsey called principles of "faithfulness" and "loyalty" not to abandon caring for their patients, particularly those who are dying. Ramsey also argued forcibly, however, that we "need . . . to discover the moral limits properly surrounding efforts to save life" (Ramsey 1970, p. 118). With this conviction, we think that he would have joined us in questioning the enactment of the principle of faithfulness in the unremitting efforts of transplant surgeons to prevent the death of their patients by doing numerous retransplants if the donor organ "fails for any reason," because they believe that "once a patient has had a transplant [they] have made a commitment that cannot be abandoned" (Park 1989, p. 30).

Rereading Ramsey's *The Patient as Person*, 20 years after it was first published, we were deeply impressed by how prophetic it has proved to be with respect to our social and cultural problems in accepting limits on organ replacement and the care of dying patients. Culturally, Ramsey argued persuasively, we need to "recover a religious sense that death is not an evil that ought always to be opposed."

> If it is not possible for modern men, when the one "lone hope" is gone, to believe that this is not the end of hope, perhaps we might share the conviction of Socrates, who said, "Now it is time that we were going, I to die and you to live, but which of us has the happier prospect, is unknown to anyone but God." That outlook, too, might save men and doctors today from the triumphalist temptation to slash and suture our way to eternal life." (Ramsey 1970, p. 238)

Two recollections come to mind. The first is our wry memory of the fact that during the early 1970s, when we were trying to find a title for the first edition of *The Courage to Fail*, sociologist Erving Goffman suggested *Spare Parts* to us as a possibility. Although we appreciated the ironic wittiness of his suggestion, at that time we considered it too cynical for us to adopt. Viewed retrospectively, this Goffmanesque title now seems prescient because we feel it captures some of the essences of the evolution that organ replacement and our relation to it have undergone during the past decade.

The second memory is of a field trip that one of us (RCF) made during the late 1970s to a dialysis center located on a small, 3.5 square mile atoll in the Marshall Islands that was supervised from afar by the Institute of Renal Diseases of St. Francis Hospital in Honolulu, Hawaii. For both of us, that coral atoll symbolizes the antithesis of a palm-fringed tropical paradise. It represents the unromantic specter of a world in which every island, no matter how small or remote, will some day have its own machines and personnel to which all persons in end-stage organ failure will be given unconditional access, until death releases them from this form of treatment, or they can be airlifted to a medical center such as St. Francis for transplantation.

As we look back, we realize that it is not only we who have been changed by the cumulative effects that our field research has had on us. The field itself has changed, especially during the 1980s, in certain ways that have influenced our decision to exit it. Above all, it is the intensity and expansion of the drive to sustain life and "rebuild people" through organ replacement that has progressively alienated us, particularly the unquestioning and even celebratory way in which the transplanting and retransplanting of virtually every organ of the human body is creating larger and larger numbers of "patchwork men and women," (Altman 1989c) whose quality of life is dubious at best. "Our culture," Ramsey observed, "is already prepared for technocratizing the bodily life into collections of parts in which consciousness somehow has residence for a time" (Ramsey 1970, p. 193).

In addition, the determination to procure organs has become so powerful that we believe there is an almost predatory obliviousness to "where [the] organs come from, and how [the] donors died" (Annas 1989, p. 34). We share George Annas' indignation over what he termed the "denial of reality" that underlies the current policy of avidly promoting organ donation and transplantation without publicly acknowledging the kinds of death—from vehicular accidents, homicides, suicides—on which they are based (Annas 1988, p. 621).

However, we disagree with what Annas goes on to say: namely, that it is not only important and right that "we all should know the stories of donors" (Annas 1988, p. 621), but also that the donor's family, the recipient, and the recipient's family should know each other's identity. In his view, the norm of confidentiality that transplant teams have established does more to protect their own emotional equilibrium than that of donors, recipients, and their families. Here we part company with Annas because, like so many analysts commenting on organ transplants during the 1980s, he has not sufficiently taken into account the importance of the gift-exchange dimensions of organ donation, the stresses and burdens that the obligations of giving, receiving, and repaying it impose on donors and donees, or how the policy of confidentiality developed out of transplanters' desire to reduce the "tyranny" of this unrepayable, symbolically charged gift. It seems to us that what Annas has overlooked is a specific instance of a more general trend during the 1980s that is another factor propelling us out of the field. It is the present tendency to minimize the importance of the "theme of gift" and of the gift relation in organ transplantation and to systematically ignore, forget, or deny what was previously known about them. Such disregard for the dynamics and meaning of the gift exchange involved has characterized most of the live-donor liver, lung, and pancreas transplants conducted during the last few years.

Nowhere is the tendency to discount the gift dimension more patently (and to us distressingly) apparent than in the movement toward the "commodification" and "marketification" of the organs. This deveopment was one theme in a 1988 symposium on organ transplantation policy, in which proponents of a market economy for human body parts wondered why transplantation has not joined the "mainstream" of American medicine.

> Does the difference in policy prescription in the organ transplantation arena reflect a kind of sub rosa, underground ground rejection of the trend toward greater competition, pluralism, and decentralization in the health care industry, or are there certain peculiar characteristics of the organ transplantation enterprise that suggest the inapplicability of competition, pluralism, and decentralization in this specific industry? (Blumstein and Sloan 1989, pp. 1–2)

Arguing, as this representative passage does, that organ transplantation, like health care in general, is analogous to a commercial industry and product and that its nonconformity to a market model is not only curious but possibly subversive makes it difficult for us to identify with the way that transplants, and medicine more generally, are now being conceived and interpreted.

The "de-gifting" of transplantation that this market approach entails has been accompanied and reinforced by the progressive "biologization" of donated organs that has occurred during the 1980s and early 1990s. Increasingly, organs are being thought of as "just organs," rather than as living parts of a person, offered in life or death to sustain known or unknown others, that resonate with the symbolic meaning of our relation to our bodies, our selves, and to each other, and with the more than fleshly significance of what has been given and received. We believe that this biological reductionism (which as sociologist Howard L. Kaye pointed out is not confined to transplantation but pervades modern biology) has insidious implications for "how we conceive of ourselves as human beings," of our connectedness with others, "and thus how we conceive of a good and proper life" (Kaye 1986, 1991, p. 13).

We are deeply troubled by the subtle but powerful tendency to redefine ourselves and others "as essentially biological beings" (Kaye 1991, p. 16) that is being displayed in current attitudes toward the transplantation of solid organs, tissues, and other body parts. Not only has this living matter been terminologically reduced to "HBPs," but what we regard as something approaching the plundering of the newly deceased person's body is taking place. In May 1991, when the news surfaced that a young organ donor (22-year-old William Norwood, who had been fatally shot in a gas station holdup) had been infected with the AIDS virus, and a search was launched for the recipients of his organs and tissues, we were struck by the fact that some 56 of his body parts went to people in different regions of the country. On the one hand, we are impressed by the magnitude of such gifts and by the number of persons who could be helped by them. On the other hand, we wonder if our avidness to procure as many organs and tissues as possible is leading us to unreflectively disassemble and dehumanize the body.

One of the most urgent value questions that has emerged from our long professional immersion in the world of "spare parts" medicine is whether, as poverty, homelessness, and lack of access to health care increase in our affluent country, it is justifiable for American society to be devoting so much of its intellectual energy and human and financial resources to the replacement of human organs. We realize that in terms of the ways our society provides, allocates, and expends resources within the "medical commons," the aggregate volume and costs of organ replacements are a relatively small portion of medical care activities and expenditures. Nor, given the benefits that many patients may derive from transplants and artificial devices, do we suppose that all organ replacement endeavors should—or conceivably would—cease. We do believe, however, that all the professional and public consideration given to transplants and pursuits such as a permanent artificial heart and the societal value commitments that organ replacement epitomizes are helping to divert attention and human and financial resources away from far more basic and widespread public and individual health care needs in our society.

We still believe that the ultimate significance of these therapeutic modalities lies in their relation to metamedical themes: uncertainty, scarcity, and generosity; the just distribution of material and nonmaterial resources; solidarity and community; life, death, and meaning; and intervention in the human condition. We also share health policy analyst Emily Friedman's passionate conviction that a "silent, largely invisible epidemic [of] medical indigence" has become the most tragically serious health care problem in the United States; that "the non-coverage of the uninsured poor and their resultant lack of access [to health care] affect every American"; that ignoring or accepting this situation puts us "all at risk," because "a society that forces its most vulnerable and needy members to beg for crumbs of care, or to go without care until they are dying, harms itself [and its moral fabric] even more than it harms the victims of its cruelty" (Friedman 1989). Allowing ourselves to become too caught up in such problems as the shortage of transplantable organs while health care continues to be defined as a private consumption rather than a social good in American society, with the consequence that millions of people do not have adequate or even minimally decent care, speaks to a values framework and a vision of medical progress that we find medically and morally untenable. The predicament of these deprived and fragile members of our society has changed the ethical context of transplantation and artificial organs for us; and it is one of the most morally compelling reasons for our leaving the field.

By happenstance, the time we chose to write about organ replacement during the 1980s coincided with a marked escalation of biomedical and technological developments, and of social attention to them. At first, we thought that the ground swell of activity we perceived in the organ replacement sphere was a kind of optical illusion caused by our heightened awareness of the field from which we were taking leave and our ambivalence about doing so. Sheer "observer effect," however, cannot account for the remarkable concatenation of events that took place from July 1989 to August 1991, when we were writing this book. During that interval, for example, the volume of transplants and the audible concern about the scarcity of organs and tissues, their procurement, and allocation mounted appreciably. An array of cluster transplants gained momentum and prominence; their chief performer and promoter, Thomas Starzl, did the first human heart–liver–kidney multiple transplant in December 1989 in a 26-year-old woman who died in March 1990 of complications from hepatitis. Professional and public debate about the feasibility and ethicality of using anencephalic infants as organ donors flared up in response to the Loma Linda Medical Center's program and their subsequent decision to suspend it. Clinical trials were conducted with the transplantation of cadaver organs from persons generally regarded as too biologically old to be donors and with using "flawed" organs for temporary transplants. In October 1989, FK 506, a powerful antirejection agent, burst on the scene. In December 1989, accompanied by considerable fanfare, the first two American transplantations of liver lobes from live donor parents to infants with biliary atresia were performed at the University of Chicago Medical Center, followed by the first parent-to-child lung lobe transplants and the beginning of professional and public debate about the morality of parents conceiving a baby to serve as a bone marrow donor for another of their children. January 1990 brought the announcement that researchers were preparing for their first human tests of a temporary artificial lung, developed by a company in Salt Lake City (Altman 1990b). Simultaneously, the Jarvik-7 artificial heart made headlines again when the FDA officially withdrew approval of the device's continued experimental use because of deficiencies in its manufacture and quality control and in the monitoring of its clinical use. A year later the artificial heart again began to attract attention, as researchers moved toward their goal of the first human tests with a new generation of electrically powered devices to replace the functions of the human heart on a long-term basis.

In the final analysis, our departure from the field in the midst of such events is not only impelled by our need and desire to distance ourselves from them emotionally. It is also a value statement on our part. By our leave-taking we are intentionally separating ourselves from what we believe has become an overly zealous medical and societal commitment to the endless perpetuation of life and to repairing and rebuilding people through organ replacement—and from the human suffering and the social, cultural, and spiritual harm we believe such unexamined excess can, and already has, brought in its wake.

Notes

Introduction

1. Writing *Spare Parts* and reexamining *The Courage to Fail* has made us more mindful of the fact that the research on which they are based has been conducted primarily in American milieux. We recognize that, as a consequence, some of the concrete facts and empirical details described through our participant observation, interview materials, and files of professional and mass media documents are so specifically American they do not have exact counterparts in other settings. Furthermore, we are highly appreciative of the more general fact that the distinctive history, organization, and cultural tradition of a society influence and structure the particular ways in which medical science, technology and care are expressed and effected within its orbit (Fox 1986).

Since we began our research together in 1968, however, we have tried to follow, albeit from an ethnographic distance, the manner in which these therapeutic innovations have evolved in various European countries, especially Belgium and France. This work has been facilitated by the fact that one of us (RCF) has been doing sociological field research in Belgium since 1959, which has involved a trip to Europe virtually every year during that period of time. Our research also has taken us, more briefly, to locales ranging from England to the People's Republic of China to a dialysis facility on Majuro, a small atoll in the Marshall Islands. Based on these research experiences, we believe that in broad outline, the major phenomena and themes on which the book is centered are connected with scientific, medical, and social features that are intrinsic enough to transplantation and artificial organs to make them cross-culturally applicable, even though how they are patterned and played out may vary considerably from one society to another.

2. It was at the Brigham Hospital, in December 1954 (at the end of RCF's study of a metabolic research ward during the years 1951–54) that Dr. Joseph E. Murray performed the first successful human kidney transplants between two men who were identical twins, followed by a transplant between two women who were identical twins. In 1990 Dr. Murray received the Nobel Prize in Physiology or Medicine for this procedure, the experimental work that led to it, and the transplantation of other organs that followed from it.

The corecipient of this 1990 Nobel Prize was E. Donnall Thomas, who pioneered the transplanting of bone marrow from one person to another.

Chapter 1

1. This analysis of the patterned characteristics of the way in which cyclosporine was reported in the medical literature is based on an extensive content analysis of a wide range of medical journals published in English, especially American and British publications. (For a fuller analysis of "The 'Advent' of Cyclosporine and the Therapeutic Innovation Cycle," see Fox et al. 1984.)

2. "Should Cyclosporine Be Continued Indefinitely?" was a topic addressed at the August 1990 meeting of the International Congress of the Transplantation Society in San Francisco through the presentation of several studies on this issue funded by the Medical Research Council of Canada.

3. From 1963 to 1982 Thomas E. Starzl personally performed virtually all of the liver transplantations in the United States. He attempted the world's first four human liver transplants in 1963 at the University of Colorado. In September 1963 and January 1964 other experimental liver transplants were conducted by surgeons in Boston and Paris. The postoperative survival time of all these patients was so short they were deemed "failures," and a moratorium was called on any further liver transplants until October 1966, when Starzl tried again. From 1966 until the early 1980s, most of the liver transplants in the world were performed by either Starzl, at Colorado and then beginning in 1981 at the University of Pittsburgh to which he moved, or by Roy Y. Calne at Addenbrook's Hospital in Cambridge, England, and Kings College Hospital in London. Beginning in January 1982 Starzl turned over organized procurement procedures to "organ harvest teams" that had been formed and trained during 1981, and he delegated responsibility for performing 40 percent of the liver transplant operations to young faculty members or fellows whom he had taught to do the procedure. In 1982 Starzl's team alone performed 80 liver transplants and in 1983 more than 100. Although this operation is now carried out at numerous medical centers in the United States, almost all the surgeons who head these liver transplant programs and a great many of the surgeons on their staffs were originally trained by Starzl. (For a fuller account of this history, see Markle and Chubin 1987; Starzl et al. 1982, 1988).

4. The consensus conference is an organized process of publicly assessing the current state of biomedical technologies and therapies and of facilitating the transfer of clinical research more rapidly into medical and health care practice; it was invented and launched by the NIH in 1977. It takes the form of a preplanned, two-and-a-half day assemblage that combines elements of a collegial meeting of scientific experts, a judicial, "science court" kind of hearing, a town meeting, and a mass media event. The liver transplantation conference was the 36th such meeting held by the NIH (Markle and Chubin 1987; Mullan and Jacoby 1985; Wortman et al. 1982).

5. In addition to the references cited, this account of the consensus conference on liver transplantation is based on the observations made by one of us (RCF) at the meeting. Other features of the conference she observed that added to its intense emotional and

political pressures were the fact that a procession of children and young people who had received successful liver transplants and their families were present at the meeting. They had followed their famous transplant surgeon, Dr. Thomas E. Starzl, to Bethesda to celebrate him at the conference, to give witness to the therapeutic benefits of liver transplantation, and to campaign for its wide application and funding. The conference audience also included mothers holding in their arms crying babies afflicted with incurable, life-threatening liver diseases. The directors of the American Liver Foundation and the Children's Liver Foundation, both ⌐f whom were mothers who had lost a child from liver disease, were given official time on the program to make statements about the "life-giving" and "life-saving" surgery that liver transplantation represents and to plead for governmental and private insurance for this operation.

6. Although this case was the first time cardiac xenotransplantation was performed on an infant, three other clinical cardiac xenografts had been done previously. The first was the transplantation of a chimpanzee heart into a 68-year-old man performed by James Hardy at the University of Mississippi Medical Center in 1964. The other two xenografts were done by Christiaan Barnard in Capetown, South Africa, in 1967: One involved transplanting a baboon heart in a 25-year-old woman and the other a chimpanzee heart in a 60-year-old man (American Medical Association 1985).

7. Our use of the terms "multiple" and "singleton" was suggested to us by Robert K. Merton's essay, "Singletons and multiples in scientific discovery" (Merton 1961).

8. Until August 1990, Starzl's group at Pittsburgh was the only one in the United States authorized by the FDA to conduct clinical trials with FK 506 through an investigational new drug permit the FDA granted to the Fujisawa Company. As a consequence, a joke that circulated widely in the transplantation community referred to FK 506 as "a unique drug" that "only works in Pittsburgh" (Werth 1990, p. 35). In September 1990 the next two American medical centers licensed to test the drug—the University of California at Los Angeles and the University of California at San Francisco—were enrolling patients in clinical trials of FK 506 to be conducted under their aegis, but were still awaiting FDA approval to begin them.

According to a Fujisawa official, the Japanese firm decided to focus its research on FK 506 in the United States because this country does the most transplants and therefore is the largest user of antirejection drugs. In addition, he noted, along with the scientific expertise of Starzl and colleagues, another important determinant of the firm's decision to test the drugs in the United States was the significant degree to which "cultural factors limit the number of transplants that are performed in Japan" (Altman 1989a, p. B7; Ohnuki-Tierney 1984).

Chapter 3

1. According to the *Journal*'s executive editor, Dr. Marcia Angell, the possibility of writing an editorial to accompany the article was considered, but it was decided not to publish one at that time, as it was still uncertain whether the Chicago team would go forward with the procedure, and if so, when they would actually perform it (personal communication).

2. The largest organ procurement system in Europe, and the second largest in the world, is the Eurotransplant Foundation, which serves Germany, Austria, and the Benelux countries (Prottas 1985).

3. Medical professionals tend to be as reluctant as laypersons to broach the subject of death with their families, to talk about arrangements they would like to have made on their behalf when their own deaths occur, and to openly consider the option of organ donation under those circumstances. In a study of the attitudes of health professionals and hospital administrators involved in procurement, for example, all the neurosurgeons interviewed said that they would be willing to donate their own or a family member's organs, but only half of them actually discussed the matter with their families (Prottas and Batten 1988).

4. The pool of potential healthy young donors was further reduced by the progress made in many states during the 1980s in lowering automobile and motorcycle accident fatality rates through the passage of new seat belt, motorcycle helmet, maximum speed, and drunk driving safety laws.

5. Largely because organ donations have been defined as a voluntary gift, there has never been a strong movement in the United States to increase the supply of transplantable organs by the types of "presumed consent" laws that exist in several European countries, such as Belgium and France. The laws permit the routine harvesting of organs unless an individual has stipulated his or her objection to this practice prior to death.

6. Approximately 89 percent of all donors are pronounced dead in intensive care units (Darby et al. 1989, p. 2222). In addition to medical and surgical intensive care unit nurses and physicians, a neurologist usually participates in the medical management of potential organ donors because of the need to diagnose and pronounce brain death before organ retrieval is permissible. Surgeons, operating room nurses, and anesthesiologists are involved in removing organs from cadaver donors.

7. For a survey and analysis of statutes on the determination of death and of judicial decisions "defining" death, see Appendices C and D in the President's Commission for the Study of Ethical Problems in Medicine and Biomedical and Behavioral Research's 1981 report on *Defining Death*.

8. If a deceased person's wishes are not known, the Act provides that the next of kin has the right to decide whether organs are to be donated.

9. Ethical and legal questions about an individual's ownership of or property rights to his or her body and bodily parts, including cells, tissues, organs, and secretions, arose in several contexts during the 1980s. The development of biotechnology and of a flourishing industrial complex in this area brought several complicated issues to the forefront: Do patented and commercially valuable cell lines belong to the medical scientists or company who developed them or to the persons who were the sources of the tissues from which the cell lines were created? Do individuals hold property rights to their genetic identity, or do these rights adhere to the human species? Related issues concerning the ownership of body parts, in the context of artificial reproduction (sperm, eggs, and embryos) and the right to receive compensation for them, also arose. A number of cases concerning cell lines and frozen embryos, their identity, ownership, and economic matters associated with them became the foci of legal disputes, some of which were heard in the courts.

Chapter 5

1. The first phase of our study of the artificial heart was supported by a 1983–84 grant from The James Picker Foundation as part of its project on The Human Condition of Medical Professionals. From July 1, 1985 to December 30, 1988, the study was supported by grant BBS 8418894 from The National Science Foundation and the National Heart, Lung, and Blood Institute. Additional support during 1988–89 was provided by a grant-in-aid from Medicine in the Public Interest, Inc. Material in this chapter draws in part on our final project report to the NSF and NHLBI (Swazey et al. 1989). Any opinions, findings, conclusions, or recommendations are those of the authors and do not necessarily reflect the views of the National Science Foundation or the National Heart, Lung, and Blood Institute. For our previous publications about the artificial heart experiment, see Fox 1984; Swazey 1986, 1987, 1988; Swazey et al. 1986.

2. Time, research, and experience have repeatedly shown that the natural biological heart is functionally more complex than the model of a simple muscular pump (Cantin and Genest 1986), and that it is not as amenable to safe, effective, and long-lasting man-made replication as the engineering model has assumed. Biomaterial-tissue compatibility and power source problems, durability, and other sometimes unanticipated shortcomings of various devices have led to increasing recognition of the fact that much of the knowledge and technique needed to replace the human heart have yet to be adequately developed. Hence several generations of artificial hearts, including the Jarvik models, have come and gone. Knowledge and perhaps some wisdom have been gained, and the experts have recurrently predicted that a safe, effective artificial heart will be in clinical use within a decade.

3. The history of the NIH artificial heart program in terms of how it approached its objectives of developing a variety of partial and total mechanical circulatory assist devices, the bioengineering and medical problems encountered in those efforts, the reasons for its giving priority at different times to total and partial artificial hearts, and assessments of the social, ethical, and financial as well as medical implications of clinically proved devices has been detailed in a series of program-based reports (Hittman 1966; National Heart, Lung, and Blood Institute 1982, 1984, 1985a–c, 1986; National Institutes of Health 1973).

4. Kolff has pointed out, somewhat ironically, that none of the many artificial models developed over the years in his laboratories at the Cleveland Clinic, the University of Utah, and Kolff Mdical Associates has ever borne his name (Kolff 1983a).

5. One option the Utah group was considering as it designed its animal experiments was to implant the Jarvik heart as a temporary bridge device in patients awaiting a heart transplant donor. Dr. Donald Olsen conducted a series of twin-calf experiments, implanting an artificial heart in one twin, removing it after 1.5 to 3.0 months, and in its place transplanting a heart from the twin. "Charles and Diana" were the third set of twins in this series. Unlike most of his fellow experimental animals, Charles was not sacrificed to enable the researchers to study the effects of the implant/transplant. Instead he was kept alive in part so the investigators could learn how well his transplanted heart worked as he grew—which he did rapidly, from 220 to more than 1,800 pounds. When he outgrew the

animal barn facilities, Charles went as a herd sire to a commercial dairy farm, where he lived for more than three prolific years, siring some 60 calves. After Charles finally went to the slaughterhouse, his organs were returned to the artificial heart laboratories for analysis (D. Olsen, personal interview).

Because heart transplants were not being performed at the University of Utah during the 1980s, the artificial heart group's plan for using the Jarvik heart as a bridge device involved an arrangement to fly the patient to Stanford, California after the implant for a heart transplant by Dr. Norman Shumway's team. Two surgeons from the Stanford program, Dr. Bruce Reitz and Dr. Phillip Oyer, assisted with the calf heart transplants at Utah (Total artificial heart development at U of U 1982, p. 6). According to Olsen, the hoped-for Utah–Stanford collaboration foundered for want of a plane. To test the feasibility of flying a patient with a Jarvik heart and its cumbersome drive system from Salt Lake City to San Francisco, the investigators wanted to make one or more trial flights with an artificial heart calf such as Charles. They could not find an airline willing to undertake such a potentially risky trip with a calf, however, much less a patient, and so the long-distance implant–transplant venture was abandoned (personal interview).

6. That the ambivalence about testing the Jarvik heart on a human subject was not expressed in professional articles is due, in part, to the norms of writing for modern scientific and clinical journals. Those norms involve a degree of conciseness and reductionism that truncates and simplifies the complex nature of research, often contributing to an inadvertent retrospective falsification of the nature of research and related decision-making. For a case study that illustrates this point in more detail, see Barber and Fox 1958.

7. Strong feelings of nationalistic competitiveness and pride concerning development and use of an artificial heart have not been confined to the United States. Our media files, for example, include an extensive series of articles from French newspapers, particularly *Le Monde* and *Le Figaro*, that chronicle the bridge-to-transplant implantation of artificial hearts by French surgeons Alain Carpentier and Christian Cabrol and the efforts by several French groups to develop "original" and "unique" new types of devices that would enable France to enter the "international race" for a totally implantable artificial heart. The development and use of artificial hearts in France during the 1980s, as detailed in press accounts, was supported by a variety of nongovernmental sources. They included funding from the Lions Clubs of France for the development of an implantable prototype heart by a group in Marseilles; support by Bayer Laboratories for Dr. Carpentier's work; and a 2.5 million franc fundraising drive by *Le Fiagaro* and *Figaro* magazine (to which King Hussein of Morocco was a major contributor) to enable Dr. Cabrol, using the Jarvik-7, to "give France its first artificial heart."

8. For details of the pre- and postoperative medical history of Dr. Clark and the other permanent artificial heart recipients, see Berenson and Grosser 1984; DeVries 1988; DeVries and Joyce 1983; DeVries et al. 1984.

9. An insight into DeVries' disorganization and the often chaotic state of record-keeping for the artificial heart experiment is provided by the case of Barney Clark's missing medical records. His chart, some 18 inches thick and containing more than 1,000 pages of his day-to-day course after the implant, was reported missing by DeVries in August

1984 as he prepared to leave Utah. After several months of investigation had failed to locate the records, news of their disappearance was released to the press in March 1985. Presumably, medical center spokesman John Dwan told the *Deseret News*, "the document had been stolen by a souvenir hunter," and if the thief was found he or she would be prosecuted by the university. Two months later, the *Deseret News* reported that DeVries had found "portions" of the records, packed away in boxes in his new offices in Louisville, after the University of Utah had made "renewed inquiries" to him about their whereabouts (Medical record of Barney Clark is missing 1985; DeVries finds portions of lost medical records 1985).

10. The major controversy about so-called paycheck journalism involved a contract that Mrs. Clark had signed with *Reader's Digest* for an exclusive book-length story about Dr. Clark's participation in the artificial heart experiment. Many reporters were distressed about this arrangement because it precluded their gaining access to people, information, and opinions about the case after Dr. Clark's death. Altman also voiced his concern about "what kind of precedent . . . the University of Utah [has] set for medical research" by endorsing such commercial exclusivity and "secrecy" (Altman 1984a, pp. 123–25; Peterson 1984, pp. 134–35).

On our first visit to Salt Lake City in June 1983, we heard much discussion about the *Reader's Digest* book and its two writers, and Dr. Chase Peterson explained to participants in the implant that they could and should talk with us, despite the Clark family's contract because we were social scientists conducting a scholarly study. During that visit Dr. Kolff was the only key figure in the artificial heart story who declined to talk with us because of the book. The book contract eventually was canceled, however, and we did talk with Dr. Kolff later in our research.

11. A number of people in Salt Lake City, including DeVries and nurses involved in Dr. Clark's care, told us that because of media coverage and images of Dr. Clark's deteriorating condition and death cardiac patients were worrying about becoming experimental subjects for the artificial heart if they were referred to Dr. DeVries. When one of us (JPS) later went on rounds with DeVries at Humana Hospital Audubon, she heard several of his patients scheduled for operations make joking but anxious comments to their surgeon about not wanting "to wake up with one of those artificial hearts."

12. Humana was founded in 1961 by two Louisville lawyers, David Jones and Wendell Cherry, when the two friends decided to open a nursing home. By 1970 the company had expanded its holdings to more than 50 nursing homes and had also begun buying hospitals. In 1972 Humana sold its nursing homes to concentrate on hospital acquisitions. At the time of DeVries' move to Louisville, the Humana Corporation owned a chain of 89 acute-care hospitals with about 17,000 beds in the United States and three foreign countries, and it had posted revenues of approximately $2.3 billion and a net income of approximately $160,649 million for its 1983 fiscal year. Over the years the company had "won praise from Wall Street analysts for shrewd management and unorthodox marketing ploys" (Barron 1984).

13. This description of the FDA hearing is based on field notes by JPS, who attended both the morning and afternoon session, and copies of the statements by speakers at the morning session.

14. On December 2–4, 1989, the Humana Corporation and the Humana Heart Institute hosted an international conference in Louisville on "1989 Cardiovascular Science and Technology: Basic and Applied." In terms of the history of the Jarvik-7 permanent artificial heart experiment, two aspects of the conference agenda are significant. First, the opening welcome was delivered by Dr. John C. Norman, a veteran and distinguished artificial heart researcher, who is now affiliated with the Humana Heart Institute. Dr. Norman's move from the Texas Heart Institute in Houston to Louisville indicated that Humana's work on artificial hearts was continuing, but without William DeVries. Second, the names of William DeVries and Robert Jarvik were conspicuously absent from the dozens of presenters at the conference, suggesting that they were no longer seen as significant figures in the professional community of those involved with the development of artificial hearts and may even have been unofficially ostracized from it.

Chapter 6

1. There are suggestively interesting parallels between Jarvik's and DeVries' search for self-identity through the medium of the artificial heart and the first-hand observations that sociologist and psychologist Sherry Turkle made of the kind of relationship with the computer formed by many American adolescents. In her book *The Second Self: Computers and the Human Spirit*, Turkle devoted a chapter to these observations, which she entitled "Adolescence and Identity: Finding Yourself in the Machine" (Turkle 1984, ch. 4).

2. As we discuss at various points in Chapters 5, 6, and 7, the clinical implantation of artificial hearts, particularly the series of permanent implants performed by William DeVries, attracted extensive print and electronic media coverage. Collecting and analyzing such media materials was an important part of our research. We videotaped or audiotaped a convenience sample of television and radio programs dealing with the artificial heart. Popular weekly and monthly magazines providing coverage of news, health, science, and opinion-type columns related to the artificial heart were identified through computer searches and print indexes. Our files of popular periodical literature include approximately 180 articles. We also collected a file of more than 1,300 newspaper stories published between 1980 and 1990, which were maintained chronologically and within a chronological order by major events. Selected blocks of the media stories were analyzed and coded in relation to key issues and themes, including comparisons between national coverage and local coverage and between coverage in Salt Lake City and Louisville. This information was logged into a computer file developed by research librarian Judith C. Watkins, our project research associate. For purposes of analyzing the media's treatment of the artificial heart, emphasis was placed on obtaining comprehensive files of stories from major national papers (*The New York Times, The Washingtoin Post*, and *The Boston Globe*) and from the chief local papers in Salt Lake City and Louisville.

Our efforts to compile a nationally representative sample of popular press coverage of the artificial heart and comprehensive files of national and local newspapers was greatly facilitated by the cooperation of Humana Hospital Audubon's Public Relations Director, Donna Hazle, who generously gave us access to her media files; by Michael King and Gideon Gil of the *Louisville Courier-Journal*, Twila Van Leer of the Salt Lake City *Deseret News*, and Joann Jacobsen-Wells of the *Salt Lake City Tribune*, who provided us with copies of the stories about the artificial heart that they authored and of those written by their colleagues.

3. The Mormon Church is divided into wards of about 600 people. These are congregations that are similar to Roman Catholic parishes. Each ward is headed by a lay bishop and several counselors. Several wards are grouped together to form a stake, which is a larger administrative unit in the church that has some comparability to Catholic dioceses.

4. The principal reason for which all the recipients of the Jarvik-7 artificial heart implants were men is that the device was too large to fit in most women's chests.

5. These conceptions of the human heart have deep roots in the Judeo-Christian religious tradition of American society and culture (Meslin 1987).

6. When analyzing public discussion of the artificial heart experiment, particularly the media's reportage of and commentaries on Barney Clark's implant, we have been struck by what seems to us to have been the "structured silence" surrounding the role of Mormonism. A comparable silence occurred in the extensive media coverage of a "happening" such as Dr. Leonard Bailey's transplantation of a baboon heart into "Baby Fae" at Loma Linda Medical Center in California, an institution sponsored by the Seventh Day Adventist Church, as well as Loma Linda's donor program for anencephalic organ donors that we discussed in Chapter 1. The reasons there was almost no mention, much less discussion, of the Mormon and Seventh Day Adventist context of these events, we believe, have to do with far more than the fact that the two religions are not in the American mainstream. Apart from some attention to the religious dimensions of particularly controversial topics such as the "pro-life/pro choice" debates about the beginning and end of life, we have long noted a pattern of avoiding or ignoring the religious dimensions of health and illness and medical research and care in United States. This pattern occurs in medical professional and bioethical milieux as well as in the media. There are exceptions, such as the work of The Park Ridge Center and its journal dealing with matters of "health, faith, and ethics," *Second Opinion*. The nursing profession is also notably more inclined to address what it explicitly refers to as "spiritual" aspects of care than is the medical profession.

7. A number of the members of the large University of Utah Medical Center team who participated in Barney Clark's implant and in his care afterward traveled to Seattle, Washington to attend his funeral. In addition to Willem Kolff, these persons included William DeVries; Robert Jarvik; Chase Peterson; Lyle Joyce, DeVries' first surgeon-assistant; Margaret Miller, the social worker who acted as the Clark family's advocate; Helen Kee, assistant administrator for nursing; Linda Gianelli, head nurse in the intensive care unit; Larry Hastings and Steve Nelson, who were involved in the design and operation of the artificial heart's support system; and F. Ross Woolley, Vice Chairman of the Utah Medical Center's Institutional Review Board and Chairman of its artificial heart subcommittee. According to the detailed article about the funeral that medical writer Twila Van Leer published in the *Deseret News*, this contingent from the University of Utah was given places of honor on the podium at the Federal Way Stake Center of The Church of Jesus Christ of Latter-day Saints, where the funeral services were held (Van Leer 1983). Although Kolff deliv-

ered a eulogy to Barney Clark and his wife and family on behalf of the Utah group, he himself is not a Mormon.

8. There is a striking fit between the aphorisms William DeVries enjoyed quoting, cited earlier in this chapter, and these Mormon images, historical associations, and values.

9. Brigham Young University, located in Provo, Utah, was founded in 1875 and is still maintained by the Mormon Church.

10. The University of Utah, originally called the University of Deseret, founded in 1850, is 25 years older than Brigham Young University. The name Deseret, which was what the Mormons who settled Utah originally called the state, is from the *Book of Mormon*, where the word means "honey bee."

11. As Thomas O'Dea stated in his book *The Mormans*: "Health of the body [is] a central religious concern in Mormonism, valued for itself and also as a necessary means for accomplishment and progress in the present life" (O'Dea 1957, p. 144).

Chapter 7

1. Because our first visits to the University of Utah and Humana Hospital Audubon were made with funding from a private foundation, we did not submit protocols to those institutions' IRBs for permission to conduct interviews and make observations. As is required by federal regulations, however, we did contact the IRBs in January 1985 about the need to submit protocols when we applied for funding from the National Science Foundation. The Audubon Hospital IRB informed us that, in their judgment, our research did not "come under [their] purview" and therefore did not "require [IRB] approval or disapproval."

The University of Utah Medical Center IRB did require us to submit a protocol and consent forms to conduct a final round of interviews, including meetings with members of the IRB who had been involved with the Jarvik-7 protocols; we also indicated that, if possible, we would like to review IRB documents concerning the experiment. Our protocol was submitted in May 1985, and after extensive correspondence with both the university and medical center IRBs and the Vice President for Health Sciences it was approved in late October 1985. The major concerns about our research plans involved our acquiring "hearsay information" or "privileged information" through interviewing IRB members and being given access to IRB documents, and how we would "protect the privacy and confidentiality of third parties." Approval to conduct our field work was granted once we had satisfied the IRB on these matters, including the stipulation that we would examine only publicly available IRB documents, such as the minutes of meetings.

When we did hold a group interview with IRB members in August 1986, we distributed the consent forms for them to sign that the IRB had approved when it acted on our protocol and explained that they would have an opportunity to review the transcript of the session in light of the concerns about hearsay and privileged information. As we had found before when physicians are the subjects of research, there was much hesitancy and confusion on the part of the physician-members of the IRB when they read their consent forms. Most of them, to everyone's amusement, at first signed their names on the line for the investigator's signature and had to be reminded that in this instance we were the researchers and they were the subjects.

2. Three points about this statement merit emphasis. First, such a judgment is not unique to the case of the artificial heart. Second, sociologically, explanations for what transpired do not involve casting the various actors in the roles of villains or heroes. Third, the issues and patterns in the artificial heart experiment involved many factors other than social controls. As we discussed in Chapter 6, for example, dimensions such as the meanings of the heart and the American sociocultural context of efforts to develop artificial hearts were significant elements in the way the story unfolded.

3. The possible research pitfalls created by the powerful capacities of telemetry, data storage, and masses of computer-generated data analyses are scarcely unique to the artificial heart experiment. Here again, this case study illustrates more generic issues: In this instance, the ways the quality of clinical (or other) research can be compromised by a Sorcerer's Apprentice-like churning out of data, without a clear sense of what is being produced, and why, and too little running analysis of the information being gathered.

4. The three moratoria on the use of the Jarvik heart illustrate several of the ways moratoria can take place. The moratorium invoked by the Utah IRB after Barney Clark's implant was an internal and private one. That is, the decision was made within the confines of the institution and indeed within the confines of the IRB itself. Except for some media leaks, speculative reporting, and the always-present institutional grapevine discussions, it was a private affair, bounded by the confidentiality of IRB deliberations. The moratorium called by the FDA Advisory Panel, in contrast, was an externally imposed and public moratorium that involved regulatory decision-making, official records, and media coverage. The moratorium that was in effect from 1985 until the FDA recalled the Jarvik heart in 1990, finally, was de facto in the sense that there had not been an explicit decision by the device's manufacturer, investigator, corporate sponsor, IRB, or FDA that the experiment should stop.

References

Aaron, H., and Schwartz, W. B. 1990. Rationing health care: the choice before us. *Science* 247(26 January):418–447.

Abraham, L. 1988. Anencephalic organ donation system stymied by controversy. *American Medical News* (23/30 September):1, 10.

ACT Newsline. July 1989. Alexandria, Va.: American Council on Transplantation.

Ad Hoc Committee of the Harvard Medical School to Examine the Definition of Brain Death. 1968. A definition of irreversible coma. *Journal of the American Medical Association* 205(5 August):337–340.

Altieri, F. D., Watson, J. T., and Taylor, K.D. 1986. Mechanical support for the failing heart. *Journal of Biomaterials Applications* 1(July):106–156.

Altman, L. K. 1984a. After Barney Clark: reflections of a reporter on unresolved issues. In *After Barney Clark*, ed. M. W. Shaw, pp. 113–128. Austin: University of Texas Press.

————. 1984b. Surgeon's move highlights controversial trends. *New York Times* (7 August):C3.

————. 1984c. U. S. grants Utah team approval for 2nd test of an artificial heart. *New York Times* (20 June):A19.

————. 1984d. Utah surgeon moving heart implant program to Kentucky. *New York Times* (1 August):A19.

————. 1985a. Cause of heart recipient's death is undetected until too late. *New York Times* (26 April):A20.

————. 1985b. Publicity and medicine: the human factors. *New York Times* (1 January):A1.

————. 1986. A hero of medicine. *New York Times* (10 August):A1, A26.

————. 1987. 4,000 in U. S. now live with another's heart. *New York Times* (1 December):C3.

————. 1988. Artificial heart in turmoil. *New York Times* (17 May): C1, C3.

————. 1989a. Great success with drug in transplants of organs. *New York Times* (18 October):A1, B7.

————. 1989b. The limits of transplantation: how far should surgeons go? *New York Times* (19 December):C3.

————. 1989c. Tracking a new drug from the soil in Japan to organ transplants. *New York Times* (31 October):C3.

————. 1989d. With new boldness, surgeons create patchwork patients. *New York Times* (12 December):C1, C14.

————. 1990a. A question of ethics: should alcoholics get transplanted hearts? *New York Times* (April 3):C3.

————. 1990b. Researchers prepare for first human tests of an artificial lung. *New York Times* (9 January):C3.

————. 1990c. U.S. halts use of Jarvik heart. *New York Times* (12 January):A20.

————. 1991. FDA approves use in tests of pump to aid failing hearts. *New York Times* (4 January):A1, 15.

American Council on Transplantation. 1989. Miss Pennsylvania's participation in 1989 Miss America pageant is a real family affair. August press release.

American Medical Association. 1984. Judicial Council Statement. [Guidelines for experimental or clinical research on the artificial heart and animal organ transplants.] *American Medical News* 14 December.

————. 1985. Council on Scientific Affairs, Division of Evaluation and Nomenclature. Xenografts: review of the literature and current status. *Journal of the American Medical Association* 254(20 December):3355–3357.

Andrews, L. B. 1986. My body, my property. *Hastings Center Report* 16(October):28–38.

Annas, G. J. 1984. *Report of the Massachusetts Task Force on Organ Transplantation*. Boston: Boston University School of Public Health.

————. 1985a. No cheers for temporary artificial hearts. *Hastings Center Report* 15(October):27–28.

————. 1985b. The Phoenix heart: what we have to lose. *Hasting Center Report* 15(June):15–16.

————. 1986a. Death and the magic machine: informed consent to the artificial heart. *Western New England Law Review* 9:89–112.

————. 1986b. Legal and ethical issues in artificial heart experimentation. Testimony presented before the Subcommittee on Investigations and Oversight, Committee on Science and Technology, U. S. House of Representatives, 5 February.

————. 1987. From Canada with love: anencephalic infants as organ donors. *Hastings Center Report* 17(December):36–38.

————. 1988. The paradoxes of organ transplantation (editorial). *American Journal of Public Health* 78(June):621–622.

————. 1989. Feeling good about recycled hearts. *Second Opinion* 12(November):33–39.

Artificial heart recipient dies in Sweden. 1985. *Boston Globe* (22 November):8.

Asimov, I. 1976. The bicentennial man. In *The Bicentennial Man and Other Stories*. pp. 519–557. New York: Ballantine.

Atsumi, K. 1986. Research and development on the total artificial heart—from the engineering aspects. *Artificial Organs* 10:12–19.

Bailey, L. L., Nehlsen-Cannarella, S. L., Concepcion, W., et al. 1985. Baboon-to-human cardiac xenotransplantation in a neonate. *Journal of the American Medical Association* 254(20 December): 3321–3329.

Ballantyne, C. M., Podet, E. J., Patsch, W. P., et al. 1989. Effects of cyclosporine therapy on plasma lipoprotein levels. *Journal of the American Medical Association* 262(7 July):53–56.

Barber, B., and Fox, R. C. 1958. The case of the floppy-eared rabbits: an instance of serendipity gained and serendipity lost. *American Journal of Sociology* 64:128–136.

Barnette, M. 1984. Audubon gives preview of heart implant. *Louisville Times* (19 November).

Barron, J. 1984. Humana focus: technology. *New York Times* (14 August):D3,D4.

Bass, A. 1989. New liver surgery: pressure on parents. *Boston Globe* (17 December):1,75.

Baumgartner, W. A., Traill, T. A., Cameron, D. E., et al. 1989. Unique aspects of heart and lung transplantation exhibited in the "domino-donor" operation. *Journal of the American Medical Association* 26(2 June):3121–3125.

Bazell, R. 1985. Hearts of gold: winners and losers in the celebrity surgery sweepstakes. *New Republic* (18 February):17–20.

Bellah, R. N. 1970. Civil religion in America. In *Beyond Belief: Essays in Religion in a Post-traditional World.* pp. 168–189. New York: Harper & Row.

Berenson, C. K., and Grosser, B. I. 1984. Total artificial heart implantation. *Archives of General Psychiatry* 41(September):910–916.

Bernstein, B. J. 1981. The artificial heart program. *Center Magazine* 14 (May/June):22–23, discussion 34–41.

———. 1983. The artificial heart: is it a boon or a high-tech fix? *Nation* (22 January):7–12.

———. 1984. The misguided quest for the artificial heart. *Technology Review* (November/December):12–19, 62–63.

———. 1985. A moratorium on heart implants? *Discover* (July):87.

———. 1986. The pursuit of the artificial heart. *Medical Heritage* (March/April):80–100.

Bevan, W. 1971. On stimulating the gift of blood (editorial). *Science* 173(13 August):583.

Bewley, M. 1970. The land of Oz: America's great good place. In *Masks and Mirrors: Essays in Criticism.* pp. 255–267. New York: Atheneum.

Billingham, R. E. 1969. Basic genetical and immunological considerations. *Proceedings of the National Academy of Science* 63(August):1020–1025.

Blakeslee, S., ed. 1986. *Human Heart Replacement: A New Challenge for Physicians and Reporters.* Washington, D.C.: Foundation for American Communications and The Gannett Foundation.

Blumstein, J. F., and Sloan, F. A., eds. 1989. *Organ Transplantation Policy: Issues and Prospects.* Durham, N.C.: Duke University Press.

Boffey, P. M. 1988a. Battling with Congress over priorities on heart. *New York Times* (8 July):B7.

———. 1988b. Federal agency, in shift, to back artificial heart. *New York Times* (13 July):1, 12.

————. 1988c. Panel appeals for funds in artificial heart work. *New York Times* (20 May):A12.

Bok, S. 1978. *Lying: Moral Choices in Public and Private Life.* New York: Pantheon Press.

Booth, W. 1988. A change of heart. *Science* 240(20 May):976.

Bosk, C. L. 1979. *Forgive and Remember: Managing Medical Failure.* Chicago: University of Chicago Press.

————. 1985. The fieldworker as watcher and witness. *Hastings Center Report* 15:10–14.

Bosso, J. A. 1984a. Considerations of the institutional review board in artificial organ development. *Journal of Contemporary Law* 11:61–65.

————. 1984b. Deliberations of the Utah Institutional Review Board concerning the artificial heart. In *After Barney Clark,* ed. M. W. Shaw, pp. 139–145. Austin: University of Texas Press.

Breo, D. L. 1989. Two surgeons who dared are still chasing their dreams. *Journal of the American Medical Association* 262(24 November):2904, 2910–2911, 2916.

Broad, W. J. 1991. Cold-fusion claim is faulted on ethics as well as science. *New York Times* (17 March):1, 30.

Browne, M. W. 1988. U. S. halts funds to develop artificial hearts for humans. *New York Times* (13 May):A1, A32.

Buckley, M. J. 1985. [American College of Cardiology] Testimony before the Food and Drug Circulatory System Advisory Panel Hearing on Artificial Heart Implants, December 20.

Busuttil, R. W. 1991. Living-related liver donation: CON. *Transplantation Proceedings* 23(February):43–45.

Calabresi, G., and Bobbit, P. 1978. *Tragic Choices.* New York: Norton.

Callahan, D. 1989. *What Kind of Life. The Limits of Medical Progress.* New York: Simon & Schuster.

————. 1990a. Modernizing mortality: medical progress and the good society. *Hastings Center Report* 20(January/February): 28–32.

————. 1990b. Rationing medical progress: the way to affordable health care. *New England Journal of Medicine* 322(21 June):1810–1813.

Cancila, C. 1986. Health care's McDonald's? Humana starts ambitious new marketing campaign. *American Medical News* (20 June):3, 29.

Cantin, M., and Genest, J. 1986. The heart as an endocrine gland. *Scientific American* 254(February):76–81.

Caplan, A. L. 1982. The artificial heart. *Hastings Center Report* 12(February):22–24.

————. 1984a. Ethical and policy issues in the procurement of cadaver organs for transplantation. *New England Journal of Medicine* 311(11 October):981–983.

————. 1984b. Organ procurement: it's not in the cards. *Hastings Center Report* 14(October):9–12.

————. 1984c. Should doctors move at a gallop? *New York Times* (17 August):25.

————. 1988. Professional arrogance and public misunderstanding. *Hastings Center Report* 18(April/May):34–37.

Carpenter, C. B. 1990. Immunosuppression in organ transplantation. *New England Journal of Medicine* 322(26 April):1224–1226.

Carter, M. N. 1983. The business behind Barney Clark's heart. *Money* (April):130–144.

Case studies: in organ transplants, Americans first? 1986. *Hastings Center Report* 16(October):23–25.

Casscells, W. 1986. Heart transplantation: recent policy developments. *New England Journal of Medicine* 315(20 November):1365–1368.

Cate, F. H., and Laudicina, S. S. 1991. Transplantation white paper: current statistical information about transplantation in America. Washington, D.C.: The Annenberg Program in Communication Policy Studies of Northwestern University and the United Network for Organ Sharing.

Centers of Excellence. 1986. Louisville, Ky.: Humana, Inc.

Chengappa, R. 1990. The organs bazaar. *India Today* (31 July):30–37.

Childress, J. F. 1986. The implications of major western religious traditions for policies regarding human biological materials. Contract paper prepared for U.S. Congress, Office of Technology Assessment.

————. 1987. Some moral connections between organ procurement and organ distribution. *Journal of Contemporary Health Law and Policy* 3:85–110.

————. 1989. Ethical criteria for procuring and distributing organs for transplantation. In *Organ Transplantation Policy: Issues and Prospects*, eds. J. F. Blumstein and F. A. Sloan, pp. 87–113. Durham, N.C.: Duke University Press.

Clark, M. 1984. A surgical star jumps ship. *Newsweek* (13 August):65.

Close, F. 1991. *Too Hot to Handle. The Race for Cold Fusion.* Princeton, N. J.: Princeton University Press.

Cohen, C., and Benjamin, M. 1991. Alcoholics and liver transplantation. *Journal of the American Medical Association* 265(13 March):1299–1301.

ConFusion in a jar. 1990. Transcript of "NOVA" program no. 1802, April 30.

Control of life. Pt 3 (Rebuilt people). 1965. *Life* 59(24 September):66–84.

Cooley, D. A., Akutsu, T., Norman, J. C., et al. 1981. Total artificial heart in two-staged cardiac transplantation. *Cardiovascular Diseases: Bulletin of the Texas Heart Institute* 8:305–319.

————, Liotta, D., Hallman, G. L., et al. 1969. Orthotopic cardiac prosthesis for two-staged cardiac replacement. *American Journal of Cardiology* 24(November):723–730.

Copeland, J. G., Levinson, M. M., Smith, R., et al. 1986. The total artificial heart as a bridge to transplantation. *Journal of the American Medical Association* 256(5 December):2991–2998.

Cotton, P. 1990. Living-donor liver transplants cap surgical research for decade of 1980s. *Journal of the American Medical Association* 263(5 January):13–14.

Council of The Transplantation Society. 1985. Commercialisation in transplantation: the problems and some guidelines for practice. *Lancet* 2(28 September):715–716.

Cowart, V. S. 1987. Artificial heart implants began five years ago. *Journal of the American Medical Association* 258:305.

Crammond, W. A. 1967. Renal homotransplantation: some observations on recipients and donors. *British Journal of Psychiatry* 113:1223–1230.

Crawshaw, R., and Garland, M. 1985. *Society Must Decide: Ethics and Health Care Choices in Oregon.* Salem, Ore.: Oregon Health Decisions.

Culliton, B. 1988. Politics of the heart. *Science* 241(15 July): 283.

Cummings, N. B. 1989. Social, ethical, and legal issues involved in chronic maintenance dialysis. In *Replacement of Renal Function by Dialysis*, ed. J. F. Maher, pp. 1141–1158. Dordrecht, The Netherlands: Kluwer Academic Publishers.

Daniels, N. 1986. Why saying no to patients in the United States is so hard: cost containment, justice, and provider autonomy. *New England Journal of Medicine* 314(22 May):1380–1393.

―――. 1991. Is the Oregon rationing plan fair? *Journal of the American Medical Association* 265(1 May):2232–2235.

Danovitch, G. 1986. Letter to the editor. *New England Journal of Medicine* 315(11 September):714.

Darby, J. M., Stein, K., Grenvik, A., et al. 1989. Approach to management of the heart-beating "brain dead" organ donor. *Journal of the American Medical Association* 261(21 April):2222–2228.

DeBakey, M. E., Hall, C. W., Hellums, J. D., et al. 1969. Orthotopic cardiac prosthesis: preliminary experiments in animals with biventricular artificial heart. *Cardiovascular Research Center Bulletin* 7(April/June): 127–142.

DeVries finds portions of lost medical records. 1985. *Deseret News* (12 June):B2.

DeVries, W. C. 1985. The artificial heart. Presentation at Conference on Transplantation and Artificial Organs: Issues Along the Experiment-Therapy Spectrum. Sponsored by The Acadia Institute, Medicine in the Public Interest and PRIM&R. Boston, November 4–5.

―――. 1988. The permanent artificial heart: four case reports. *Journal of the American Medical Association* 259(12 February):849–859.

―――, and Joyce, L. D. 1983. The artificial heart. *Ciba Clinical Symposia*, 35(6):1–32.

―――, and Symbion, Inc. 1983. Special patient consent for the implantation of the total artificial heart and related procedures (unpublished).

―――, Anderson, J. L., Joyce, L. D., et al. 1984. Clinical use of the total artificial heart. *New England Journal of Medicine* 310(2 February):273–278.

―――, Kwan-Gett, C. S., and Kolff, W. J. 1970. Consumptive coagulopathy, shock, and the artificial heart. *ASAIO Transactions* 16:29–36.

Didisheim, P., Olsen, D. B., Farrar, D. J., et al. 1989. Infections and thromboembolism with implantable cardiovascular devices. *ASAIO Transactions* 35:54–70.

Doctor says it's time to resume using permanent artificial hearts. 1989. *Bangor Daily News* (July 22–23):30.

Dracula of medical technology (editorial) 1988. *New York Times* (21 May):A16.

Dubos, R. 1987. *Mirage of Health. Utopias, Progress, and Biological Change.* New Brunswick, N.J.: Rutgers University Press.

Edson, L. 1979. The search for a "bionic" heart. *New York Times Magazine* (21 October):36ff.

Egan, T. 1990. Oregon lists illnesses by priority to see who gets medicaid care; aid to be tied to cost and how many can benefit. *New York Times* (3 May):A1, B10.

Eggers, P. 1988. Effect of transplantation on the medicare end-stage renal disease program. *New England Journal of Medicine* 318(28 January):223–229.

Eichwald, E. J., Woolley, F. R., Cole, B., et al. 1981. Insertion of the artificial heart. *IRB* (August-September):4–5.

Evans, R. W. 1986. The heart transplant dilemma. *Issues in Science and Technology* 2(3):91–101.

————, and Broida, J. H. 1985. *The National Heart Transplantation Study*. Seattle, Wash.: Battelle Human Affairs Research Centers.

————, Manninen, D. L., Overcast, T. D., et al. 1984. *The National Heart Transplantation Study: Final report*. Seattle, Wash.: Battelle Human Affairs Research Centers.

Federal Register 1980. Medical devices, procedures for investigational device exemptions. 45(January 18):3732–3759. Amended, 1980. 45(September 5):58841–58843.

Federal Register 1985. Guidance for the emergency use of unapproved medical devices; availability. 50(October 22):42866–42867.

Fellner, C. H., and Marshall, J. R. 1968. Twelve kidney donors. *Journal of the American Medical Association* 206(16 December): 2703–2707.

————, and Marshall, J. R. 1970. Kidney donors: The myth of informed consent. *American Journal of Psychiatry* 126(March): 1245–1251.

————, and Schwartz, S. H. 1971. Altruism in disrepute: medical versus public attitudes toward the living organ donor. *New England Journal of Medicine* 284(18 March):582–585.

Fields, A., Harasaki, H., Sands, D., et al. 1983. Infection in artificial blood pump implantation. *ASAIO Transactions* 29:532–58.

Fineberg, H. V. 1983. *Final Report of the Task Force on Liver Transplantation*. Boston: Department of Public Health, Commonwealth of Massachusetts.

Fox, R. C. 1959. *Experiment Perilous*. Glencoe, IL: Free Press; University of Pennsylvania Press [paperback edition, 1974].

————. 1978. Organ transplantation: sociocultural aspects. In *Encyclopedia of Bioethics* (Vol. 3), ed. W. T. Reich, pp. 1166–1169. New York: Free Press.

————. 1984. "It's the same, but different": a sociological perspective on the case of the Utah artificial heart. In *After Barney Clark*. ed. M. W. Shaw, pp. 68–90. Austin: University of Texas Press.

————. 1986. A preface. The cultural shaping of biomedical science and technology [entire issue]. *International Journal of Technology Assessment in Health Care* 2(2):189–194.

————, 1989. The sociology of bioethics. In *The Sociology of Medicine: A Participant Observer's View*. pp. 224–276. Englewood Cliffs, NJ: Prentice-Hall.

————, and Swazey, J. P. 1974. *The Courage to Fail: A Social View of Organ Transplants and Dialysis*. Chicago: University of Chicago Press.

————, and Swazey, J. P. 1978a. *The Courage to Fail. A Social View of Organ Transplants and Dialysis* (2nd ed. rev.). Chicago: University of Chicago Press.

————, and Swazey, J. P. 1978b. Kidney dialysis and transplantation. In *Encyclopedia of Bioethics* (Vol. 2), ed. W. T. Reich, pp. 811–816. New York: Free Press.

————, and Swazey, J. P. 1982. Critical care at Tianjin's First Central Hospital and the fourth modernization. *Science* 217(20 August):700–705.

————, and Swazey, J. P. 1984. Medical morality is not bioethics—medical ethics in China and the United States. *Perspectives in Biology and Medicine* 27(3):336–360.

————, Swazey, J. P., and Cameron, E. M. 1984. Social and ethical problems in the treatment of end-stage renal disease patients. In *Controversies in Nephrology and Hypertension*, ed. R. G. Narins, pp. 45–70. New York: Churchill Livingstone.

Freidson, E. 1975. *Doctoring Together. A Study of Professional Social Control.* New York: Elsevier.

Friedman, E. 1989. The torturer's horse (Commentary/Caring for the poor). *Journal of the American Medical Association* 261(10 March):1481–1482.

Gallup Organization. 1985. *The U. S. Public's Attitude Toward Organ Transplants/Organ Donation.* Princeton, N.J.: Gallup.

Gil, G. 1987. Anatomy of a transplant. *Louisville Courier-Journal* (20 December):1ff.

————. 1988. Infection kills Walton Jones, oldest man to get temporary artificial heart. *Louisville Courier-Journal* (18 January):A1, A8.

————, King, M., and Cross, A. 1986. Schroeder dies after 620 days on Jarvik-7. *Louisville Courier-Journal* (7 August):1, 8–9.

Gill, T. J., and Lund, R. D. 1989. Implantation of tissue into the brain. *Journal of the American Medical Association* 261(12 May):2674–2676.

Gladwell, M. 1990. FDA recalls artificial heart used in historic transplants. *Washington Post* (January 11):1.

Glaser, R. J. 1985. The artificial heart—show business or science? (editorial) *Pharos* (Summer):38.

Goetz, C. G., Olanow, C. W., and Koller, W. C. 1989a. Letter to the editor. *New England Journal of Medicine* 321(3 August):326–327.

————, Olanow, C. W., Koller, W. C., et al. 1989b. Multicenter study of autologous adrenal medullary transplantation to the corpus striatum in patients with advanced Parkinson's disease. *New England Journal of Medicine* 320(9 February):337–341.

Goldsmith, M. F. 1988. Anencephalic organ donor program suspended; Loma Linda report expected to detail findings. *Journal of the American Medical Association* 260(23/30 September):1671–1672.

————. 1989. New visceral transplants invigorate cancer victims. *Journal of the American Medical Association* (10 March):1397.

————. 1991. First implant of portable heart-assist device. *Journal of the American Medical Association* 265(12 June):2930, 2933.

Gonzales, L. 1986. The rock 'n roll heart of Robert Jarvik. *Playboy* (April):84ff.

Gore, Senator Albert, Jr. 1986. [Public] Letter to Frank E. Young, Commissioner, Food and Drug Administration, February 5.

Gorovitz, S. 1984. Against selling bodily parts. *QQ: Report from the Center for Philosophy and Public Policy* 4(2):9–12.

Gray, B. H., ed. 1983. *The New Health Care for Profit: Doctors and Hospitals in a Competitive Environment.* Washington, D.C.: Institute of Medicine/National Academy Press.

Gréen, K., Liska, J., Egbert, N., et al. 1987. Hemostatic disturbances associated with implantation of an artificial heart. *Thrombosis Research* 48(3):349–362.

Greene, G. 1983. *Monsignor Quixote.* New York: Pocket Books, Washington Square Press.

Griffith, B. P., Hardesty, R. L., Kormos, R. L., et al. 1987. Temporary use of the Jarvik-7 total artificial heart before transplantation. *New England Journal of Medicine* 316(15 January):130–134.

Gutkind, L. 1988. *Many Sleepless Nights.* New York: W. W. Norton & Company.

Hadorn, D. 1991. Setting health care priorities in Oregon: cost effectiveness meets the rule of rescue. *Journal of the American Medical Association* 265(1 May):2218–2224.

Hallowell, C. 1985. Charles Lindbergh's artificial heart. *American Heritage of Technology and Invention* (Fall):58–62.

Hansmann, H. 1989. The economics and ethics of markets for organs. In *Organ Transplantation Policy: Issues and Prospects,* ed. J. F. Blumstein and F. A. Sloan, pp. 57–85. Durham, N.C.: Duke University Press.

Hardin, G. 1968. The tragedy of the commons. *Science* 162(13 Dec.):1243–1248.

Hastings, W. L., Aaron, J. L., Deneris, J., et al. 1981. A retrospective study of nine calves surviving five months on the pneumatic total artificial heart. *ASAIO Transactions* 27:71–76.

Havighurst, C. C., and King, N.M.P. 1989. Liver transplantation in Massachusetts: public policymaking as morality play. In *Organ Transplantation Policy: Issues and Prospects,* ed. J. F. Blumstein and F. A. Sloan, pp. 229–260. Durham, N.C.: Duke University Press.

Haydon best hope yet. 1985. *Bangor Daily News* (18 February):1–2.

Hazle, D. 1987. Mr. Walton Jones. Humana Hospital Audubon press advisories, December 4–28.

Heart of gold. 1983. *The Progressive* (12 February):12.

Heart patient steps forward grateful for extended life. 1985. *New York Times* (20 July):8.

Heart of the experiment (editorial). 1985. *New York Times* (7 January):A16.

Herskowitz, L. 1986. With latest death, criticism of artificial-heart program. *Philadelphia Inquirer* (8 August):7A.

Hiatt, H. 1975. Protecting the medical commons: who is responsible? *New England Journal of Medicine* 293(31 July):235–241.

Hittman Associates. 1966. *Final Summary Report on Six Studies Basic to the Consideration of the Artificial Heart Program.* Baltimore, Md.: Hittman Associates.

Hogness, J. R., and VanAntwerp, M., eds. 1991. *The Artificial Heart. Prototypes, Policies, and Patients.* Committee to evaluate the Artificial Heart Program of the National Heart, Lung, and Blood Institute. Institute of Medicine. Washington, D.C.: National Academy Press [prepublication edition].

Holder, A. 1980. The FDA's final regulations: IRBs and medical devices. *IRB* 2(June/July):1–4.

Hostetler, A. J. 1991. Calf sets record with Penn State Heart. *Philadelphia Inquirer* (21 July):5-B.

Humana Heart Institute International News Release. November 23, 1984. Artificial heart patient selected. Surgery scheduled for Sunday, November 25.

Humana Heart Institute International. 1985. *First report.*

Humana Inc. 1985. *Humana and the Artificial Heart.*

Iglehart, J. K. 1983. Transplantation: the problem of limited resources. *New England Journal of Medicine* 309(14 July):123–128.

Irvine, R. B. 1987. *When You Are the Headline: Managing a Major News Story.* Homewood, Ill.: Dow Jones-Irwin.

Jacobsen-Wells, J. 1987. Heart research beating strongly. *Deseret News* (17 October):B1–B2.

Jarvik, R. K. 1981. The total artificial heart. *Scientific American* 244(1):74–80.

Jiao, S., Zhang, W. C., Ding, M. C., et al. 1987. The clinical study of adrenal medullary tissue transplantation to striatum in parkinsonism. Presented at the Schmitt Neurological Sciences Symposium, Rochester, N.Y., June 30–July 3.

Jonas, H. 1970. Philosophical reflections on experimenting with subjects. In *Experimentation with Human Subjects,* ed. P. A. Freund, pp. 1–31. New York: George Braziller.

Jonsen, A. 1986. Bentham in a box: technology assessment and health care allocation. *Law, Medicine, and Health Care* 14:172–174.

Joyce, L. D., DeVries, W. C., Hastings, W. L., et al. 1983. Response of the human body to the first permanent implant of the Jarvik-7 total artificial heart. *ASAIO Transactions* 29:81–84, 87.

———, Johnson, K. E., Pierce, W. S., et al. 1986. Summary of the world experience with clinical use of total artificial hearts as heart support devices. *Journal of Heart Transplantation* 5(May/June):229–235.

Kahan, B. D. 1981. Cosmas and Damian in the 20th century? (editorial). *New England Journal of Medicine* 305(30 July):280–281.

———. 1989. Cyclosporine. *New England Journal of Medicine* 321(21 December):1725–1738.

Kaye, H. L. 1986. *The Social Meaning of Modern Biology.* New Haven, Conn.: Yale University Press.

———. 1991. Cultural being or biological being: the "implications" of modern biology. Unpublished.

Kearney, W., and Caplan, A. L. 1991. Parity for the donation of bone marrow: ethical and policy considerations. In A. Bonnicksen and R. Blank, eds. *Emerging Issues in Biomedical Policy,* pp. 262–285. New York: Columbia University Press.

King, M. 1984a. AMA officials criticize Humana heart project. *Louisville Courier-Journal* (6 December):B1.

———. 1984b. Artificial heart gets go-ahead at Audubon. *Louisville Courier-Journal* (9 November):A1, A8.

————. 1984c. Artificial heart plans get quick approval from Audubon board. *Louisville Courier-Journal* (21 September):A1f.

————. 1984d. Delays in Utah led heart surgeon to Louisville. *Louisville Courier-Journal* (5 August):A1, A20.

————. 1984e. DeVries adjusts to added spotlight on his operating room. *Louisville Courier-Journal* (12 August):A1.

————. 1984f. Doctors dominate panel deciding on artificial-heart operation. *Louisville Courier-Journal* (21 September).

————. 1984g. Research money attracted heart surgeon. *Louisville Courier-Journal* (1 August):A1, A10.

————. 1984h. Surgeon defends procedure for implant. *Louisville Courier-Journal* (9 November):A1, A8.

————. 1985a. Artificial-heart project stymied while DeVries waits for right patient. *Louisville Times* (20 October):1.

————. 1985b. FDA panel to discuss artificial heart's future. *Louisville Courier-Journal* (2 December):B1.

————. 1986a. Artificial heart surgery to become commonplace soon, DeVries says. *Louisville Courier-Journal* (18 September): B1, B3.

————. 1986b. Experts question increased use of Jarvik-7 as temporary tool. *Louisville Times* (12 February):A1.

————. 1986c. Haydon remains tied to machines after year on artificial heart. *Louisville Courier-Journal* (17 February):A1.

————. 1986d. Medicine and the media. *Louisville Medicine* (October):17.

————. 1986e. Regulations hampering research on artificial heart, DeVries says. *Louisville Courier-Journal* (6 February):B1.

————. 1986f. Schroeder family unity shines through funeral. *Louisville Courier-Journal* (10 August):A1, A4.

————. 1987a. Heart surgeon DeVries severs ties with Lansing. *Louisville Courier-Journal* (2 June):1.

————. 1987b. Jarvik fired as chairman of mechanical-heart firm. *Louisville Courier-Journal* (28 April):B6.

————. 1987c. Jarvik-7 put in man whose heart failed. *Atlanta Journal-Constitution* (5 December):4A.

————. 1988. Transplants: a shadow is cast over the century's medical miracle. *Atlanta Journal-Constitution* (17 July):1ff.

————, and Gil, G. 1986. The end to Schroeder's struggle touched many. *Louisville Courier-Journal* (8 August):A1, A4.

Kirkman, R. L., and Ferry, J. A. 1991. A 56-year-old woman with pneumoperitoneum three months after receiving a renal transplant: Case 29–1991. Case records of the Massachusetts General Hospital. *New England Journal of Medicine* 325(18 July):183–195.

Kitzhaber, J. A. 1988. Health care rationing. *State Government News* (June):22–23.

————. 1990. Rationing health care: the Oregon model. *The Center Report* [The Center for Public Policy and Contemporary Issues. University of Denver] 2(1):3–4.

Kjellstrand, C. M. 1988. Age, sex, and race inequality in renal transplantation. *Archives of Internal Medicine* 148:1305–1309.

Kluge, E. H. 1989. Designated organ donation: private choice in social context. *Hastings Center Report* 19(September/October):10–16.

Knox, R. 1984a. State opposes a heart transplant. *Boston Globe* (4 January):1.

————. 1984b. Task force debates arrangements for heart transplants. *Boston Globe* (13 April):25.

————. 1984c. Transplant insurance expanded. *Boston Globe* (2 February):25.

Kolata, G. 1989a. Complication occurs in liver transplant. *New York Times* (28 November):C10.

————. 1989b. First U.S. liver transplant from a living donor. *New York Times* (27 November):A1, B9.

————. 1991a. Lungs from parents fail to save girl, 9, and doctors assess ethics. *New York Times* (20 May):A11.

————. 1991b. More babies being born to be donors of tissues. *New York Times* (4 June):A1,C3.

Kolff, J. 1982. The heart that Temple has. *Temple M.D.* Winter/Spring:7–13.

————. 1984. Artificial heart substitution: the total or auxiliary artificial heart. *Transplantation Proceedings* 16(June):898–907.

Kolff, W. J. 1983a. Artificial organs—forty years and beyond. *ASAIO Transactions* 29:6–24.

————. 1983b. Words spoken at the funeral service for Dr. Barney Clark (29 March). Unpublished.

Korcok, M. 1985. The business of ethics. *Canadian Medical Association Journal* 132(15 March):676–687.

Kwan-Gett, C. S., DeVries, W. C., and Kolff, W. J. 1969. Performance of an autoregulatory cardiac prosthesis (abstract). *Circulation* (suppl. III):128.

Langone, J. 1986. The artificial heart is really very dangerous. *Discover* (June):38–48.

Lawrie, G. M. 1988. Permanent implantation of the Jarvik-7 total artificial heart: a clinical perspective. *Journal of the American Medical Association* 259(12 February):892–893.

Leaf, A. 1980. The MGH trustees say no to heart transplants. *New England Journal of Medicine* 302(8 May):1087–1088.

Levey, A. S., Hou, S, and Bush, H. L., Jr. 1986. Kidney transplantation from unrelated living donors: time to reclaim a discarded opportunity. *New England Journal of Medicine* 314(3 April):914–916.

Levine, C. 1985. Why Blacks need more kidneys but donate fewer. *Hastings Center Report* 15(August):3.

Levinsky, N. G., and Rettig, R. A., eds. 1991a. *Kidney Failure and the Federal Government*. Washington, D.C.: National Academy Press.

————, and Rettig, R. A. 1991b. The Medicare end-stage renal disease program: a report from the Institute of Medicine. *New England Journal of Medicine* 324(18 April):1143–1148.

Lewin, R. 1987. Dramatic results with brain grafts. *Science* 237(17 July):245–247.

Lin, H. S., Rocher, L. I., McQuillan, M. A., et al. 1989. Cyclosporine-induced hyperuricemia and gout. *New England Journal of Medicine* 321(August):287–292.

Lindsey, P. A., and McGlynn, E. A. 1988. State coverage for organ transplantation: a framework for decision making. *Health Science Research* 22(6):881–927.

Lubeck, D. P. 1986. The artificial heart: costs, risks, and benefits—an update. *International Journal of Technology Assessment in Health Care* 2(3):369–386.

———, and Bunker, J. P. 1982. *The Artificial Heart: Costs, Risks, and Benefits: Case Study #9*. U.S. Congress, Office of Technology Assessment. Washington, D.C.: U.S. Government Printing Office.

MacNeil/Lehrer News Hour. 1984. Dr. William DeVries: a change of heart (1 August, Transcript 2308).

Madrazo, I., Drucker-Colin, R., Diaz, V., et al. 1987a. Open microsurgical autograft of adrenal medulla to the right caudate nucleus in two patients with intractable Parkinson's disease. *New England Journal of Medicine* 316(2 April):831–834.

———, Drucker-Colin, R., Leon, V., et al. 1987b. Adrenal medulla transplanted to caudate nucleus for treatment of Parkinson's disease: report of 10 cases. *Surgical Forum* 38:510–512.

Mallove, E. F. 1991. *Fire from Ice. Searching for the Truth Behind the Cold-Fusion Furor*. New York: John Wiley & Sons.

Manninen, D. L., and Evans, R. W. 1985. Public attitudes and behavior regarding organ donation. *Journal of the American Medical Association* 253(7 June):111–115.

Markle, G. E., and Chubin, D. E. 1987. Consensus development in biomedicine: the liver transplant controversy. *Milbank Quarterly* 65:1–24.

Marshall, E. 1991. Artificial heart: the beat goes on. *Science* 253(2 August):500–502.

Martyn, S., Wright, R., and Clark, L. 1988. Required request for organ donation: moral, clinical, and legal problems. *Hastings Center Report* 18(April/May):27–34.

Marx, L. 1964. *The Machine in the Garden*. New York: Oxford University Press.

Mauss, M. 1954. *The Gift: Forms and Functions of Exchange in Archaic Societies*. Trans. Ian Cunnison. Glencoe, Ill.: Free Press.

Mayfield, M. 1986. DeVries believes in more "Bionic Bills." *USA Today* (7 August):1,2.

McDonald, J. C. 1988. The national organ procurement and transplantation network. *Journal of the American Medical Association* 259(5 February):725–726.

McIntosh, C. L. 1986. Statement by [the] Chairman, Circulatory System Devices Advisory Panel, U.S. Food and Drug Administration, before the Subcommittee on Investigations and Oversight, Committee on Science and Technology, U.S. House of Representatives, February 5.

McMurran, K. 1987. There's nothing artificial about the way Robert Jarvik's heart beats for his brainy bride-to-be. *People* (27 July):47–50.

Mead, M. 1977. *Letters from the Field, 1925–1975*. New York: Harper & Row. [volume 52 in the World Perspectives series, ed. Ruth Nanda Anshen]

Medical record of Barney Clark is missing from the U. 1985. *Deseret News* (4 March):3.

Medical Task Force on Anencephaly. 1990. The infant with anencephaly. *New England Journal of Medicine* 322(8 March):669–674.

Medicare to cover some liver transplants. 1990. *New York Times* (10 March):8.

Medicare coverage is approved for liver transplant operations. 1991. *New York Times* (14 April):A24.

Melville, H. 1924. *Billy Budd, Sailor.* Chicago: University of Chicago Press, ed. 1962.

Mendelsohn, E., Swazey, J. P., and Taviss, I. eds. 1971. *Human Aspects of Biomedical Innovation.* Cambridge, Mass.: Harvard University Press.

Merton, R. K. 1961. Singletons and multiples in scientific discovery. *Proceedings of the American Philosophical Society* 105(October):470–486.

Merz, B. 1990. FDA cites deficiencies, withdraws approval for Jarvik-7 artificial heart. *American Medical News* (26 January):1, 31.

Meslin, M. 1987. Heart. Tr. K. Anderson. In *The Encylopedia of Religion* (Vol. 6), Mircea Eliade, editor in chief, pp. 234–237. New York: Macmillan and Free Press.

Miller, A. 1949. *Death of a Salesman.* New York: Viking Press.

Mills, D. 1988. Artificial-heart researchers see red over loss of funds. *Washington Times* (31 May):E1, E12.

Mims, R. 1987. DeVries departure fails to daunt U. of U. heart researchers. *Salt Lake City Tribune* (29 November).

Miscellanea Medica. 1990. *Journal of the American Medical Association* 263(23/30 May):2721.

Moore, F. D. 1964. New problems for surgery. *Science* 144(24 April):388–392.

––––––. 1968. Medical responsibility for the prolongation of life. *Journal of the American Medical Association* 206(7 October):384–386.

––––––. 1989. The desperate case: CARE (costs, applicability, research, ethics). *Journal of the American Medical Association* 261(10 March):1483–1484.

Morrow, L. 1991. When one body can save another. *Time* (17 June):54–58.

Moss, A. H., and Siegler, M. 1991. Should alcoholics compete equally for liver transplantation? *Journal of the American Medical Association* 265(13 March):1295–1298.

Mullan, F., and Jacoby, I. 1985. The town meeting for technology: the maturation of the consensus conference. *Journal of the American Medical Association* 254(23/30 August):1068–1072.

Murray, K. D., Hughes, S., Bearnson, D., et al. 1983. Infection in total heart recipients. *ASAIO Transactions* 29:539–545.

––––––, and Olsen, D. B. 1984. The Utah artificial heart: success in the laboratory and its application to man. *Journal of Contemporary Law* 1:4–28.

National Heart, Lung, and Blood Institute. 1984. *Devices and Technology Branch Contractors Meeting, 1983. Summary and Abstracts.* Cleveland: ISAO Press.

––––––. 1985a. *Devices and Technology Branch Contractors Meeting, 1984. Summary and Abstracts.* Washington, D.C.: U.S. Government Printing Office. 1985-461-338-814/36014.

––––––. 1985b. *Devices and Technology Branch Contractors Meeting, 1985. Program and Abstracts.* Washington, D.C.: U.S. Government Printing Office. 1985-491-313-814/44703.

––––––. 1986. *Devices and Technology Branch Contractors Meeting, 1986. Program and Abstracts.* Washington, D.C.: U.S. Government Printing Office. 1986-0-167-449:QL 3.

————. Division of Heart and Vascular Diseases. 1982. *Devices and Technology Branch Contractors Meeting. Program.* Washington, D.C.: U.S. Government Printing Office. 381–132:706.

————. Working Group on Mechanical Circulatory Support. 1985c. *Artificial Heart and Assist Devices: Directions, Needs, Costs, Societal and Ethical Issues.* U.S. Dept. HHS Publ. (NIH) 85–2723.

National Institutes of Health. 1973. *The Totally Implantable Artificial Heart: Economic, Ethical, Legal, Medical, Psychiatric, and Social Implications.* Bethesda, Md.: National Institutes of Health.

————. 1983a. *Liver Transplantation.* NIH Consensus Development Conference Summary 4(7).

————. 1983b. *Liver Transplantation: Speakers' Presentations.* Washington, D.C.: NIH.

Neu, S., and Kjellstrand, C. M. 1986. Stopping long-term dialysis: an empirical study of withdrawal of life-supporting treatment. *New England Journal of Medicine* 314(2 January):14–20.

New liver transplant recipient in "outstanding" recovery. 1989. *New York Times* (28 November):49.

O'Dea, T. F. 1957. *The Mormons.* Chicago: University of Chicago Press.

Ohnuki-Tierney, E. 1984. *Illness and Culture in Contemporary Japan. An Anthropological View.* New York: Cambridge University Press.

Olsen, D. 1987. ISAO international registry: bridge-to-transplant experience with the Jarvik-7 and the Jarvik-7-70 artificial heart. *Artificial Organs* 11:63–68.

Oregon rationing plan: inspired or misguided? 1990. *Healthweek* (21 May):18

Pae, W. E., and Pierce, W. S. 1987. Combined registry for the clinical use of mechanical ventricular assist pumps and the total artificial heart: first official report—1986. *Journal of Heart Transplantation* 6:68–70.

Park, P. M. 1989. The transplant odyssey. *Second Opinion* 12(November):27–32.

Patient a father, a neighbor and a "fighter." 1985. *New York Times* (17 February):20.

Peabody, J. L., Emery, J. R., and Ashwal, S. 1989. Experience with anencephalic infants as prospective organ donors. *New England Journal of Medicine* 321(10 August):334–350.

Pellegrino, E. D. 1991. Families' self-interest and the cadaver's organs: what price consent? *Journal of the American Medical Association* 265(13 March):1305–1306.

Pennington, G. 1985. [Society of Thoracic Surgeons] Testimony before the Food and Drug Circulatory System Advisory Panel Hearing on Artificial Heart Implants, December 20.

Pennock, J. L., Pierce, W. S., Campbell, D. B., et al. 1986. Mechanical support of the circulation followed by cardiac transplantation. *Journal of Thoracic Cardiovascular Surgery* 92:994–1004.

Peters, D. A. 1986. Protecting autonomy in organ procurement procedures: some overlooked issues. *Milbank Quarterly* 64(2):241–270.

Peters, T. G. 1991. Life or death: the issue of payment in cadaveric organ donation. *Journal of the American Medical Association* 265(13 March):1302–1305.

Peterson, C. N. 1983. Terminal events. Unpublished news conference about Barney Clark's death (24 March).

————. 1984. A spontaneous reply to Dr. Lawrence Altman. In *After Barney Clark*, ed. M. W. Shaw, pp. 129–138. Austin: University of Texas Press.

Pierce, H. W. 1985. Presby has new transplants policy. *Pittsburgh Post Gazette* (18 July):1, 14.

Pierce, W. S. 1988. Permanent heart substitution: better solutions lie ahead (editorial). *Journal of the American Medical Association* 259(12 February):891.

Pirsch, J. D., Sollinger, H. W., Kalayoglu, M., et al. 1988. Living-unrelated renal transplantation: results in 40 patients. *American Journal of Kidney Diseases* 12(December):499–503 [in Domestic abstracts, *Journal of the American Medical Association* 262(21 July, 1989):404].

Pittsburgh surgeon seeks hiatus on multiple-organ transplants. 1989. *Philadelphia Inquirer* (15 January).

Poole, R. 1989. How cold fusion happened—twice! *Science* 244(28 April):420–423.

President's Commission for the Study of Ethical Problems in Medicine and Biomedical and Behavioral Research. 1981. *Defining Death: Medical, Legal and Ethical Issues in the Determination of Death*. Washington, D.C.: U.S. Government Printing Office.

————. 1983. *Securing Access to Health Care: The Ethical Implications of Differences in the Availability of Health Services* (Vol. 1: Report). Washington, D.C.: U.S. Government Printing Office.

Preston, T. A. 1983. The case against the artificial heart. *The Weekly* (Seattle) 30 March–5 April:25ff.

————. 1985a. The artificial heart controversy: research, rationing, and regulation. *Medical World News* (11 February):37.

————. 1985b. Who benefits from the artificial heart? *Hastings Center Report* 15(February):5–7.

————. 1986. Public relations and public policy. *Medical World News* (13 October):37.

————. 1987. Organ rationing: jumping the queue. *Medical World News* (12 January):31.

————. 1988. The artificial heart. In *Worse than the Disease: Pitfalls of Medical Progress*, ed. D. B. Dutton. New York: Cambridge University Press.

Prottas, J. M. 1983. Encouraging altruism: public attitudes and the marketing of organ donation. *Milbank Memorial Fund Quarterly/Health and Society* 61(2):278–306.

————. 1985. Organ procurement in Europe and the United States. *Milbank Memorial Fund Quarterly/Health and Society* 63(1):94–126.

————. 1988. Shifting responsibilities in organ procurement: a plan for routine referral. *Journal of the American Medical Association* 260(12 August):832–833.

————. 1989. The organization of organ procurement. In *Organ Transplantation Policy: Issues and Prospects*, eds. J. F. Blumstein and F. A. Sloan, pp. 41–55, Durham, N.C.: Duke University Press.

————, and Batten, H. L. 1988. Health professionals and hospital administrators in organ procurement: attitudes, reservations, and their resolutions. *American Journal of Public Health* 78(June):642–645.

————, and Batten, H. L. 1991. The willingness to give: the public and the supply of transplantable organs. *Journal of Health Politics, Policy, and Law* 16:121–134.

Quindlen, A. 1991. The heart's reasons. *New York Times* (6 June):A25.

Ramsey, P. 1970. *The Patient as Person: Explorations in Medical Ethics.* New Haven, Conn.: Yale University Press.

Randall, T. 1990. Cyclosporine: vital in today's transplantation, but questions remain about tomorrow. *Journal of the American Medical Association* 264(10 October):1794, 1797.

————. 1991. Too few human organs for transplantation, too many in need . . . and the gap widens. *Journal of the American Medical Association* 265(13 March):1223, 1227.

Reed, J. D. 1970. Organ transplant. *The New Yorker* (26 September):126.

Reimer, L. G. 1989. The power of the individual's story. *Second Opinion* (12 November):40–45.

Reiser, S. J. 1984. The machine as means and end: the clinical introduction of the artificial heart. In *After Barney Clark*, ed. M. W. Shaw, pp. 168–175. Austin: University of Texas Press.

Relman, A. S. 1980. The new medical-industrial complex. *New England Journal of Medicine* 303(23 October):963–970.

————. 1984. Privatizing artificial-heart research. (letter to the editor). *Wall Street Journal* (26 December).

————. 1986. Artificial hearts: permanent and temporary. *New England Journal of Medicine* 314(6 March):644–645.

————. 1990. Is rationing inevitable? (editorial). *New England Journal of Medicine* 322(21 June):1809–1810.

Rettig, R. A. 1976. The policy debate on patient care financing for victims of end-stage renal disease. *Law and Contemporary Problems* 40(4):196–230.

————. 1980. The politics of health cost containment: end-stage renal disease. *Bulletin of the New York Academy of Medicine* 56:115–137.

————. 1989. The politics of organ transplantation: a parable of our time. In *Organ Transplantation Policy: Issues and Prospects*, ed. J. F. Blumstein and F. A. Sloan, pp. 191–228. Durham, N.C.: Duke University Press.

Rice, L. B., and Karchmer, A. W. 1988. Artificial heart implantation: what limitations are imposed by infectious complications? *Journal of the American Medical Association* 259 (12 February):894–895.

Rosenberg, C. E. 1961. *No Other Gods: On Science and American Thought.* Baltimore, Md.: Johns Hopkins University Press.

Sachar, D. B. 1989. Cyclosporine treatment for inflammatory bowel disease: a step backward or a leap forward? *New England Journal of Medicine* 321(28 September):894–895.

Saltus, R. 1985. Burcham's artificial heart hid massing of clots, doctor says. *Boston Globe* (26 April):28.

Scheck, A. 1991. Permanent heart pump to be tested. *Internal Medicine News & Cardiology News* (1–14 February):1, 17.

Scheier, R. 1987. Robert Jarvik, MD. Inventor, lecturer, 'hero.' *American Medical News* (22 December):9–10.

Schneider, A., and Flaherty, M. P. 1985a. Favoritism shrouds Presby transplants. *Pittsburgh Press* (May 12):A1, A10–11.

———, and Flaherty, M. P. 1985b. Foreigners get kidneys with flaws. *Pittsburgh Press* (8 July):A1–A2.

———, and Flaherty, M. P. 1985c. Selling the gift [six articles in the Challenge of a Miracle series]. *Pittsburgh Press* November 3–8.

———, and Flaherty, M. P. 1985d. U.S. kidneys sent overseas as Americans wait. *Pittsburgh Press* (6 November):A1, A24.

———, and M. P. Flaherty. 1985e. Woman passed over after 3-year wait. *Pittsburgh Press* (12 May):A10.

Schroeder, J. S., and Hunt, S. A. 1991. Chest pain in heart-transplant recipients. *New England Journal of Medicine* 324(20 June):1805–1807.

Schroeder, M. 1985. An affair of the heart. *People* (16 December):58–61.

Schroeder Family with Martha Barnette. 1987. *The Bill Schroeder Story*. New York: William Morrow.

Schuck, P. H. 1989. Government funding for organ transplants. In *Organ Transplantation Policy: Issues and Prospects*, eds. J. F. Blumstein and F. A. Sloan, pp. 169–190. Durham, N.C.: Duke University Press.

Scouting. October 1989. [Donor awareness patch advertisement.]

Scouting. September 1990. [Donor awareness patch advertisement.]

Selzer, R. S. 1990. Whither thou goest. *Yale Medicine* (Spring):23–30. (Reprinted in R. S. Selzer. 1990. *Imagine a Woman and Other Tales*. pp. 1–28. New York: Random House.)

Shaw, M. W., ed. 1984. *After Barney Clark. Reflections on the Utah Artificial Heart Program*. Austin: University of Texas Press.

Shem, S. 1978. *The House of God*. New York: Dell Books.

Shewmon, D. A., Capron, A. M., Peacock, W. J., et al. 1989. The use of anencephalic infants as organ sources, a critique. *Journal of the American Medical Association* 261(24/31 March):1773–1781.

Shortell, S. M., and McNerney, W. J. 1990. Criteria and guidelines for reforming the U.S. health care system. *New England Journal of Medicine* 322(15 February):463–466.

Siebert, C. 1990. The rehumanization of the heart. *Harper's Magazine* 280(February):53–60.

Simmons, R. G., Klein, S. D., and Simmons, R. I. 1977. *Gift of Life: The Effect of Organ Transplantation on Individual, Family, and Societal Dynamics*. New York: John Wiley & Sons.

Singer, P. A., Siegler, M., Whitington, P. F., et al. 1989. Ethics of live transplantation with liver donors. *New England Journal of Medicine* 321(31 August):620–622.

Smith, H. 1989. *The Power Game: How Washington Really Works*. New York: Ballantine Books.

Southwick, K. 1990. Oregon blazing a trail with plan to ration health care. *Healthweek* (12 March):30, 33.

Spital, A., and Spital, M. 1990. The ethics of liver transplantation from a living donor (correspondence). *New England Journal of Medicine* 322(22 February):549–550.

————, ————, and Spital, R. 1986. The living kidney donor, alive and well. *Archives of Internal Medicine* 146(October):1993–1996.

Starr, P. 1982. *The Social Transformation of American Medicine.* New York: Basic Books.

Starzl, T. E. 1989. Reply to letter to the editor. *Journal of the American Medical Association* 262(1 September):1184.

————. 1990. Comments on the death of Stormie James. Unpublished.

————, and Fung, J. J. 1990. Transplantation. *Journal of the American Medical Association* 263(16 May):2686–2687.

————, Demetris, A. J., and Van Thiel, D. 1989a. Liver transplantation (Part 1). *New England Journal of Medicine* 321(12 October):1014–1022.

————, Groth, C-G., and Makowka, L., eds. 1988. *Liver Transplantation.* Clio Chirugica. Austin, Tex.: Silvergirl, Inc.

————, Hakala, T. R., and Tzakis, A., et al. 1987. A multifactorial system for equitable selection of cadaver kidney recipients. *Journal of the American Medical Association* 257(12 June):3073–3075.

————, Shunzaboro, I., Van Thiel, D., et al. 1982. The evolution of liver transplantation. *Hepatology* 2:614–636.

————, Todo, S., Fung, J., et al. 1989b. FK-506 for liver, kidney and pancreas transplantation. *Lancet* 2(28 October):1000–1004.

————, Towe, M. I., Todo, S., et al. 1989c. Transplantation of multiple abdominal viscera. *Journal of the American Medical Association* 261(10 March):1449–1457.

————, VanThiel, D., Tzakis, A., et al. 1988. Orthotopic liver transplantation for alcoholic cirrhosis. *Journal of the American Medical Association* 260(4 November):2542–2544.

Stason, E. 1968. The uniform anatomical gift act. *Business Lawyer* 23(4):919–929.

Stevens, R. 1989. *In Sickness and in Wealth: American Hospitals in the Twentieth Century.* New York: Basic Books.

Strauss, M. J. 1984. The political history of the artificial heart. *New England Journal of Medicine* 310(2 February):332–336.

Surgeon gets federal approval for 2nd artificial heart transplant. 1984. *Bangor Daily News* (9 November):13.

Swazey, J. P. 1974. *Chlorpromazine in Psychiatry. A Study of Therapeutic Innovation.* Cambridge, Mass.: MIT Press.

————. 1978. Protecting the "animal of necessity": limits to inquiry in clinical investigation. *Daedalus* 107:129–145.

————. 1980. Professional protectionism rides again: a commentary on responses of social and behavioral science researchers to IRB review and informed consent. *IRB* 2:4–6.

————. 1986. Transplants . . . the gift of life. *Wellesley* (alumnae magazine) 70(summer):13–15.

————. 1987. Ethical issues of artificial and transplanted organs. *American Scientist* (March/April):192–196.

————. 1988. The social context of medicine: lessons from the artificial heart. *Second Opinion* 8(July):45–65.

————, and Fox, R. C. 1970. The clinical moratorium: a case study of mitral valve surgery. In *Experimentation with Human Subjects,* ed. P.A. Freund, pp. 315–357. New York: George Braziller.

————, and Scher, S. R., eds. 1982. *Whistleblowing in Biomedical Research. Policies and Procedures for Responding to Reports of Misconduct.* President's Commission for the Study of Ethical Problems in Medicine and Biomedical and Behavioral Research. Washington, D.C.: U.S. Government Printing Office.

————, and Scher, S. R., eds. 1985. *Social Controls and the Medical Profession.* Boston: Oelgeschlager, Gunn & Hain.

————, Fox, R. C., and Watkins, J. C. 1989. *The Artificial Heart: A Case Study of Social and Ethical Issues Posed by Advanced Medical Technology.* Final report to the National Science Foundation and the National Heart, Lung and Blood Institute. Grant BBS 8418894.

————, Watkins, J. C., and Fox, R. C. 1986. Assessing the artificial heart: the clinical moratorium revisited. *International Journal of Technology Assessment in Health Care* 2(3):387–410.

Symbion board ousts Jarvik. 1987. *New York Times* (27 April):D7.

Szycher, M. 1986. The human heart: vault of the soul or pump? *Journal of Biomaterials Applications* 1(July):3–13.

Tanner, C. M., Watts, R. L., Bakay, R.A.E., et al. 1989. Letter to the editor. *New England Journal of Medicine* 321(3 August): 325.

Task Force on Organ Transplantation. 1986. *Organ Transplantation: Issues and Recommendations.* Washington, D.C.: Department of Health and Human Services.

Terasaki, P. I. 1989. A proposal to increase donations of cadaveric organs. *New England Journal of Medicine* 321(31 August):618–619.

Theodore, J., and Lewiston, N. 1990. Lung transplantation comes of age. *New England Journal of Medicine* 322(15 May):772–774.

Thiru, S., Collier, S. T. and Calne, R. 1987. Pathologic studies in canine and baboon renal allograft recipients immunosuppressed with FK 506. *Transplantation Proceedings* 19(Suppl. 6):98–99.

Thorwald, J. 1971. *The Patients.* New York: Harcourt Brace Jovanovich.

Top 10 finish in Miss America pageant gives Miss Pennsylvania unique forum to promote importance of organ/tissue donation. 1989. American Council on Transplantation Newsline, November.

Total artificial heart development at U of U 1982. *University of Utah News* (press release), December 22.

Transplants and miracles (editorial). 1989. *Boston Sunday Globe* (22 October):A26.

Trucco, T. 1989. Sales of kidneys prompt new laws and debate. *New York Times* (1 August):C1, C6.

Truog, R. D., and Fletcher, J. C. 1989. Anencephalic newborns: can organs be transplanted before death? *New England Journal of Medicine* 321(10 August):388–391.

Turkle, S. 1984. *The Second Self: Computers and the Human Spirit.* New York: Simon & Schuster.

Turkle, S. 1987. Hero of the life cycle. *New York Times Book Review* (5 April):36. (Review of Erikson, E. 1987. *A Way of Looking at Things*, ed. S. Schlein. New York: W. W. Norton.)

Un pionnier du coeur artificielle est suspendu de ses fonctions. 1987. *Le Monde* (24 January):23.

United Network for Organ Sharing. 1988a. *Policy Proposal Statement: UNOS Policies Regarding Transplantation of Foreign Nationals and Exportation and Importation of Organs.* Richmond, Va.: UNOS.

————. 1988b. *Policy Proposal Statement: UNOS Policy Regarding the Listing of Patients on Multiple Transplant Waiting Lists.* Richmond, Va.: UNOS.

U.S. Department of Health and Human Services. Office of Analysis and Inspections, Office of Inspector General. 1986. *The Access of Foreign Nationals to U.S. Cadaver Organs.* Washington, D.C.: U.S. DHHS. Publ. no. P-01-86-00074.

————. 1987. *The Access of Dialysis Patients to Kidney Transplantation.* Washington, D.C.: U.S. DHHS. Publ. no. OAI-01-86-00107.

Van Leer, T. 1983. Dr. Barney B. Clark eulogized for his "2nd salute to God." *Deseret News* (30 March):A1.

————, and Jacobsen-Wells, J. 1987. The beat goes on. *Deseret News* (29 November):B1–B2.

Vitez, M. 1988. A marriage of minds. *The Philadelphia Inquirer* (26 June):1L, 7L.

Voelker, R. 1989. Surgeons urge caution on repeating live-donor liver tissue transplant. *American Medical News* (15 December):2, 34.

Wallis, C. 1985. Another setback in Louisville. *Time* (6 May):64.

Weiner, W. J., Sanchez-Ramos, J. S., and Singer, C. 1989. Letter to the editor. *New England Journal of Medicine* 321(3 August):326.

Welch, H. G., and Larson, E. B. 1988. Dealing with limited resources: the Oregon decision to curtail funding for organ transplantation. *New England Journal of Medicine* 319(21 July):171–173.

Werth, B. 1990. The drug that works in Pittsburgh. *New York Times Magazine* (30 September):35, 58, 60.

Wheelwright, J., Haupt, D., and Strode, W. 1985. Bill's heart: the troubling story behind a historic experiment. *Life* (May):33–43.

Wikler, D., and Weisbard, A. J. 1989. Appropriate confusion over 'brain death' (editorial). *Journal of the American Medical Association* 261(21 April):2246.

Williams, J. W., Sankary, H. N., Foster, P. F., et al. 1989. Splanchnic transplantation: an approach to the infant dependent on parenteral nutrition who develops irreversible liver disease. *Journal of the American Medical Association* 261(10 March):1458–1462.

Winsten, J. A. 1985. Science and the media: the boundaries of truth. *Health Affairs* 4(Spring):5–23.

Wolfe, A. 1989. *Whose Keeper? Social Science and Moral Obligation.* Berkeley: University of California Press.

Wolfe, S. M. 1985. Statement before the Food and Drug Circulatory System Advisory Panel Hearing on Artificial Heart Implants (20 December).

Woolley, F. R. 1984. Ethical issues in the implantation of the total artificial heart. *New England Journal of Medicine* 310(2 February):292–296.

Wortman, P. M., Vinokur, A., and Sechrest, L. 1982. *Evaluation of NIH Consensus Development Process: Phase 1: Final Report.* Ann Arbor, Mich.: Institute for Social Research.

Wrenn, M-C. 1982. The heart has its reasons. *Utah Holiday* (July):32–47.

Yalof, I. 1990. *Life and Death: The Story of a Hospital.* New York: Ballantine Books.

Youngner, S. J., Allen, M., Bartlett, E. T., et al. 1985. Psychosocial and ethical implications of organ retrieval. *New England Journal of Medicine* 313(1 August):321–324.

———, Landefeld, S., Coulton, C. J., et al. 1989. 'Brain death' and organ retrieval: a cross-sectional survey of knowledge and concepts among health professionals. *Journal of the American Medical Association* 261(21 April):2205–2210.

Zenger, G. H. 1985a. No "Roman circus" at Humana (letter). *New York Times* (19 January):20.

———. 1985b. Proprietary hospital good place for research—Humana official. *American Medical News* (19 April):28.

Index

		DATE DUE	

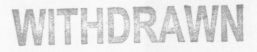